THE
GOOD CARB
COOKBOOK

SECRETS OF EATING LOW ON THE GLYCEMIC INDEX

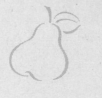

THE GOOD CARB COOKBOOK

SECRETS OF EATING LOW ON THE GLYCEMIC INDEX

Sandra Woodruff, M.S., R.D.

Avery
A MEMBER OF
PENGUIN PUTNAM INC.
NEW YORK

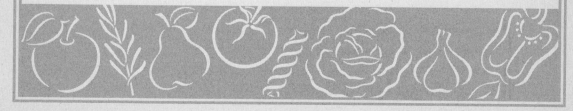

a member of
Penguin Putnam Inc.
375 Hudson Street
New York, NY 10014
www.penguinputnam.com

Copyright © 2001 by Sandra Woodruff, M.S., R.D.

Library of Congress Cataloging-in-Publication Data
Woodruff, Sandra L.
The good carb cookbook : secrets of eating low
on the glycemic index / Sandra Woodruff.
p.   cm.
Includes bibliographical references and index.
ISBN 1-58333-084-4
1. Cookery.   2. Low-carbohydrate diet—Recipes.   I. Title.

TX714.W654   2000   00-046430
641.5'638—dc21

Printed in the United States of America
10 9 8 7 6 5 4 3 2 1

BOOK DESIGN BY JILL WEBER

Acknowledgments

I am grateful for the guidance offered by the team of professionals at Penguin Putnam, whose input at every stage of development has made this book possible. Special thanks go to John Duff for providing the opportunity to publish this book and to my editor, Dara Stewart, whose excellent suggestions and diligent attention to detail have added so much.

Thanks also go to my husband, Tom, and to my friends and family members for their long-term support and encouragement. And last but not least, I would like to express my gratitude to the many clients, coworkers, colleagues, and readers whose questions, ideas, and suggestions have been a constant source of inspiration.

THIS BOOK IS DEDICATED TO MY FAVORITE TASTE TESTERS,

Wiley, C.D., and Belle.

CONTENTS

Introduction

*T*he *Good Carb Cookbook* is about choosing healthful foods that have a minimal impact on blood sugar and insulin levels. It is based on the *glycemic index,* a ranking of carbohydrate-containing foods according to their potential to raise blood sugar levels.

Why eat low on the glycemic index? In recent years, the glycemic index has emerged as one of the foremost predictors of health. Choosing foods that maintain lower levels of blood sugar and insulin has been found to help protect against obesity, cardiovascular disease, and diabetes and may be instrumental in treating a number of other health problems.

Though many Americans have only recently become aware of the glycemic index, it is not new. Twenty years of scientific research support its health-protective benefits. The glycemic index has been used in Canada, Australia, and parts of Europe for many years. A 1998 report issued by World Health Organization (WHO) and Food and Agricultural Organization (FAO) also emphasizes the importance of using the glycemic index in guiding food choices.

The first part of *The Good Carb Cookbook* introduces you to this revolutionary way of looking at carbohydrates and explains why all carbohydrates are not created equal. It then provides guidelines for choosing the best low-GI foods and explains how eating low on the glycemic index can facilitate weight loss and promote optimal health. *The Good Carb Cookbook* next delves into the practical aspects of transforming your diet by providing a wealth of tips for meal planning, snacking smart, eating in restaurants, grocery shopping, and cooking the low-GI way.

The remainder of the book features over 200 delicious user-friendly recipes that prove that eating low on the glycemic index can be both easy and immensely enjoyable. Each chapter focuses on a specific meal of the day or type of dish. Need some ideas for starting your day the low-GI way? "Breakfast and Brunch Favorites" presents a wide selection of dishes, from Light Eggs Benedict and Broccoli Frittata to Sunrise Smoothie and Morning Müesli. Or perhaps you are looking for some palate-pleasing appetizers to liven up your next party without wreaking havoc on your healthy lifestyle. "Hors D'Oeuvres with a Difference" will lead the way with choices like Sausage-Stuffed Mushrooms and Crab and Artichoke Dip. Still other chapters will show you how to make satisfying soups and stews like Sicilian Meatball Soup, refreshing salads like Greek Grilled Shrimp Salad, hearty sandwiches like Turkey-Bacon Club Sandwiches, wholesome side dishes like Rosemary Roasted Sweet Potatoes, comforting pasta dishes like Slim Spaghetti Pie, hearty homestyle entrées like Chicken Breasts with Savory Apple Stuffing, and even something to satisfy the sweet tooth like Peach-Almond Crisp and Chocolate-Covered Strawberries.

Besides featuring low-glycemic-index ingredients, the recipes in this book also have been designed to provide maximum nutrition without excessive fat or calories. The emphasis is on getting a healthy balance of fats by limiting ingredients that are high in saturated and trans fats, and instead using small amounts of healthful fats like olive and canola oils, as well as moderate amounts of nuts and seeds. Lean meats and low-fat dairy products are featured in many recipes; and vegetables, fruits, and whole grains are used in generous amounts. Most of the recipes in this book are compatible with a diet that gets 20 to 25 percent of calories from fat and is rich in fiber, vitamins, minerals, and health-promoting phytochemicals and antioxidants. In addition, sugar has been kept at a low to moderate level, and I strove to limit the use of salt and high-sodium ingredients when possible.

You will be pleased to know that each recipe is presented in a straightforward, easy-to-follow format, and every effort has been made to keep the number of pots, pans, and utensils to a minimum. This will save you time and will make cleanup a breeze—important considerations for most people today. Finally, a complete nutrition analysis accompanies each recipe so you know exactly what you are getting, enabling you to plan meals that match your nutrition goals.

Through your food choices, you have the tremendous power to determine your health. The information presented in this book can be instrumental in helping you make the right choices. It is my hope that *The Good Carb Cookbook* will prove to you that a low-GI lifestyle is enjoyable, practical, and easy to maintain anywhere, anytime, and anyplace.

PART I

The Secrets of the Glycemic Index

1. All Carbohydrates Are Not Created Equal

I f you're confused about carbohydrates, you're not alone. Over the past several years, opinions about the role of carbohydrates in a healthy diet have ranged from "eat more for optimal health" to "nothing could be worse for your health." The truth about carbohydrates, however, lies somewhere in between. The fact is the type of carbohydrates that we eat is one of the foremost predictors of health. As you will see, a diet high in the wrong kinds of carbohydrates can lead to obesity, insulin resistance, diabetes, cardiovascular disease, and many of the other health problems that are so pervasive today. On the other hand, a diet that includes the right carbohydrates can help prevent these same diseases and put you on the road to excellent health.

Over the past couple of decades, the medical establishment has paid little attention to the impact of carbohydrates on health and wellness. But a growing body of evidence has made this a topic that can no longer be ignored. The fact is there are good and bad carbohydrates, and making the right choices is crucial to your pursuit of a healthy body weight and optimal health.

What makes some carbohydrate-containing foods better choices than others? One of the most important factors is the rate at which they raise blood sugar levels—or their glycemic index. This chapter will introduce you to this revolutionary way of looking at carbohydrates and show you why all carbs are not created equal. The following chapters will help you apply the glycemic index to your everyday life and create simple and satisfying meals that will enhance your health for years to come.

A Brief History of Carbohydrates

To truly understand how carbohydrates affect our health, it's important to look at how the carbohydrates we eat have changed over time. Throughout most of history, the only carbohydrate foods that were available were the wild roots, tubers, fruits, vegetables, and nuts that people foraged for. These foods were loaded with fiber and nutrients, and they were slowly digested and absorbed to provide a slow-release, sustained form of energy.

With the advent of agriculture about 10,000 years ago, people learned to cultivate grains such as wheat, rice, corn, oats, and barley. These foods, which quickly became mainstays in the human diet, were consumed in their natural unprocessed forms. Whole, cracked, or coarsely ground grains were made into porridges or baked into hearty whole-grain breads. These foods, too, were high in fiber and nutrients.

While the introduction of cereal grains substantially changed the human diet, the past 200 years have had an even greater impact on the types of carbohydrates available in the food supply—starting with the invention of high-speed grain mills in the early 1800s. Using this technology, millers learned to remove the fibrous bran and nutritious germ from grains and to make finely ground flour from just the starchy endosperm portion of the grain. People eagerly adopted this new flour, which had a very long storage life and made softer and lighter breads, cakes, and pastries. Unfortunately, this new white flour was also virtually devoid of the vitamins, minerals, and fiber found in whole grains. And its superfine texture makes it quickly digested and absorbed in the body, causing a rapid release of glucose and insulin into the blood. The past fifty years have brought the most dramatic changes of all to our food supply. For instance:

- Products made from quickly digested white flours—such as breads, bagels, crackers, pretzels, and baking mixes—have become staples in most people's diets.

- New technologies for processing grains—such as explosion puffing, extruding, and flaking—have been developed. Products made using these technologies, including breakfast cereals, snack foods, and a wide variety of "instant" and "quick-cooking" foods, are also rapidly digested, causing a fast rise in blood glucose and insulin levels. Like white-flour products, these foods make up a large part of many people's diets.

- Consumption of refined sugars is at an all-time high.

- The serving sizes of refined-carbohydrate foods like muffins, bagels, candy bars, and sodas have grown to enormous proportions.

This deluge of quickly digested nutrient-poor carbohydrates represents much of what's wrong with today's diets. Currently, about 85 percent of all grain products eaten by Americans are refined. And together, refined grains and sugars compose close to 40 percent of all calories eaten! What can you do to bring your diet back into balance? Learning about the glycemic index is a great place to start.

What Is the Glycemic Index?

The glycemic index (GI) is a ranking of foods based on their potential to raise blood sugar levels. The higher the GI of a food, the faster the resultant rise in blood sugar after eating it. And the higher

> ### Trends in Carbohydrate Consumption over the Past Twenty Years*
>
> Consumption of grain products has increased steadily since the late 1970s. Unfortunately, most of the increase has come from highly refined and processed snack foods, sugary sodas, white-flour products, and sweets instead of minimally processed whole-grain foods. Currently, most people eat less than one serving of a whole-grain food per day.
>
> | | |
> |---|---|
> | Snack foods (crackers, pretzels, chips, etc.) | ⇧ 200% |
> | Sugar-sweetened sodas | ⇧ 160% |
> | Grain mixtures (pizza, lasagna, burritos, etc.) | ⇧ 110% |
> | Pasta | ⇧ 51% |
> | Breakfast cereals | ⇧ 51% |
> | Dairy desserts | ⇧ 29% |
> | Cakes, cookies, pastries, and pies | ⇧ 15% |
>
> *Source: USDA Economic Research Service 1999

the GI, the higher the body's insulin response tends to be. Why is this important? High levels of blood sugar and insulin in the body have been linked to many of the health problems that are so common today.

The glycemic index has been the subject of scientific research for over twenty years. It was originally developed as a dietary strategy to help people with diabetes gain better control over their blood sugar levels. Today the GI is widely accepted in Canada, Australia, and much of Europe, and its use has expanded to include roles in treating obesity, cardiovascular disease, and various other health problems. Health professionals in the United States have been slow to adopt this revolutionary way of classifying carbohydrates. However, this is rapidly changing as mounting evidence on the benefits of the GI make this a topic that can no longer be ignored. The health effects of high- versus low-GI foods are summarized below:

High-GI Foods	Low-GI Foods
• Are quickly digested, causing a rapid rise in blood sugar and insulin levels.	• Are slowly digested, allowing for a gradual rise in blood sugar and insulin.
• Provide short bursts of energy that may be quickly followed by hunger and a roller-coaster pattern of overeating.	• Provide a slow-release form of energy that sustains you between meals and promotes a healthy body weight.
• Promote excess insulin secretion, which may increase the risk for diabetes, cardiovascular disease, and some types of cancer and may contribute to a variety of other health problems.	• Protect the body from the harmful effects of too much insulin.

You might look at this comparison and deduce that you should eliminate entirely foods that have a high glycemic index and eat only low-GI foods. Fortunately, going to extremes is not necessary. And as you will discover, just because a food has a low GI does not necessarily mean it is a healthful choice. However, replacing some of the high-GI carbohydrates in your diet with healthful lower-GI carbohydrates should be a primary strategy for anyone who wants to achieve a healthy body weight and maximize his or her health.

Ranking Foods on the Glycemic Index

Determining the GI of a food is a fairly complicated process (see the inset "How Do Researchers Determine the GI of a Food?" on page 11 for details), so the GI of every food is not known. However, researchers have tested a variety of common foods, some of which are shown on page 9. A more extensive listing of the GI values of foods can be found in the appendix. These tables list the glycemic indexes of foods when compared to pure glucose, which has a GI of 100. When comparing foods, the following scale will help you put the GI in perspective:

* Very low G1 = 39 or lower
* Low GI = 40 to 54
* Moderate GI = 55 to 69
* High GI = 70 or higher

A look at Table 1.1 may surprise you. Many foods that are often thought of as "health foods"— rice cakes and baked potatoes, for instance—have very high indexes, while "junk foods" like potato chips and chocolate have relatively low indexes. Is there any rhyme or reason to the glycemic index?

TABLE 1.1. THE GLYCEMIC INDEX OF SOME COMMON FOODS[1,2]
VERY LOW GI = ≤39   LOW GI = 40–54   MODERATE GI = 55–69   HIGH GI = ≥70

Breakfast Cereals
All Bran (av)	42
Bran Chex	58
Cheerios	74
Corn flakes (av)	84
Crispix	87
Grape Nuts Nuggets	67
Grape Nuts Flakes	80
Just Right	60
Life	66
Müesli (av)	56
Oat Bran (Quaker)	50
Oats, quick-cooking	65
Oats, old-fashioned (av)	49
Puffed wheat (av)	74
Rice Chex	89
Rice Krispies	82
Shredded Wheat (av)	69
Special K	54

Breads
Bagel (white)	72
Baguette	95
Chapati (av)	57
Croissant	67
Kaiser roll	73
Linseed (flax) rye bread	55
Oat-bran bread (50% oat bran) (av)	47
Pita bread	57
Pumpernickel (whole-grain)	46
Rye flour bread (av)	65
Rye kernel bread (80% kernels) (av)	46
Sourdough rye bread	57
Stone-ground whole-wheat bread	60
White bread (av)	70
Whole wheat bread (av)	69

Vegetables
Beets	64
Carrots (av)	71
Corn, sweet (av)	55
Lima beans, baby	32
Parsnips	97
Peas, green (av)	48
Potatoes, baked (av)	85
Potatoes, French-fried	75
Potatoes, instant (av)	83
Potatoes, new (av)	62
Pumpkin	75
Rutabaga	72
Sweet potatoes (av)	54

Fruits
Apple (av)	36
Apricots, dried (av)	31
Banana (av)	53
Cantaloupe	65
Cherries	22
Grapefruit	25
Grapes	43
Kiwi fruit (av)	52
Mango (av)	55
Orange (av)	43
Papaya (av)	58
Peach	28
Pear (av)	36
Pineapple	66
Plum	24
Raisins	64
Watermelon	72

Dairy
Ice cream, low-fat	50
Milk, skim	32
Milk, whole (av)	27
Fruit yogurt, sugar-free	14
Fruit yogurt, with sugar	33

Crackers
Melba toast	70
Rice cakes	82

Rye crisp bread (av)	65		Grapefruit juice	48
Saltines	74		Soft drink	68
Water crackers (av)	72			

Grains

Barley (av)	25
Buckwheat groats (av)	54
Bulgur wheat (av)	48
Couscous	61
Rice, basmati	58
Rice, long-grain brown (av)	55
Rice, long-grain white (av)	56
Rice, short-grain white (av)	88
Rice, wild	57
Wheat berries (av)	41

Pasta

Egg fettuccine	32
Linguine (av)	46
Macaroni	45
Spaghetti (av)	41
Spaghetti (whole-wheat) (av)	37
Star pastina	38
Tortellini, cheese	50
Vermicelli	35

Legumes

Baked beans (av)	48
Black-eyed peas (av)	42
Butter beans (av)	31
Chickpeas (av)	33
Kidney beans (av)	27
Lentils (av)	29
Navy beans (av)	38
Pinto beans	39
Soybeans (av)	18
Split peas	32

Beverages

Apple juice (av)	41

Snack Foods

Corn chips (av)	73
Peanuts (av)	14
Popcorn	55
Potato chips (av)	54
Pretzels	80

Sweets and Desserts

Banana bread	47
Cake, angel food	67
Cake, pound	54
Cake, sponge	46
Cookies, oatmeal (av)	55
Custard	43
Donut, cake-type	76
Graham crackers	74
Vanilla wafers	77

Candy and Candy Bars

Chocolate	49
Jellybeans	80
Life Savers	70
M&M's (peanut)	33
Mars Bar	62
Skittles	70
Snickers Bar	41
Twix Cookie Bars (caramel)	44

Sugars and Sweeteners

Fructose (av)	23
Glucose	100
Honey	58
Lactose (milk sugar) (av)	46
Maltose	105
Sucrose (white sugar) (av)	65

1. *In some studies, researchers use white bread as the reference food instead of glucose. This will cause the GI of a food to be different from the values shown above. If you should run across this situation, you can convert a GI based on white bread to a GI that uses glucose as the reference simply by multiplying the white bread–referenced GI by 0.7.*
2. *(av) denotes a GI value that is an average of 2 or more studies.*

How Do Researchers Determine the GI of a Food?

Researchers at universities in Canada and Australia have compiled the vast majority of the information currently available on the glycemic indexes of foods. Here's how they test specific foods:

- ◆ Researchers measure out a portion of the food to be tested that contains 50 grams of available (digestible) carbohydrate. For instance, 4½ slices of whole-wheat bread, 1¼ cups of cooked brown rice, 1½ pounds of carrots, and 3 medium apples each supplies about 50 grams of available carbohydrate. They then serve the measured portion of food to a group of volunteers.

- ◆ The researchers draw blood samples from the volunteers every fifteen to thirty minutes for up to three hours after they ate the food in question to determine their blood sugar levels. The blood sugar levels are plotted on a graph, and the curve is calculated so the researchers can determine the magnitude of the volunteers' blood sugar responses.

- ◆ The volunteers' blood sugar responses to the test food are compared with their responses to eating 50 grams (about 3 tablespoons) of pure glucose. For instance, if the test food is apples, and the apples raise blood sugar only 36 percent as much as glucose does, then apples are assigned a GI of 36.

Researchers will undoubtedly discover simpler ways to estimate the GI of foods in the future. This will broaden our knowledge of how foods affect health and make it easier to apply the GI to everyday life.

Yes. The GI of a food is influenced by a variety of factors, including the degree to which the food is processed; how long the food is cooked; the kind of starch, sugar, or fiber the food contains; and the food's acidity. In general, anything that speeds the rate at which a food is digested and absorbed will increase the GI of a food. The section "Factors That Affect the Glycemic Index of a Food" on page 13 provides more details about what factors can raise or lower the GI of a food.

Of course, the glycemic index cannot be the only factor that determines which foods you should eat. As you can see from looking at Table 1.1, just because a food has a low GI does not necessarily mean it is good for you. It's important to consider all the nutritional qualities of a food when planning your diet. This book will help you make the best choices based on this philosophy.

While the GI should not be the only criterion used for choosing foods, some generalities can be drawn from Table 1.1 that can help guide you in choosing foods:

FOODS THAT RAISE THE GLYCEMIC INDEX OF YOUR DIET	FOODS THAT LOWER THE GLYCEMIC INDEX OF YOUR DIET
◆ Bread	◆ Vegetables
◆ Potatoes	◆ Fruits
◆ Breakfast cereals	◆ Legumes
◆ Processed snack foods like chips, crackers, and pretzels	◆ Minimally processed whole grains
	◆ Pasta
	◆ Dairy products

Realize that some variation exists within these lists. For instance, not all kinds of bread and potatoes have a high GI. The remaining chapters of this book will help you make these distinctions and help you to plan varied and satisfying meals and snacks.

What effect do sweets have on the glycemic index of your diet? Many candies, cakes, cookies, and sodas have a moderate GI. However, these foods are very concentrated sources of carbohydrate, and the workload they place on the pancreas is considerable. Since sweets are often high in calories and low in nutritive value, they should be eaten with your total carbohydrate and nutrition goals in mind.

Perspective on Portions

How do portion sizes affect the glycemic index? The more carbohydrate you eat in a meal, the more insulin your pancreas must secrete to process the carbohydrate. For instance, eating a 4-ounce bagel will cause twice the insulin response as eating a 2-ounce bagel. Choosing low-GI foods will minimize the amount of insulin that you secrete when you eat carbohydrates, but portions are still important. Chapter 2 will give you an idea of how much carbohydrate is right for you.

GLYCEMIC INDEX VERSUS GLYCEMIC LOAD

Recognizing that both the *GI* of the carbohydrate-containing food and the *amount* of carbohydrate eaten affect blood insulin levels, researchers have coined the term *glycemic load* to describe these two factors considered together. Glycemic load is a better indicator of total insulin demand and the workload of the pancreas than just glycemic index by itself. This term is becoming more popular in the scientific literature, so when you see it, just realize that it reflects both the type and the amount of dietary carbohydrate.

Insulin—Friend or Foe?

While insulin is often portrayed as a harmful, toxic substance and the underlying cause of many diseases, you should also know that insulin is essential to life. This hormone, which is produced by the pancreas, regulates the storage and release of energy throughout the body.

To understand how insulin works, it is helpful to know a little bit about the process of digestion. When we eat, food moves from the mouth to the stomach and through the intestines where it is systematically broken down into glucose, amino acids, and fatty acids that the body can absorb and use. Glucose entering the bloodstream from digested carbohydrates is the most potent stimulator of insulin secretion.

As blood glucose levels rise, insulin ushers it into the cells where it is used for energy. Any glucose that is not immediately used for energy is stored in the muscles and liver for later use. Once the muscle cells and liver are filled with all the glucose they can hold, any leftover glucose is made into fat and stored in fat cells. Besides directing glucose into storage, insulin also guides amino acids into muscle cells and fatty acids into the fat cells.

About two to three hours after you eat a meal, your blood sugar and insulin levels start to gradually fall. This signals the body to release some of its stored carbohydrate and fat to provide a constant supply of energy between meals and during sleep.

As you can see, we need insulin, in the right amounts, to stay alive. However, a problem can arise when we eat too many high-GI carbohydrates. Because these foods are quickly absorbed, they overstimulate the pancreas, which must work harder to handle the rush of sugar entering the bloodstream. Researchers believe that over a long period of time, a high-GI diet can lead to pancreatic exhaustion and type-2 diabetes in some people. Long-term exposure to high levels of insulin can also increase the risk of heart disease, high blood pressure, and other health problems. On the other hand, slowly absorbed low-GI carbohydrates require less insulin and reduce the workload of the pancreas.

Factors That Affect the Glycemic Index of a Food

Table 1.1, which lists the glycemic index of a variety of common foods, reinforces the statement that all carbohydrates are not created equal. However, at first glance, the glycemic index may not seem to make much sense. Why do two starchy foods like pasta and potatoes have such different indexes? And why does fruit have a lower GI than bread? Differences in cooking and processing methods; the chemical structure of the starches, sugars, and fibers in foods; and the presence of fat, protein, or acid can all markedly affect the GI of a food. Knowing more about how these factors affect the digestibility of foods will help you make sense of the GI.

MILLING, GRINDING, AND PROCESSING OF GRAINS

Modern food-processing techniques, such as grinding, pulverizing, puffing, extruding, and otherwise destroying the natural intact form of whole grains, make whole grains easier to digest and absorb. This is why most breads, breakfast cereals, snack chips, and crackers have such a high glycemic index. This is also why thinly cut instant oats have a higher GI than thicker cut old-fashioned oats.

COOKING

During cooking and baking, the starches in foods like grains, pasta, breads, and muffins absorb water. This causes the starch granules to swell and rupture, a process known as *gelatinization*. Gelatinized starch is readily attacked by digestive enzymes and very quickly digested and absorbed. Bread has a high GI partly because the starch in the finely ground flour used to make bread is easily gelatinized. And soft, overcooked pasta has a higher GI than firm, al dente pasta because the overcooked pasta absorbed more water during cooking.

Many of the processing methods used to make extruded, flaked, or puffed cereals and snack foods involve steam-cooking at very high temperatures and pressures. This fully gelatinizes the starch in these foods and contributes to their high glycemic indexes.

THE TYPE OF STARCH PRESENT

Starch is a storage form of glucose found in plant foods. Because starch is composed of hundreds or thousands of glucose molecules that are strung together in chains, it is often referred to as *complex carbohydrate*. Scientists have long believed that because starch has a complex structure, it is more slowly digested than simple sugars. However, the glycemic index has proven this notion to be false.

There are two main kinds of starch present in plant foods—*amylose* and *amylopectin*. When these starches are digested, their glucose molecules are liberated and absorbed, causing a rise in blood sugar. However, because of the differences in their chemical structures, these two starches have very different effects on blood sugar.

Amylopectin's structure resembles the branches of a tree and so it is easily attacked by digestive enzymes. Starchy foods that contain a high proportion of amylopectin—like baking potatoes and sticky short-grain rice—are quickly digested and produce rapid rises in blood sugar levels. Amylose, on the other hand, consists of a long, straight chain of tightly packed glucose molecules that resists digestion. Foods high in amylose—such as new potatoes and basmati rice—are absorbed more slowly and have lower glycemic indexes.

THE TYPE OF SUGAR PRESENT

Many people are surprised to learn that with the exception of glucose (GI = 100), most sugars have low to moderate glycemic indexes. Fructose, the sugar that occurs naturally in fruits, is very slowly absorbed, giving it a GI of only 23. Lactose, the sugar naturally present in milk and dairy products, has a GI of 46. This is one reason why most fruits and dairy products have such low glycemic indexes. Sucrose (white table sugar), a combination of equal parts fructose and glucose, has a GI of 65. The fact that sucrose is part fructose is one reason why many sweets have a moderate GI.

ACID

The naturally occurring acids in fruits, as well as the acids in fermented foods like yogurt, buttermilk, and sourdough bread, slow the rate of digestion and contribute to the low GI of these foods. Likewise, adding just 4 teaspoons of vinegar or lemon juice to a meal can lower the GI of the meal by about 30 percent. For this reason, using vinegar and lemon juice to flavor foods can be a powerful way to lower the GI of your diet.

FIBER

Oats, barley, legumes, and many fruits and vegetables are rich in soluble fibers, which form a thick gel when mixed with water. This slows their passage through the digestive tract and contributes to the low GI of these foods. The insoluble fibers that form the outer bran layers of whole grains also slow digestion by making it more difficult for digestive enzymes to attack the starches within these foods. However, when whole grains are ground into fine flours this effect is lost.

FAT

The presence of fat lowers the GI of a food or meal by slowing the rate at which it leaves the stomach. This is why potato chips and French fries have lower indexes than a plain baked potato. This does not mean that high-fat chips and fries are better choices than plain baked potatoes or that you should add butter to bread to lower its GI. When you turn a potato into chips or fries, the added fat doubles the calories. And the fat used to make these foods is usually the hydrogenated artery-clogging type. There are far better ways to lower the GI of your diet than adding fat.

Applying the GI to Everyday Life

In real life, people eat mixed meals containing several different foods. So how do you know what the GI of your entire meal is? While protein, fat, and other food constituents can influence the GI of a meal, the type and amount of carbohydrate present in the meal is by far the major determinant of the meal GI. In fact, researchers have shown that the carbohydrate portion of the meal predicts 80 to 90 percent of the meal GI and insulin response, even for meals that contain some protein and fat. This knowledge makes it possible to estimate the GI of mixed meals based on the GIs of the carbohydrate foods in the meal instead of performing cumbersome laboratory tests.

Suppose you are having a sandwich made with turkey, mustard, and whole-wheat bread, along with an apple and a glass of milk. Here's how a dietitian or researcher might estimate the GI of the meal:

1. Figure out how much carbohydrate the meal contains. In this meal, the bread in the sandwich supplies 26 grams of carbohydrate, the apple 21 grams, and the milk 12 grams, for a total of 59 grams of carbohydrate in the meal.

2. Determine what percentage of the total carbohydrate content of the meal is supplied by each food. In this meal, the bread supplies 44 percent of the carbohydrate (26/59 = 44%), the apple supplies 36 percent of the carbohydrate (21/59 = 36%), and the milk supplies 20 percent of the carbohydrate (12/59 = 20%).

3. Multiply the percentage of carbohydrate supplied by each food by its GI to see how much of the meal GI is attributed to each food. For instance, the whole-wheat bread, which supplies 44 percent of the carbohydrate in the meal, has a GI of 69, so multiply 0.44 x 69, and you will find that the bread contributes 30 points to the meal GI. The apple, which supplies 36 percent of the carbohydrate in the meal, has a GI of 36 and so contributes 13 points to the meal GI (0.36 x 36 = 13). The milk, which supplies 20 percent of the carbohydrate in the meal, has a GI of 32, and contributes 6 points to the meal GI (0.20 x 32 = 6).

4. Add up the number of points that each food contributes to the meal GI. In this case, the bread contributes 30 points, the apple 13 points, and the milk 6 points for a total meal GI of 49. See Table 1.2.

TABLE 1.2. CALCULATING THE GLYCEMIC INDEX OF A MIXED MEAL

FOOD	% of Total Carbs Contributed to Meal (# of grams in food/ total grams in meal)	Contribution to Meal GI (% of carb contribution × the food's GI)
2 SLICES WHOLE-WHEAT BREAD (Carbs—26 g, GI—69)	26/59 = 44%	.44 × 69 = 30
MEDIUM APPLE (Carbs—21 g, GI—36)	21/59 = 36%	.36 × 36 = 13
1 CUP SKIM MILK	12/59 = 20%	.20 × 32 = 6
MEAL TOTALS (Carbs—59 g, GI—49)		

Realize that it is not necessary or recommended that you try to calculate the GI of your meals. Just know that this is how researchers estimate the GI of mixed meals, diets, and recipes and that this method offers a very good prediction of how a meal will affect blood sugar and insulin levels. The two key points to take from this are:

- The GI of a meal reflects the types and amounts of all the carbohydrate-containing foods in the meal.
- You can reduce the impact of a high-GI food in a meal by balancing it out with lower-GI foods in the same meal.

The glycemic index can be an effective tool for choosing foods that minimize fluctuations in blood glucose and insulin levels and thus maintaining good health and optimal weight. A variety of factors affect the glycemic response of individual foods and mixed meals, and becoming familiar with these will help you apply the glycemic index to your everyday life.

A large selection of foods can be enjoyed on a low-GI eating plan, and choosing more foods that are both high in nutrients and low on the glycemic index can put you on the road to excellent health.

2. A Matter of Balance

As mentioned in Chapter 1, both the type and amount of carbohydrate eaten are important determinants of blood insulin levels and overall health. In addition, carbohydrates must be balanced properly with protein and fat to assure adequate nutrition and foster optimal health. This chapter takes a closer look at carbohydrates, proteins, and fats; offers guidelines for making the best choices within each group; and presents some recommendations for determining how much of each is right for you.

How Much Carbohydrate Should You Eat?

In recent years, recommendations for carbohydrate intake have ranged from 40 percent of calories to as high as 75 percent of calories. And at the extreme end of the spectrum, proponents of high-protein diets recommend almost no carbohydrate at all. It's easy to see why people are confused.

The truth is the human body can adapt to a wide range of carbohydrate intake. However, carbohydrate is the body's preferred fuel, especially for the brain and nervous system. This is why people feel weak, tired, and irritable when they cut too much carbohydrate from their diet. For the past 10,000 years, most of the world has depended on carbohydrate-rich foods for their very existence, and they thrived exceedingly well until processed, high-GI carbohydrates became the norm. So how much carbohydrate should you eat? A diet that supplies 50 to 60 percent of calories as carbohydrate is a healthy amount for most people—if you choose mostly unprocessed, low-GI carbs.

Table 2.1 shows some recommended ranges for carbohydrate intake based on a variety of body weights. (If you are over- or underweight, use the weight you would like to be as your guideline.) The intent of this table is not to have you obsess about counting carbohydrate grams, but rather just to give you an idea of what a healthy amount of this nutrient would be. This will help you make wise choices when reading food labels and preparing foods. Realize that everyone is different and that calorie and carbohydrate needs can vary greatly among people, depending on age, gender, body weight, and activity level. Some experimentation may be required to find out what proportions of carbohydrate intake are best for you. A registered dietitian or licensed nutritionist can help you plan a diet that suits your individual needs.

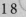

Body Weight (in pounds)	Recommended Daily Calorie Intake (13–15 calories per pound)	Recommended Carbohydrate Intake–50 Percent of Calorie Intake (grams/day)	Recommended Carbohydrate Intake–60 percent of calorie intake (grams/day)
		TABLE 2.1. DAILY RANGES FOR CALORIE AND CARBOHYDRATE INTAKE	
100	1,300–1,500	162–187	195–225
110	1,430–1,650	179–206	215–247
120	1,560–1,800	195–225	234–270
130	1,690–1,950	211–243	253–292
140	1,820–2,100	227–262	273–315
150	1,950–2,250	243–281	292–337
160	2,080–2,400	260–300	312–360
170	2,210–2,550	276–319	331–382
180	2,340–2,700	292–337	351–405
190	2,470–2,850	308–356	370–427
200	2,600–3,000	325–375	390–450

A Closer Look at Carbohydrates

Just about all foods except unprocessed meats and fats contain carbohydrate in the form of sugar or starch. This section takes a closer look at foods, starting with those that are the most concentrated sources of carbohydrate, including their nutritional qualities and their effects on your glycemic load. Table 2.2 shows you the average amount of carbohydrates found in different foods.

SUGAR

Sugar is the most concentrated source of carbohydrate there is, and its use has almost doubled over the past century. The average American diet currently supplies a record-breaking 32 teaspoons of refined sugar daily, and refined sugars now compose 16 to 18 percent of all calories eaten!

Type of Food	Serving Size	Average Amount of Carbohydrate and Calories
SUGAR	1 tablespoon sugar, honey, jam, maple syrup, molasses, etc.	12–15 g carb 45-60 calories
GRAIN PRODUCTS (BREAD, RICE, CEREAL, PASTA)	1 slice bread (about 1 ounce) ½ cup ready-to-eat breakfast cereal ½ cup cooked grain (about 2½ tablespoons dry) ½ cup cooked pasta (about 1 ounce dry)	15 g carb 100 calories
HIGH-CARBOHYDRATE (STARCHY) VEGETABLES	½ cup corn, lima beans, peas, white potatoes, sweet potatoes, winter squash	15 g carb 100 calories
LEGUMES	½ cup cooked dried beans, split peas, lentils	15 g carb 100 calories
FRUITS	1 small piece of fresh fruit ¾ to 1 cup berries or cut fresh fruit ½ cup canned fruit in juice ⅓ to ½ cup fruit juice 3 tablespoons dried apricots or prunes 2 tablespoons raisins	15 g carb 60 calories
DAIRY PRODUCTS	1 cup milk or plain yogurt (low fat)	12 g carb 90 calories
LOW-CARBOHYDRATE	½ cup artichokes, asparagus, broccoli, Brussels sprouts, cabbage, carrots,	5 g carb 25 calories

TABLE 2.2. AVERAGE CARBOHYDRATE AND CALORIE CONTENT OF FOODS

(NONSTARCHY) VEGETABLES	cauliflower, eggplant, green beans, greens, okra, onions, bell peppers, snow peas, spinach, yellow squash, tomatoes, turnips, zucchini, etc.	
SALAD VEGETABLES	1 cup lettuce/spinach and celery, cucumbers, mushrooms, radishes, etc.	<5 g carb 10 calories
NUTS	¼ cup almonds, Brazil nuts, cashews, peanuts, pecans, pumpkinseeds, sunflower seeds, walnuts, and other nuts and seeds	5–8 g carb 200 calories
MEATS, POULTRY, AND SEAFOOD	3 ounces lean meat, skinless poultry, seafood	0–4 g carb (only processed meats like lunchmeats and sugar-cured ham contain carbohydrate)

Where is all this sugar coming from? Soft drinks are, by far, the biggest contributor, providing about 10 teaspoons of sugar per 12-ounce can. Next in line are sweets such as cookies, cakes, pastries, pies, ice cream, and candies. Sugar is also added to foods like breakfast cereals, cereal bars, hot dogs, side dish mixes, soups, spaghetti sauce, canned vegetables, ketchup, mayonnaise, salad dressings, and peanut butter. In fact, sugar is the number-one additive to our food supply.

Most sugars have a low to moderate GI. For instance, fructose (fruit sugar) has a GI of only 23. Sucrose (table sugar) has a moderate index of 65. You may be surprised to learn that sucrose has a lower GI than the starches found in most breads, cereals, and potatoes, which yield pure glucose when they are digested. Does this mean that sugar can be part of a low-GI diet? Yes, but in reasonable amounts. Bear in mind that most sugary foods are high in calories and low in nutrients, so they should be consumed with your weight-management and health goals in mind.

The remaining chapters of this book provide tips for cutting back sugar in your favorite recipes and offer some recipes for satisfying lower-sugar treats. Use the following tips to guide you in budgeting your sugar intake.

- Limit your intake of added sugars to no more than 24 to 48 grams (6 to 12 teaspoons) of sugar per day. Most women should stay on the lower end of this range, while most men and very active people can be a little more liberal.

- Check food labels for sugar content. Bear in mind that 4 grams of sugar is the equivalent of 1 teaspoon of sugar.

- When reading labels for products that contain milk or fruit, realize that the sugar content listed lumps the added refined sugars together with the naturally occurring sugars from milk and fruit. This makes it impossible to determine exactly how much added refined sugar the product contains.

GRAIN PRODUCTS

Throughout most of history, cereal grains were virtually absent from the human diet. And when they were introduced about 10,000 years ago, they were available only in their whole, unprocessed forms. Today, grain products are often referred to as the "staff of life," and they form the foundation of the United States Department of Agriculture (USDA) Food Guide Pyramid.

The role that grain products should play in the diet has been the subject of intense controversy. Recommendations range from "avoid them completely" to "eat some at every meal." What should you do? Realize that most of the grain products eaten today—such as breakfast cereals, breads, and white-flour products—rank very high on the glycemic index. Replacing these foods with grainy breads, pasta, oats, barley, bulgur wheat, and brown rice can go a long way toward lightening your glycemic load while adding fiber and vital nutrients to your diet.

As for amounts, grain products are fairly concentrated sources of carbohydrates and calories (though they are not nearly as high in calories as fatty foods). If you are an active person who burns a lot of calories, you would likely have trouble keeping enough weight on if you did not eat some grain products at every meal. On the other hand, if you are a small person, are unable to do much exercise, or tend to gain weight easily, you would be wise to make vegetables and fruits the foundation of your diet and give grains a less prominent role. The low-GI foods pyramids on pages 29–31 illustrate some diet-planning approaches that meet different needs.

LEGUMES

Dried beans, peas, and lentils are among the lowest-GI foods available, so include them in your diet often. High in protein and rich in fiber and nutrients, legumes make an excellent alternative to meat. Use legumes often in entrées, soups, salads, and side dishes, and dips and spreads.

STARCHY VEGETABLES

Starchy vegetables like white potatoes, sweet potatoes, corn, peas, and lima beans contain about the same amount of carbohydrate and calories as grain products. For this reason, many health professionals believe these foods should be thought of as bread substitutes instead of vegetables. And, in fact, diabetes educators have been categorizing starchy vegetables as bread substitutes for many years.

Where do starchy vegetables rank on the glycemic index? Most people are surprised to learn that within this group, only white potatoes rank high on the glycemic index. Unfortunately, the potato is also the number-one eaten vegetable in America, making up over one-quarter of our national vegetable intake—often served as French fries, baked potatoes, mashed potatoes, and potato chips. Cutting back on potatoes or substituting lower-GI alternatives like new potatoes, sweet potatoes, corn, or pasta salad can go a long way toward lightening your glycemic load. Watching your weight? You can trim calories from your diet by substituting lower-calorie green vegetables, salads, or fruit for potatoes.

FRUITS

Most fruits, like apples, citrus fruit, grapes, cherries, berries, and peaches, rank very low on the glycemic index. Tropical fruits and melons rank higher, but most still fall within the low to moderate range. Most people are surprised to learn that even bananas have a moderately low GI. Learn to enjoy the taste of fresh ripe fruit and have several servings daily—it's a great way to satisfy a sweet tooth for very few calories. One of the most effective ways to lower the GI of your diet is to substitute fruit for high-GI snacks like snack crackers, chips, and pretzels.

DAIRY PRODUCTS

Excellent sources of calcium and protein, dairy foods have very low GIs, so if you like dairy products, do include them in your diet. In fact, snacking on low-fat yogurt, milk, cottage cheese, or cheese instead of high-GI crackers, chips, and pretzels can go a long way toward lightening your glycemic load. And if you are watching your weight, you will be interested to know that preliminary studies indicate that people who consume plenty of calcium weigh less than people who consume low-calcium diets, even when calorie intakes are similar. For this reason, for each recipe in the latter portion of this book, I provide information on the amount of calcium along with the rest of the nutritional information.

LOW-CARBOHYDRATE VEGETABLES

Exceptionally low in calories, nonstarchy vegetables like asparagus, broccoli, cabbage, cauliflower, summer squash, and salad vegetables fill you up but not out. And since they are so low in carbohydrate and high in fiber, they have very favorable effects on blood sugar and insulin levels. Even carrots, which are much maligned by proponents of low-carb diets, have a minimal impact on blood sugar.

Vegetables provide a wealth of anti-aging, disease-protective nutrients that are sorely lacking in most people's diets. Think of low-carb veggies as "free" foods, and eat them in generous portions at every meal—aim for a minimum of five to seven servings per day.

NUTS AND SEEDS

Rich in vitamins, minerals, health-promoting phytochemicals, and essential fats, nuts and seeds contain a small amount of carbohydrate (about 5 grams per quarter cup). Their impact on blood sugar levels is negligible. If you are watching your weight, though, do watch portions, as nuts and seeds are very high in calories (about 800 per cup!).

MEATS AND MEAT ALTERNATIVES

Fresh, unprocessed meats, poultry, and seafood contain no carbohydrate. Some processed meats, like sugar-cured ham, lunchmeats, and marinated meats, may contain a few grams of sugar but not enough to have a significant impact on your diet. The GI of meat, poultry, and seafood is considered to be zero. Be sure to choose lean meats and skinless poultry to keep calories under control.

Meat alternatives like veggie burgers are high in carbohydrate, but the carbohydrate usually comes from low-GI ingredients like vegetables, brown rice, oats, bulgur wheat, legumes, soy, and dairy products. Tofu and tofu hamburger substitutes are low in carbohydrate.

The Power of Protein

Getting enough protein is critical for maintaining lean body mass, muscular strength, and a strong immune system. But many people who have been following low-fat, high-carbohydrate diets do not eat enough protein. In an effort to reduce fat and cholesterol, many people choose to eat less meat or even to give it up entirely. And while you don't have to eat meat to get enough protein, you *must* substitute a protein-rich alternative like dried beans, soy foods, or eggs. Unfortunately, many people do not do this.

If you are watching your weight, you should know that it is especially important to include some protein in each meal. Protein-rich foods are the most filling of all foods, so they stave off hunger and keep you feeling full and satisfied until your next meal. Eating the right amount of protein in conjunction with low-GI carbs is one of your most powerful weapons against the battle of the bulge. You can read more about this in Chapter 3.

How much protein do you need? The standard recommendations are 10 to 15 percent of calories or about .36 gram per pound of ideal body weight. This amounts to about 54 grams of protein per day for a 150-pound person. However, there is growing evidence that protein needs may be higher for people over the age of fifty. Some researchers recommend .45 to .57 gram of protein per pound for people in this age group. This means that a 150-pound person could need as much as 68 to 86 grams of protein per day. (If you are under- or over-weight, use your desired weight as a guideline for calculating your protein needs.) As Table 2.3 shows, a well-planned, balanced diet can easily provide enough protein.

While it is essential that you get adequate protein for good health, you must also avoid going overboard and eating *too much* protein. People with certain medical conditions must be especially careful to avoid excess protein, which can hasten the development of kidney disease and contribute to other health problems. For this reason, it's prudent to check with your physician or dietitian/nutritionist to see how much protein is right for you.

TABLE 2.3. PROTEIN CONTENT OF SELECTED FOODS		
FOOD	Serving Size	Amount of Protein
Chicken, fish, beef, pork	3 ounces cooked	21 g
Legumes	1 cup cooked	14 g
Tofu	3 ounces	13 g
Milk	1 cup	8 g
Cheese	1 ounce	8 g
Bread	1 piece	3 g
Rice, pasta, grains	½ cup cooked	3 g
Vegetables	½ cup cooked	2 g
Fruit	1 piece	less than 1 g

TIPS FOR CHOOSING HEALTHFUL HIGH-PROTEIN FOODS

- Choose lean cuts of red meat and skinless poultry. This will help trim saturated fat and calories from your diet. (See Chapter 6 for the best choices.)
- Choose meats that are certified to be free of hormones and antibiotics when possible.
- Substitute fish or seafood for meat at least twice a week. Choose oily cold-water fish often to boost your intake of omega-3 fat.
- Substitute legumes and soy foods for meat at least several times a week. This will boost your intake of fiber and health-promoting phytochemicals, while keeping your dietary glycemic index low.

Where Does Fat Fit In?

With the nutrition focus shifting to carbohydrates, many people are under the impression that fat intake doesn't matter and that, in fact, low-fat diets are bad news. Many diet books even recommend eating foods like high-fat meat, bacon, full-fat ice cream, and mayonnaise instead of low-fat versions. What should you do? First realize that the typical American low-fat diet *is* bad news. It's too high in quickly digested, refined carbohydrates and too low in fiber and essential nutrients. It has contributed to an epidemic of obesity, diabetes, and cardiovascular disease. But substituting mayonnaise and butter for potatoes and bread is not going to help matters.

You may be surprised to learn that despite the abundance of low-fat foods that are now available, the typical American diet contains just as much fat as ever. Fat intake has remained steady at about 100 grams per day for men and 65 grams for women since the 1970s. Many people find this confusing since it is widely publicized that the *percent of calories from fat* in the American diet has dropped from 40 percent to about 33 percent over the past couple of decades. Why the discrepancy? Fat composes a smaller percentage of our diet today only because carbohydrate and calorie intakes have increased, not because fat intake has dropped.

The fact is the kind of fat that you eat is one of the most important determinants of your overall health. If you choose the right fats, you can greatly reduce your risk of heart disease, boost your immune system, and derive many other health benefits. Furthermore, watching your fat intake is an important strategy for controlling calories. With 9 calories per gram, fat has more than twice the calories of carbohydrate or protein. This is why fried foods, untrimmed meats, and full-fat dairy products have about twice as many calories as their nonfat and low-fat counterparts.

How much fat should you eat? Thirty percent of calories is the recommended upper limit, and for most people, 20 to 25 percent would be even better. This is more than enough to provide a healthy balance of essential fat while leaving plenty of room in your diet for healthful low-GI car-

Weight (pounds)	Recommended Daily Calorie Intake (13–15 calories per pound)	Daily Fat Gram Intake (20% of calorie intake)	Daily Fat Gram Intake (25% of calorie intake)	Daily Fat Gram Intake (30% of calorie intake)
	TABLE 2.4. RECOMMENDED DAILY CALORIE AND FAT INTAKES			
100	1,300–1,500	29–33	36–42	43–50
110	1,430–1,650	32–37	40–46	48–55
120	1,560–1,800	34–40	43–50	52–60
130	1,690–1,950	38–43	47–54	56–65
140	1,820–2,100	40–46	51–58	61–70
150	1,950–2,250	43–50	54–62	65–75
160	2,080–2,400	46–53	58–67	69–80
170	2,210–2,550	49–57	61–71	74–85
180	2,340–2,700	52–60	65–75	78–90
190	2,470–2,850	55–63	69–79	82–95
200	2,600–3,000	58–66	72–83	87–100

bohydrates. Table 2.4 shows some recommended ranges for fat intake based on a variety of body weights. (If you are over- or under-weight, use the weight you would like to be as your guideline.) This will give you an idea of what a healthy amount of fat would be and will help you make wise choices when reading food labels and preparing foods.

As for the *type* of fat to eat, be sure to avoid saturated and trans (hydrogenated) fats, which are powerful promoters of heart disease. Diets high in saturated fats have also been linked to insulin resistance, and evidence is emerging that saturated fats promote weight gain more readily than unsaturated fats do. At the same time, you'll want to get enough essential fat—especially omega-3 fat, which most people are deficient in. (See "Getting a Healthy Balance of Essential Fats" on page 28 to learn more about essential fats.) This can be accomplished by doing the following:

Getting a Healthy Balance of Essential Fats

Most discussions about fat are generally aimed at eating less of it. However, two classes of polyunsaturated fats, known as *omega-3* and *omega-6* fats, are essential for life. In recent years, these fats have attracted a lot of attention, as they each have very powerful—and very different—effects in the body. For instance, omega-6 fat promotes blood clotting, while omega-3 fat inhibits clot formation. Omega-6 fat acts to raise blood pressure, while omega-3 fat helps to lower blood pressure. These fats also affect the immune system in different ways. Because of their powerful and opposing effects, the balance of these essential fats in your diet can greatly affect your susceptibility to a variety of disorders.

Humans evolved on a diet that provided about equal amounts of these two fats. But over time—and especially in the past century—our diets changed dramatically. First, technology made it possible to mass-produce vegetable oils and our food supply became inundated with vegetable oils that are concentrated sources of omega-6 fat and practically devoid of omega-3 fat. Then, farmers began feeding livestock grains, which made the animals fatter as well as higher in saturated and omega-6 fats. To make matters worse, manufacturers began using omega-6-rich oils as the main ingredient in foods like mayonnaise, margarine, and salad dressings. As a result, the ratio of omega-6 to omega-3 fats in the diet rose from about 1 to 1 to as high as 20 to 1—creating an imbalance that alters body chemistry to favor the development of heart disease, cancer, inflammatory diseases like rheumatoid arthritis, autoimmune disorders, and many other health problems.

Fortunately, it is a simple matter to bring your intake of these two fats into balance. How? Since fish is a rich source of especially potent omega-3 fatty acids, eat some at least twice a week. Also include generous amounts of green plant foods in your daily diet, as they, too, supply some omega-3 fats. For most of your cooking needs, choose oils like canola, olive, walnut, and soybean, which have a healthier balance of omega-6 to omega-3 fats than do oils like cotton seed, sunflower, and corn. When purchasing products like mayonnaise, margarine, and salad dressings, read labels to see which oils they contain.

- Choose lean meats and low-fat dairy products. This will greatly reduce your intake of saturated fat.
- Avoid foods such as margarine, baked goods, and snack foods made with hydrogenated vegetable oil or vegetable oil shortening. This will minimize your intake of trans fat.
- Make olive oil and canola oil your primary cooking oils. This will provide a healthy balance of monounsaturated and essential fats.

- Include healthful high-fat foods like avocados, olives, nuts, and seeds in your diet as your calorie budget allows.

- Eat fish at least twice a week, choosing oily cold-water fish for the most omega-3 fatty acids.

- Incorporate flaxseeds and walnuts into recipes for an omega-3 boost.

- Choose omega-3-enriched eggs.

Balancing Your Diet

For most people, meticulously counting grams of carbohydrate, fat, and protein is unnecessary and may even lead to unhealthy food obsessions. A much simpler way to bring your diet into balance is

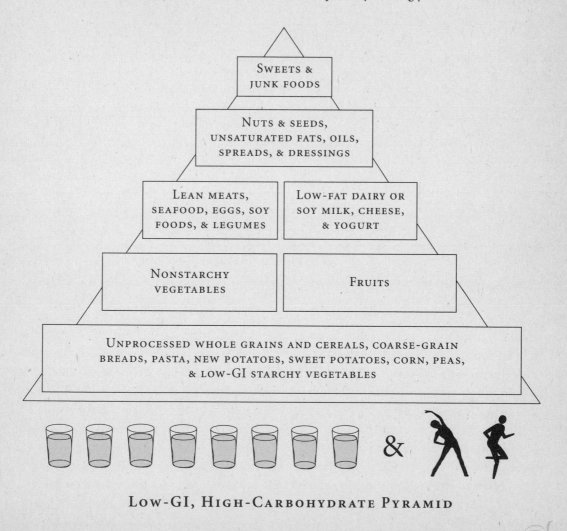

LOW-GI, HIGH-CARBOHYDRATE PYRAMID

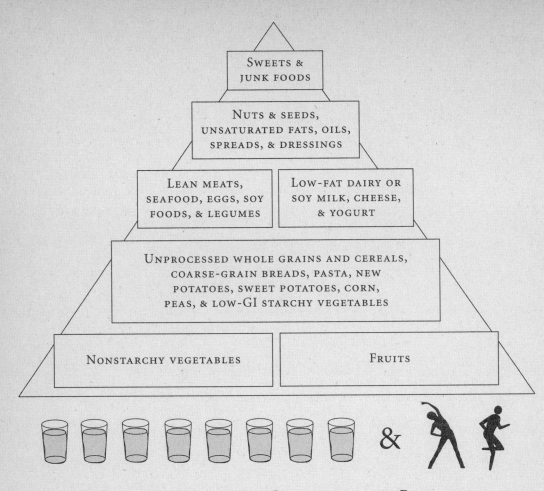

LOW-GI, MODERATE-CARBOHYDRATE PYRAMID

to use one of the food pyramid guides on pages 29 to 31 as a model for food choices. All these pyramids differ from the USDA Food Guide Pyramid in that they group starchy foods like potatoes with other starchy foods like breads and grains. These pyramids also place more emphasis on foods that are minimally processed and low on the glycemic index, and they emphasize lower-fat food choices.

The first pyramid features a high proportion of carbohydrates and is best suited for very active people who are not concerned with losing weight. The second pyramid contains a moderate amount of carbohydrate and calories and is better suited for small adults who don't burn very many calories, are unable to do much exercise, or tend to gain weight easily. The third pyramid is moderately low in carbohydrate and higher in protein—though not nearly as extreme as some of the high-protein,

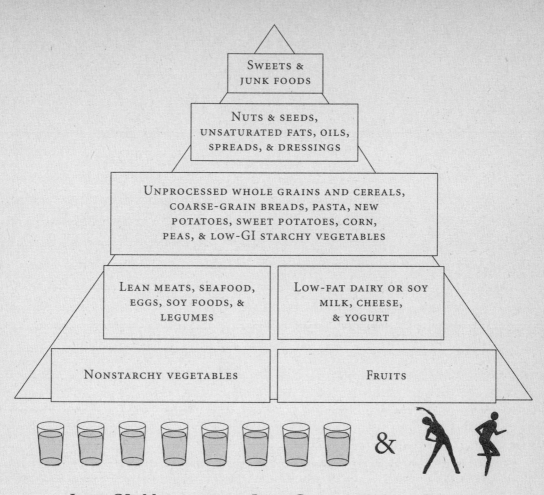

SWEETS &
JUNK FOODS

NUTS & SEEDS,
UNSATURATED FATS, OILS,
SPREADS, & DRESSINGS

UNPROCESSED WHOLE GRAINS AND CEREALS,
COARSE-GRAIN BREADS, PASTA, NEW
POTATOES, SWEET POTATOES, CORN,
PEAS, & LOW-GI STARCHY VEGETABLES

LEAN MEATS, SEAFOOD,
EGGS, SOY FOODS, &
LEGUMES

LOW-FAT DAIRY OR SOY
MILK, CHEESE,
& YOGURT

NONSTARCHY VEGETABLES

FRUITS

&

LOW-GI, MODERATELY LOW-CARBOHYDRATE PYRAMID

low-carb diets that are out there today. This moderately low-carbohydrate pyramid might be useful to someone who finds weight loss difficult on higher-carbohydrate regimens. Realize, though, that these pyramids are just general guides. Each person is unique, and one diet does not fit all.

An eating plan that emphasizes plenty of nutrient-rich unprocessed carbohydrates, lean protein foods, and a smart balance of essential fats lays the foundation for excellent health. Because requirements for calories, carbohydrate, protein, and fat can vary greatly among people, some experimentation may be necessary to find what works best for you. A registered dietitian or licensed nutritionist can help you find the eating pattern that best suits your individual needs. Read on to learn exactly what benefits you can gain from eating low on the glycemic index.

3. The Glycemic Index— What's in It for You?

*J*ust about everyone can derive health benefits from eating low on the glycemic index. Our bodies are genetically programmed to function best on slowly digested, low-GI carbohydrates, and these are the foods that have sustained humans since the beginning of time. In contrast, the fast-release, processed carbohydrates that predominate today overstimulate the pancreas, raise daylong insulin levels, and contribute to a myriad of health problems.

Although the glycemic index was originally developed as a dietary strategy for controlling diabetes, it has also proven to be a valuable tool for preventing and treating obesity, cardiovascular disease, and a variety of other health problems. The positive health effects of low-GI foods are supported by twenty years of research, and as researchers increase their focus on carbohydrates and health, evidence continues to mount at an increasing pace.

Weight Loss

Better weight control is the number-one reason why many people are making the change to a low-GI diet. How can the glycemic index help with weight loss? By helping you gain control over hunger. Because low-GI carbohydrates are slowly digested, they produce a gradual and sustained rise in blood sugar. This keeps you feeling full and satisfied and delays the return of hunger between meals. Conversely, high-GI carbohydrates provide short bursts of energy that are quickly followed by hunger and create a roller-coaster pattern of overeating.

Many people who have adopted a low-fat diet for weight loss have experienced this vicious cycle of overeating. Many of the fat-free and low-fat foods that have become so popular over the last decade—such as bagels, cereal, crackers, snack chips, cookies, and pretzels—rank high on the glycemic index. These foods are quickly digested and absorbed, causing a rapid rise in blood sugar and insulin levels. This surge of insulin puts too much of the incoming fuels into storage too soon, leaving you with not enough fuel to get you through to the next meal. This is why high-GI foods satisfy you in the short term, but soon have you going back for more. The fact is many of the low-fat foods that people have been eating for weight loss are actually making them hungry.

How powerful might the effects of a low-GI diet be? Researchers at Children's Hospital in Boston found that overweight teenagers who ate a low-GI breakfast consisting of a low-fat cheese omelet and a large serving of fruit were less hungry and ate 45-percent fewer calories later that day than they did after eating a high-GI cereal breakfast. An intermediate-GI breakfast of steel-cut oats curbed their eating by 34 percent. In another study of adult men, investigators found that a low-GI diet not only curtailed eating; it also helped to prevent the drop in metabolic rate that occurs with dieting.

There is also some evidence to suggest that low-GI foods may provide a weight-loss advantage over high-GI foods—even when calorie intakes are the same. In one study, a group of researchers compared the effectiveness of a conventional balanced weight-loss diet to a low-GI diet in a group of overweight insulin-resistant women. Both diets were identical in calories, carbohydrates, protein, and fat—only the glycemic index of the foods eaten in the two diets differed. After twelve weeks, women on the low-GI diet lost four to six pounds more than women who consumed the conventional weight-loss diet did. The low-GI diet also caused a significant drop in the women's insulin levels, while the conventional diet had no effect on insulin levels.

GETTING THE MOST FROM YOUR LOW-GI DIET

Eating low on the index is a powerful weight-loss tool, but it is not the only strategy you should use to shed pounds. Here are some other tips that can enhance the fat-burning benefits of your low-GI eating plan.

Trim the Fat

A high-fat diet poses several obstacles to your success at weight loss. First, fat has more than twice the calories of carbohydrate or protein. This is why you double the calories in a potato by turning it into French fries, triple the calories in pasta by tossing it in a creamy sauce, and increase cabbage's calories tenfold by making it into coleslaw. It's easy to see how a high-fat diet can blow your calorie budget in a hurry. Second, contrary to popular belief, fat is not very filling. Compared with protein and carbohydrate, fat is rather ineffective in satisfying hunger. This means that you end up eating a lot of calories before you feel full enough to stop. And finally, the fat in foods is readily stored as body fat. When you overeat carbohydrates, about 80 percent of the excess calories are stored as fat. However, when you overeat fat, about 95 percent of the excess calories are stored.

Although some low-fat foods, such as sweets and snack foods, can sabotage your weight-loss efforts, others—such as lean meats, low-fat dairy products, vegetables, fruits, whole grains, legumes, and low-fat spreads and dressings—are valuable additions to your low-GI diet. The fact is people who are successful at losing weight and keeping it off *do* watch their fat intake. Research shows that, on average, weight-loss maintainers consume about 24 percent of their calories as fat.

A Weight-Loss Case Study

Karen, a forty-three-year-old office manager, had been struggling with her weight for about ten years, having gained thirty pounds during that time. She was also concerned because type-2 diabetes runs in her family, and she wanted to do everything possible to avoid developing this disorder. She had been trying to lose weight for the past year with a low-fat diet. Her day usually started with a bowl of corn flakes or a bagel with nonfat cream cheese. For lunch, she would pack a sandwich made with high-GI wheat bread and a thin slice of low-fat lunchmeat, which she would have with a bag of baked chips. Dinner typically consisted of three ounces of lean meat, potato or white rice, and a salad or steamed vegetables.

Karen's main problem was that she constantly felt hungry and ended up nibbling all day on graham crackers, pretzels, cereal bars, and other high-GI and refined-carbohydrate foods. She was having no success with weight loss, and in fact, found her weight slowly creeping upward. She was also tiring of eating the "same old thing" night after night and was getting very bored with her diet. Out of frustration, she consulted a registered dietitian.

Karen's dietitian explained how her high-GI breakfast and lunch had created a vicious cycle of hunger and overeating and helped her plan some alternative meals. Here are some of the changes that Karen made:

- She replaced the corn flake or bagel breakfast with a bowl of old-fashioned oatmeal, low-fat milk, and fresh fruit. On the weekends, she would have scrambled eggs (made with two whites and one yolk) with low-fat cheese, a piece of grainy low-GI toast, and fruit. She also made some oat bran muffins and kept them in the freezer. When she needed breakfast on the run, she grabbed one of those and a glass of low-fat milk.

- She made her lunch sandwiches with grainy low-GI bread, increased the meat in the sandwiches to 2 ounces, added a slice of low-fat cheese, and piled on some vegetable toppings. Instead of chips, she switched to a cup of soup, a piece of fruit, or an assortment of fresh-cut vegetables.

- She substituted yogurt, low-fat string cheese, and fresh fruit for most of the high-GI snack foods.

- She incorporated more pasta, legumes, and vegetarian entrées into her evening meals.

Karen noticed a difference right away. Breakfast was so filling that she no longer needed a midmorning snack. Her higher-protein lunch left her feeling fuller and satisfied, as well. A piece of fruit with some string cheese or a cup of yogurt in the afternoon kept her going until dinner. Though Karen no longer felt hungry, her weight started dropping at the rate of about a pound a week. She also developed more energy and decided to increase her daily activity by taking the stairs several times a day instead of the elevator, and by increasing the length of her daily walks from fifteen to thirty minutes. She also spent more time gardening on the weekends. After six months, Karen had lost the thirty pounds, and her dietitian helped her fine-tune her diet to maintain her weight loss.

Besides losing the weight, Karen felt good knowing that she had substantially reduced her risk for developing diabetes. She had also increased her calcium intake and was getting much more of the fiber, antioxidants, and phytochemicals that would help keep her in the best of health.

Fill Up with Fiber

High-fiber foods like vegetables, fruits, whole grains, and legumes are naturally high in bulk and low in calories, so they fill you up but not out. Fibrous foods also have more texture and require more chewing than their processed counterparts, which adds to their satiety value. And since fiber slows the passage of food through the digestive tract, most high-fiber foods are also low-GI foods, which maximizes their weight-loss benefits.

The fat-fighting effects of fiber were highlighted in a 1999 study in which researchers tracked the eating habits of men and women over a ten-year period. They found that people who consumed about 28 grams of fiber per day had lower insulin levels and gained, on average, eight pounds less than people who ate half as much fiber.

Most health organizations recommend 25 to 35 grams per day—about twice what the typical American diet now supplies. However, numerous studies have demonstrated that an amount closer to 50 grams per day (obtained from natural foods, not supplements) would be even better for preventing spikes in blood sugar and insulin levels.

If you are not used to eating high-fiber foods, be sure to add them to your diet gradually. Some people experience gas and bloating when they begin a high-fiber regimen, although this usually passes in a few weeks as the body becomes accustomed to eating whole, natural foods. When following a high-fiber diet, it is also important to drink at least six to eight glasses of water per day. Fiber needs to absorb water to move smoothly through the digestive tract and exert its beneficial effects.

Pack Some Protein into Meals

High-protein foods are powerful appetite suppressants, decreasing hunger more than any other foods. So including some protein in your low-GI meals offers the best possible scenario for keeping hunger at bay. The satiating power of protein was demonstrated by a 1999 study in which a group of overweight men and women was assigned to eat all they wanted of a low-fat diet that included either 12 percent or 25 percent protein. After six months, both groups lost weight, but people on the higher-protein diet lost eight pounds more than the people who ate the lower-protein regimen. Why did the higher-protein diet produce better results? People felt less hungry, so they ate less food.

Besides filling you up, protein has an added benefit. The digestion, absorption, and processing of nutrients in a meal cause an increase in metabolic rate for several hours after eating the meal. This process is known as *dietary induced thermogenesis* (DIT). About 25 percent of protein calories eaten are burned this way. Next in line are carbohydrate calories, with a DIT of 8 to 15 percent, and last is fat, with a DIT of less than 3 percent.

One final reason to be cognizant of your protein intake is that when you lose weight, you lose not just body fat but also some muscle. Getting enough protein in conjunction with the right exercise program helps prevent loss of muscle. This is crucial to your long-term success because muscle keeps your metabolism high and helps prevent weight regain.

If protein is so great for weight loss, why not just skip the carbs and eat a high-meat, all-protein diet? In recent years, many people have been doing just this. Meat-based high-protein diets do produce rapid weight loss, but since they restrict so many foods, most people cannot happily stay on them long-term. As a result, the lost weight is quickly regained—along with the accompanying health problems. In addition, these diets pose a variety of health threats, including:

- Too much protein burdens the kidneys and liver, which have the job of excreting any excess protein that the body cannot use.

- High-protein, low-carbohydrate diets deprive the brain of glucose, its preferred fuel.

- High-fat meats and dairy products are rich in saturated fats, which raise the risk for heart disease.

- Pesticides and other environmental toxins accumulate in foods high on the food chain, so meats and dairy products (especially high-fat versions) contain higher concentrations of these substances than plant foods do.

- High-meat diets cause the consumption and pollution of far more natural resources than plant-based diets do.

- A diet high in meat and low in plant foods lacks the phytochemicals (nutrients found only in plant foods), antioxidants, vitamins, and minerals that delay aging and fight cancer, heart disease, and many other health problems.

- High-meat diets are very low in fiber and can cause chronic constipation and diseases of the colon.

Chapter 2 will guide you in meeting your protein needs without going overboard using a variety of healthful foods. Chapter 6 provides additional information on stocking your pantry with the best high-protein choices.

Exercise—Just Do It

There's no getting around it. Exercise is a must for success at losing weight and keeping it off. In fact, frequent exercising is one the strongest predictors of weight-loss maintenance—and television viewing is one of the strongest predictors of weight regain. Exercise works in several ways to banish body fat:

- It burns calories and hastens weight loss while allowing you to still eat a reasonable amount of food.

- It builds muscle mass. Since muscle needs more calories than fat does to maintain itself, over time exercise will increase your metabolic rate.

- Exercise helps reduce stress and depression, which are major causes of overeating for many people.

How much exercise is enough? The latest guidelines issued by the Surgeon General of the United States urge people to be active for at least thirty minutes on most days of the week. However, people who lose weight and keep it off do much more than this. Researchers have found that successful weight-loss maintainers burn an average of 2,800 calories a week (400 calories per day) with exercise. This is the equivalent of a 4-mile walk or about an hour of moderate activity daily, which may be performed all at once or in several smaller bouts.

And you don't have to spend tedious hours on a treadmill or join a gym to get the health benefits of exercise. When performed on a regular basis, everyday lifestyle activities, such as taking a brisk walk or bike ride, raking leaves, gardening, engaging in leisure sports, doing housework, and taking the stairs instead of the elevator can be just as effective as a structured exercise program. The

Exercise, Sunshine, and Carbohydrates

Exercise can greatly enhance the health benefits of your low-GI diet, and getting your exercise outdoors may boost these benefits even more. Why? Being deprived of natural sunlight alters the body's levels of the hormones melatonin and serotonin. This causes some people to feel lethargic, irritable, and depressed and to crave carbohydrates and gain weight.

If this sounds like you, spending more time outside may be just what the doctor ordered. Some studies show that people who regularly exercise outdoors have fewer symptoms of seasonal depression and feel more invigorated and refreshed and happier, while people who exercise indoors tend to feel more fatigued and depressed. So, when weather permits, get outside for a walk or run, spend time gardening, play a game of tennis or basketball, or go biking or canoeing. These simple activities can powerfully boost your weight-management and total-wellness programs.

important thing is to find a variety of activities that you enjoy doing and that fit your lifestyle and do them often.

Combating Insulin Resistance

Insulin resistance, also known as *syndrome X* or *metabolic syndrome*, is a form of carbohydrate intolerance in which people have a blunted response to the effects of insulin. If you are one of the 65 to 70 million Americans who are insulin resistant, your cells do not take up glucose efficiently, and glucose begins to build up in your blood. To compensate, your pancreas shifts into high gear and secretes enough extra insulin to usher glucose into the cells. This extra insulin allows you to maintain normal or near-normal blood sugar levels and protects you from developing type-2 diabetes.

While you may be saved from diabetes, all this extra insulin circulating in your blood creates a whole new set of problems—high blood pressure, increased blood fats (triglycerides), lower HDL (good) cholesterol levels, an increased tendency for blood-clot formation—all of which translates into a very high risk for heart disease. Over time, you could also go on to develop type 2-diabetes as your pancreas becomes too exhausted to compensate any longer.

Genetics and lifestyle play about equal roles in the cause of insulin resistance. A family history of heart attack, high blood pressure, or type-2 diabetes increases your risk. As for lifestyle factors—obesity (particularly abdominal obesity), lack of exercise, and a poor diet all hasten the development of this syndrome.

The good news about insulin resistance is that it is highly treatable with some very simple lifestyle changes. And a healthy lifestyle may even prevent insulin resistance from ever developing in the first place. Being active, watching your weight, and controlling the type and amount of carbohydrates that you eat are three of the most important things you can do to control insulin resistance.

Choosing low-GI carbohydrates can help control insulin resistance. Replacing high-GI foods with lower-GI alternatives will lower blood insulin levels by decreasing the amount of insulin the pancreas puts out. People with insulin resistance should work with their physician, registered dietitian, or licensed nutritionist to determine the *amount* of carbohydrate that will best control their condition, as this will vary from person to person.

Combining a program of regular exercise with your low-GI diet is also essential for controlling insulin resistance. Exercise makes your cells more sensitive to the effects of insulin. As your cells become more sensitive, this will also reduce the amount of insulin that your pancreas secretes, amplifying the benefits of your low-GI diet.

Diabetes Control and Prevention

An estimated 16 million Americans suffer from diabetes, and its incidence is skyrocketing worldwide. Type-2 diabetes, formerly known as non-insulin-dependent diabetes, is by far the most common kind of diabetes, making up about 90 percent of all diabetes cases. A family history of diabetes, being overweight, a sedentary lifestyle, and a poor diet all put you at risk for developing this disorder. Type-2 diabetes has historically been an adult-onset disease, usually affecting people over the age of forty. However, fueled by increasingly sedentary lifestyles and ever-worsening diets, this malady is now becoming common in children and adolescents too.

Like insulin resistance, type-2 diabetes is a disorder in which the body's cells cannot take up glucose efficiently. But unlike an insulin resistant person, in the case of a diabetic, the pancreas cannot compensate enough to clear sugar from the blood, and so blood sugar levels rise to dangerous levels.

Type-1 diabetes is a condition in which the beta cells of the pancreas become damaged and are no longer able to produce insulin. Less than 10 percent of people with diabetes have type-1 diabetes, which usually strikes children and adolescents.

Unless well managed, both types of diabetes can lead to a number of complications, including kidney disease, heart disease, blood vessel damage, blindness, and digit and limb amputations. These complications are caused partly by high blood sugar levels and partly by the underlying insulin resistance present in most cases of diabetes.

How can a low-GI diet benefit a person with diabetes? Since low-GI foods produce slower and smaller rises in blood sugar levels than high-GI foods do, they can be instrumental in helping people with diabetes manage their condition. And since low-GI foods produce less of an insulin response, they reduce the workload of the pancreas and may help preserve its ability to function. By keeping insulin levels down, low-GI foods can also help control the cardiovascular disease associated with diabetes.

A number of studies conducted over the past twenty years have confirmed that substituting low-GI carbohydrates (like oats, pasta, and legumes) for high-GI carbohydrates (like processed cereals, bread, and potatoes) can help lower blood glucose, insulin, and triglycerides; raise HDL (good) cholesterol; and reduce the tendency of the blood to form dangerous clots. This is why the glycemic index has been an integral part of medical nutrition therapy for diabetes in Australia, Canada, New Zealand, and Europe for many years.

There is no doubt that the right diet plus a regular exercise program can substantially lower blood sugar levels and greatly reduce the risk of developing diabetes complications. Some people will also require oral medications or insulin injections to manage their diabetes, though proper diet and exercise can reduce the need for these. People with diabetes should consult a licensed health-care professional for help with designing a diet that meets their unique requirements for calories, fat, and protein and that will complement their exercise program and use of medications.

People with diabetes who take medications or insulin sometimes experience low blood sugar or *hypoglycemia*. If not treated quickly, hypoglycemia can pose a serious health threat. Quickly digested high-GI carbohydrates will produce the fastest relief for hypoglycemia. This is why diabetics often keep glucose tablets (GI = 100) on hand. Be sure to discuss plans for dealing with hypoglycemia with your health-care provider.

While a low-GI diet can help manage diabetes, perhaps a more significant role lies in its power to help prevent type-2 diabetes from ever developing in the first place. In recent studies, researchers at Harvard University who tracked the eating habits of over 65,000 women and 43,000 men found that people whose diets are low in fiber and high in refined and high-GI carbohydrates are more than twice as likely to develop type-2 diabetes as are people who eat a fiber-rich diet with a low glycemic load. These investigators believe that because fast-release carbohydrates generate a higher insulin demand, an excessive intake of these foods can eventually lead to pancreatic exhaustion and type-2 diabetes in susceptible people.

Heart Disease Prevention

Cardiovascular disease is, by far, the leading health threat in industrialized countries, causing about half of all deaths that occur each year. A high-carbohydrate, low-fat diet has long been recommended as the first line of defense for preventing and treating heart disease. In recent years, though, it has become apparent that for many people a high-carb, low-fat diet can actually make things *worse*. How can this be? The original research that showed lowering fats and eating more carbohydrates reduced heart disease risk was based on a diet that was much different from the high-carb, low-fat diet of today.

In the 1970s and early 1980s, high-carbohydrate, low-fat diets were often called *high-carbohydrate, high-fiber* or *HCF* diets. These diets were composed of vegetables, fruits, whole grains, legumes, lean meats, skinless poultry, fish, and low-fat dairy products. HCF diets were low in calories, so they promoted weight loss, they lowered blood cholesterol levels, and they were packed with nutrients, fiber, antioxidants, and phytochemicals that protect against heart disease.

As high-carb, low-fat diets caught on in the 1980s, manufacturers began to develop many new kinds of low-fat foods. Some of these, such as leaner meats, lower-fat dairy products, and low-fat mayonnaise, were a real boon to the fat-fighter. Others, such as fat-free cookies, snack chips, and other foods made from processed grains and refined sugars started the downfall of the low-fat diet. As more and more of these foods entered the marketplace, the nutritional value of many people's diets went down—and the glycemic index of their diet went up.

The typical American high-carb, low-fat diet, as it exists today, is definitely not what the doctor ordered to prevent heart disease. In fact, researchers at Harvard University have discovered that a high dietary glycemic load from refined carbohydrates *doubles* the risk for heart disease. These foods increase blood insulin levels, which in turn contributes to a higher blood pressure, higher levels of blood fats (triglycerides), lower levels of HDL (good) cholesterol, and an increased tendency for dangerous clots to form and linger in the blood. As discussed earlier in this chapter, this is why

A Heart-Disease-Prevention Case Study

Martin, a fifty-year-old small-business owner, discovered that he was at high risk for heart disease when he failed the physical exam that was required to purchase a life insurance policy. His blood work showed that his LDL cholesterol (the so-called bad cholesterol) and triglycerides were dangerously elevated. He went to his doctor for a follow-up exam and was advised to immediately begin drug therapy to bring his cholesterol and triglycerides under control.

Martin did not like the idea of taking a drug for the rest of his life. He had always tried to stay in shape by exercising regularly and watching his fat intake. He had developed a small "spare tire" over the past few years, and needed to lose about fifteen pounds, though. He decided to forgo the drugs and see what he could do by making some changes in his diet instead.

He consulted a registered dietitian who helped him fine-tune his diet to meet his goals. Though Martin's diet was low in fat, he was prone to eating too much bread and potatoes, and his dinners often contained no vegetables at all. High-GI breakfast cereals, sugary sodas, and high-GI snack foods were other problem foods. Here are the changes Martin and his dietitian implemented:

- He prepared a smoothie made with yogurt, fruit, juice, and a heaping tablespoonful of wheat germ or flaxseed meal for breakfast. On weekends when he had more time, he would have a low-fat cheese and vegetable omelet served with turkey bacon and toast made with grainy low-GI bread.

- He cut back on the bread with his meals and ate more vegetables instead. Martin bought a microwave steamer, which he used to quickly prepare a variety of fresh vegetables in season. He also learned how to roast vegetables in the oven, and prepared them often.

- He chose more wholesome foods like fruit, low-fat popcorn, nuts (in moderation), or a half-sandwich made with grainy bread for snacks.

- He drank more water and had sodas only a couple of times a week instead of a few times a day.

Though Martin ate until he was full, he started losing weight almost immediately, and his energy level quickly increased. He liked what he was eating and realized that he had forgotten how much he enjoyed fruits and vegetables. After twelve weeks, Martin had lost twenty pounds and actually had to look for ways to add a few calories back to his diet so that he would stop losing weight. The real test, though, was getting his blood work rechecked. He was pleased at the dramatic results. Not only had his cholesterol and triglyceride levels dropped substantially, but his HDL cholesterol (the so-called good cholesterol) levels had increased. Martin had greatly reduced his risk for heart disease and eliminated the need for medications. He was motivated to continue his new eating style. Look at the differences in Martin's blood test results:

	Before (High-GI Diet)	After (Low-GI Diet)	Desirable Range
Total cholesterol	294 mg/dl	198 mg/dl	<200 mg/dl
LDL cholesterol	175 mg/dl	115 mg/dl	<130 mg/dl
HDL cholesterol	51 mg/dl	57 mg/dl	>35 mg/dl
Triglycerides	339 mg/dl	128 mg/dl	<200 mg/dl

people with insulin resistance have such a high risk for heart disease. And this is why making the change to a diet that emphasizes low-GI unrefined carbohydrates should be a primary strategy for anyone who wants to prevent heart disease.

Cancer Prevention

Scientists have long known that obesity, a sedentary lifestyle, and diets high in refined carbohydrates are linked to cancer. Just how these factors raise cancer risk is the subject of ongoing research, but compelling evidence points to insulin as the common denominator that ties these risk factors together. Positive associations have been found between insulin levels and a variety of cancers including breast, colorectal, and prostate, suggesting that lifestyle changes like maintaining a healthy body weight, exercising, and eating a healthy low-GI diet may protect against cancer, largely by decreasing insulin levels.

How might insulin hasten the development of cancer? Insulin is a cellular growth factor that can directly promote tumor formation in animals. Over the past decade, the results of numerous scientific studies have supported the notion of the association between insulin and cancer in humans. For instance, one team of researchers found that women with high blood insulin levels were nearly three times as likely to develop breast cancer as women with low insulin levels. Other researchers have found that besides raising the risk for cancer, high insulin levels can also make breast cancer more aggressive and more likely to recur. More evidence to support the insulin-cancer link comes from studies showing that people who have high intakes of refined sugar and a high glycemic load are one and one-half to three times more likely to develop colon cancer.

Measures to decrease insulin levels, including eating a low-GI diet and exercising, show great promise for preventing and slowing the progression of cancer. Besides lowering insulin levels, a healthy low-GI diet offers another cancer-fighting bonus: The nutrients, fiber, antioxidants, and phytochemicals present in low-GI foods like vegetables, fruits, unrefined whole grains, and legumes are some of the most potent cancer-fighters ever discovered. For instance, if everyone ate just five servings of vegetables and fruits a day, the incidence of cancer would drop by 20 percent.

Hypoglycemia

As described earlier in this chapter, the most common cause of hypoglycemia (low blood sugar) is as a complication of diabetes. Taking too much blood-sugar lowering medication or injecting too much insulin without eating enough food causes the diabetic reaction, which can be life threatening and must be treated quickly as prescribed by your health-care provider.

Another type of low blood sugar that is not related to diabetes is meal-related *reactive hypoglycemia*. People with reactive hypoglycemia secrete too much insulin after eating. In addition, their cells may be hypersensitive to the effects of insulin and they may not secrete enough of the hormone *glucagon*, which helps to raise blood sugar levels when they drop too low. This causes the cells to remove so much sugar from the blood that a person feels weak, shaky, irritable, headachy, unable to concentrate, and very hungry within two to five hours of eating.

Choosing low-GI carbohydrates is a key strategy for treating reactive hypoglycemia because eating foods that promote a gradual rise in blood sugar and a lower insulin response reduces the likelihood that blood sugar levels will drop too low. An equally important tactic for controlling this condition is eating small, frequent, well-balanced meals and snacks. A registered dietitian or licensed nutritionist can help you develop a meal plan that best suits your individual needs.

Polycystic Ovary Syndrome Therapy

Polycystic ovary syndrome (PCOS) is a disorder in which the ovaries enlarge and develop fluid-filled cysts. Affecting about 7 percent of reproductive-age women, PCOS symptoms include increased levels of androgens (male hormones), disturbances in the menstrual cycle, infertility, hirsutism (excessive growth of facial and body hair), and acne. Because this condition is often associated with insulin resistance, women with PCOS are also at a high risk for diabetes, high blood pressure, and coronary heart disease.

Improvement of polycystic ovary syndrome appears to be another benefit of following a low-GI diet. Measures that improve insulin sensitivity—such as weight loss and exercise—can help reverse PCOS symptoms and restore menstrual regularity and fertility. This is why a low-GI diet, which minimizes insulin secretions more than a traditional weight-loss diet, shows such potential for treating this disorder.

Diabetes drugs that improve insulin sensitivity have also become a popular treatment for PCOS. However, the right diet and exercise program may reduce or eliminate the need for drugs and provide an attractive alternative for women who wish to avoid exposing themselves to the risks that drugs can pose.

As you have seen, eating low on the glycemic index can be a powerful strategy for keeping hunger under control and promoting a healthy body weight. And by lowering blood insulin levels, a low-GI diet can be instrumental in preventing and treating some of the most common health problems that people face today—including insulin resistance, diabetes, and heart disease. All this builds a strong case for making a low-GI eating plan a way of life. The following chapters will show you how easy and enjoyable it can be to do just this.

4. Transforming Your Diet

*I*f the thought of radically changing your diet conjures up images of starvation and deprivation, you will be happy to know that these practices do not apply here. The fact is a wide variety of delicious and satisfying foods can be included in your low-GI eating plan. Living on a starvation diet and sacrificing flavor in the name of nutrition is just not necessary.

This chapter will show you how easy it can be to make the change to a low-GI lifestyle. Knowing about some simple substitutions is the first step to transforming your diet. This chapter teaches you some convenient substitutions and offers a wealth of tips for planning every meal of the day, along with some sample low-GI menus. Last but not least, you will find plenty of possibilities for smart snacking and even some ideas for satisfying a sweet tooth.

Smart Substitutions

Learning about some simple substitutions will lay the foundation for your low-GI lifestyle. The following table shows some low-GI alternatives to high-GI foods. The menu makeover that follows illustrates how you can put these principles into practice in a daily menu. (See chart on page 47)

Menu Makeover

Here is an example of how some simple substitutions can make a big difference in the glycemic index of your diet. Both of the following menus are low in fat, but like the typical American diet, the high-GI menu is too heavy in processed grain products and potatoes and too low in vegetables and fruits.

The low-GI menu features minimally processed grain products. It also substitutes vegetables, fruits, and dairy products for some of the starchy foods in the high-GI menu. The end result is not only a lower glycemic index but also a better-balanced, more nutritious diet. The low-GI diet is also slightly lower in calories even though it provides a larger amount of food.

HIGH-GI MENU (GI = 70)	LOW-GI MENU (GI=42)

Breakfast
2 ounces presweetened instant oatmeal
1 cup low-fat milk
1 slice soft wheat toast

Snack
Cereal bar

Lunch
Sandwich:
    2 ounces roast beef
    2 slices soft wheat bread
    Nonfat mayonnaise, mustard
    1 ounce low-fat potato chips

Snack
1 ounce pretzels

Dinner
3 ounces roast chicken
1 cup mashed potatoes
½ cup green beans
1 dinner roll

Snack
2 graham cracker sheets
1 cup low-fat milk

Calories: 1,842
Fat: 42 g (20%)
Protein: 91 g (20%)
Carbs: 277 g (60%)
Fiber: 21 g
Calcium: 885 mg

Breakfast
2 ounces old-fashioned oatmeal
2 tablespoons chopped dried apricots
2 tablespoons chopped walnuts or pecans
Cinnamon
1 cup low-fat milk
1 cup fresh berries

Snack
8 ounces light fruit yogurt

Lunch
Sandwich:
    2 ounces roast beef
    2 slices grainy bread
    Nonfat mayonnaise, mustard
    Lettuce, tomato, onion
    Apple

Snack
3 cups low-fat popcorn

Dinner
3 ounces roast chicken
8-ounce baked sweet potato
1 cup green beans
2 cups fresh garden salad with light olive-
    oil vinaigrette dressing

Snack
2 oatmeal cookies
1 cup low-fat milk

Calories: 1,717
Fat: 40 g (21%)
Protein: 99 g (23%)
Carbs: 247 g (57%)
Fiber: 34 g
Calcium: 1,202 mg

LOW-GI ALTERNATIVES TO HIGH-GI FOODS

Instead of . . . (High-GI Food)	Choose . . . (Lower-GI Alternatives)
Soft white and wheat breads made from finely ground flours	Hearty breads containing high proportions of grain kernels, oats, bran, and flaxseeds
Processed breakfast cereals	Unrefined cereals, such as old-fashioned oatmeal, oat bran, müesli, and All Bran; cereals made with psyllium
Baked potatoes, mashed potatoes, French fries	Sweet potatoes, small new potatoes, sweet corn, baked beans, lima beans, butter beans, legumes, or basmati or long-grain brown rice
Rice	Choose long-grain or basmati brown rice or substitute wild rice, barley, bulgur wheat, pasta, or whole-wheat couscous
Snack chips and pretzels	Popcorn, nuts (in moderation)
Crackers	Look for those made with 100-percent whole grains and containing high proportions of whole and cracked grains and seeds. Or substitute wedges of whole-grain pita bread or hearty whole-grain breads for crackers.
Cookies	Look for those made with high proportions of oats, whole grains, fruits, and nuts
Muffins and quick breads	Look for those made with high proportions of oats, flax, bran, whole grains, fruits, and nuts

When planning low-GI meals, remember that the GI of a meal is a weighted average of all the carbohydrate-containing foods in the meal (see pages 15–17 for more details). This means that if you eat a small baked potato (GI = 85) in a meal that also contains some low-GI foods like green peas (GI = 48), a fresh green salad (negligible GI), and cup of fresh peaches (GI = 28), the GI of the mixed meal will be moderate. If you dress your salad with a splash of vinegar or lemon juice, you will bring down the GI of the meal even more.

THREE WAYS TO LOWER THE GLYCEMIC INDEX OF MEALS

- Replace high-GI foods with low-GI alternatives.

- Pair a high-GI food with a low-GI food to create an intermediate GI meal.

- Add a splash of vinegar or lemon juice to meals. Four teaspoons can lower the GI of a meal by up to 30 percent.

Breakfast—Starting Your Day the Low-GI Way

Many people trying to lose weight skip breakfast because it just makes them feel hungry all morning long. If this sounds familiar, you should reevaluate what you're eating for breakfast. Typical breakfast foods—such as ready-to-eat cereals, bagels, toast, fat-free cereal bars, muffins, and toaster pastries—are often low in fiber and high in refined carbohydrates. And since many of these foods also have a high glycemic index, they provide a quick burst of energy that is soon replaced by hunger. Below you will find some tips and ideas for simple and sustaining breakfast meals. Use these as guidelines for planning your own menus and for ordering meals in restaurants.

TIPS FOR BUILDING A BETTER BREAKFAST

- Choose low-GI carbohydrates such as grainy breads, unprocessed whole-grain cereals, and fruits.

- When preparing foods like muffins, quick breads, pancakes, and waffles, look for recipes that contain a high proportion of whole grains, oats, bran, and flax. Make French toast with low-GI bread.

- Top pancakes, waffles, and French toast with fresh or canned (in juice) fruit, applesauce, or a low-sugar fruit sauce instead of syrup.

- For extra staying power, include some protein in your breakfast. Egg substitutes, eggs, low-fat milk, cheese, cottage cheese, and yogurt are all excellent sources of protein.

- Don't limit yourself to just "breakfast" foods. Some people find a morning meal of leftovers, some chicken salad and a piece of fruit, or a sandwich preferable to traditional breakfast foods.

Some Low-GI Breakfast Solutions

- Sunrise Smoothie (page 100)

- A glass of sugar-free instant breakfast made with low-fat milk. If desired, add some frozen fruit and blend into a smoothie.

- Multigrain toast topped with natural peanut butter and sliced banana; glass of low-fat milk.

- Whole-grain pumpernickel toast topped with melted low-fat cheese; apple.

- A small whole-grain bagel or pumpernickel toast topped with light cream cheese and smoked salmon; fresh mixed-fruit cup.

- A bowl of old-fashioned oatmeal topped with mixed dried fruit, a sprinkling of nuts, and low-fat milk.

- A bowl of All Bran or Bran Buds cereal topped with fresh berries and low-fat milk; hard-boiled omega-3-enriched egg.

- Blueberry Oat Bran Muffin (page 105); hard-boiled omega-3-enriched egg; and orange juice.

- Broccoli Frittata (page 92); sourdough whole-wheat toast; half grapefruit.

- Breakfast Burrito (page 93); a fresh mixed fruit cup.

- Bacon, Egg, and Cheese Breakfast Sandwich (page 99); a glass of orange or grapefruit juice.

- Scrambled eggs (made with fat-free egg substitute or omega-3-enriched eggs), extra-lean turkey bacon, whole-grain rye toast, fresh mixed-fruit cup, and a glass of low-fat milk.

- Spring Vegetable Omelet (page 91); lean smoked sausage or kielbasa; multigrain toast; and fresh strawberries.

- A parfait made with light vanilla yogurt layered with low-fat granola and chopped apples, peaches, pears, or berries.

- Low-fat cottage cheese with fresh or canned (in juice) peaches or pears and a sprinkling of almonds or toasted wheat germ.

Enjoying a Low-GI Lunch

Whether you are eating out or packing your lunch, there are plenty of low-GI lunch options to choose from. Sandwiches, soups, salads, and quiches are popular lunch dishes, and made properly, all can be part of a healthy low-GI eating plan. Following are some tips and ideas for light and healthy midday meals. Use these as guidelines for planning your own menus and for ordering meals in restaurants.

LOW-GI LUNCH TIPS

◆ Substitute low-GI sides like vegetable or bean soups, fresh vegetable salad, fruit salad, pasta salad, sliced tomatoes, or cottage cheese for high-GI sides like chips, pretzels, baked potatoes, and French fries.

◆ Choose whole-grain, low-GI breads for sandwiches.

◆ Be sure to include some protein (such as lean meat, legumes or cottage cheese) in your mid-day meal to sustain you through the afternoon.

A DOZEN LOW-GI LUNCH IDEAS

◆ Saucy Roast Beef Sandwich (page 178) with a cup of Barley-Vegetable Soup (page 135).

◆ Herbed Turkey Salad Sandwich (page 177), grapes, and a glass of low-fat milk.

◆ Whole-wheat pita bread filled with Garden Hummus (page 117), tomato, and sprouts, and Fabulous Fruit Salad (page 170).

◆ Tangy Tuna Melt (page 183) and Apple Crunch Coleslaw (page 163).

◆ A veggie burger with lettuce, tomato, onion, and mustard on a whole-grain bun with a cup of Bueno Black Bean Soup (page 141).

◆ California Wrap (page 193) with Tortellini Salad (page 168).

◆ Big Sur Turkey Salad (page 160) in a cantaloupe half and a carton of light fruit yogurt.

◆ Roasted Vegetable Salad (page 153) with a cup of Tuscan Lentil Soup (page 138).

◆ Greek Grilled Shrimp Salad (page 145) with wedges of warm whole-wheat pita bread.

◆ Quiche Lorraine (page 96), Springtime Asparagus Salad (page 168), and grapes.

◆ A bowl of Quick Chicken Chili (page 140) and Orange-Avocado Salad (page 165).

◆ A bowl of Zippy Vegetable-Beef Soup (page 132), cottage cheese, and sliced canned peaches (packed in juice).

What's for Dinner?

Low-GI living presents a wealth of dinner possibilities. Pasta; bean dishes; hearty soups and stews; and lean meat, seafood, and poultry dishes can all fit into your low-GI eating plan. For a light evening meal, a main-course salad, sandwich, omelet, frittata, or even pancakes (made the low-GI way) can also fill the bill.

You may be surprised to learn that side dishes are often the biggest obstacle to eating low on the glycemic index at dinner. Why? The evening meal in many households is heavy in high-GI starch and low in vegetables and fruits. Following are some tips and ideas for low-GI evening meals. Use these as guidelines for planning your own menus and for ordering meals in restaurants.

Low-GI Dinner Tips

* Limit high-GI starches like baked or mashed potatoes, French fries, instant rice, boxed side dish mixes, commercial stuffing mixes, and refined breads and dinner rolls.

* Choose low-GI starches like baked sweet potatoes, small new potatoes, corn, peas, long-grain brown or basmati rice, legumes, pasta, and whole-grain breads. Be careful with portions if you are watching your weight.

* Include generous portions of nonstarchy vegetables and fresh salads.

* Get in the habit of finishing dinner off with some fresh fruit instead of a sweet dessert.

A Dozen Low-GI Dinner Ideas

* Baked Chicken Dijon (page 235), baked sweet potato, Fresh Roasted Asparagus (page 195), and Spinach and Pear Salad (page 165).

* Chicken Breasts with Savory Apple Stuffing (page 236), steamed fresh vegetable medley, and a fresh garden salad.

* Citrus-Sauced Chicken (page 237), Broccoli Couscous (page 212), and Glorious Greens (page 166).

* Classic Meatloaf (page 247), Parsley New Potatoes (page 207), steamed broccoli, and sliced fresh tomatoes.

* Saucy Stuffed Cabbage (page 244), Savory Black-Eyed Peas (page 206), and steamed green beans.

* Pot Roast with Sour Cream Gravy (page 250), brown rice, fresh steamed vegetable medley, and Crunchy Layered Salad (page 163).

* Cantonese Roast Pork (page 252), Sesame Fried Rice (page 209), and Asian-Style Collard Greens (page 200).

* Pork Medallions with Sherry Mushroom Sauce (page 251), Autumn Acorn Squash (page 196), Green Beans with Toasted Almonds (page 197), and Cherry-Apple Salad (page 171).

* Grouper el Greco (page 256), Mediterranean Green Beans (page 197), whole-wheat couscous, and Glorious Greens (page 166).

* Citrus Grilled Fish (page 259), fresh corn on the cob, steamed broccoli, and Simple Pear Salad (page 169).

* Slim Spaghetti Pie (page 230), Zucchini & Mushroom Sauté (page 202), fresh garden salad.

* Portabella Pizza (page 261) with a large fresh garden salad.

Dessert Dos and Don'ts

The best advice regarding dessert is to develop the habit of finishing off a meal with some ripe sweet fruit, as is the European custom. Once you curtail your intake of concentrated sweets, you will most likely find that your taste threshold for sugar becomes much lower and you regain an appreciation for the more subtle flavors of wholesome, natural foods. However, while cutting back on sweets is sound advice, there is no need to completely eliminate them from your diet.

TIPS FOR HAVING YOUR CAKE, PUDDING, OR ICE CREAM AND EATING IT, TOO

* Fruit desserts and dairy desserts like puddings, custard, and ice cream will usually have a lower glycemic index than flour-based desserts like cakes, pastries, and cookies.

* Choose cookies and other sweet baked goods that are made with high proportions of oats, fruits, and nuts.

* Look for desserts that contain low to moderate amounts of sugar and fat.

SOME LOW-GI WAYS TO SATISFY A SWEET TOOTH

* A small piece of chocolate

* A few chocolate-covered almonds or peanuts

* A scoop of low-fat ice cream topped with fresh fruit

* Fresh fruit marinated with a little sugar and some brandy or liqueur

* Baked apples stuffed with dried fruits and nuts

* Poached fruits

* Fruit crisps and crumbles made with more fruit and less sugar, with oat toppings

* Applesauce

* Low-fat custards and puddings

* Low-sugar gelatin desserts

* A parfait made with layers of low-fat vanilla or fruit yogurt and fresh fruit

* A float made with low-fat vanilla ice cream and sugar-free root beer or orange soda

* A couple of oatmeal cookies with a glass of low-fat milk

Snacking Smart

Choosing the right snacks is one of the most powerful ways to lower your glycemic load. Traditional snack foods like chips, pretzels, crackers, cookies, sodas, and candies contribute greatly to the overload of processed starches and refined sugars in many people's diets. And besides being high in refined carbohydrates, these foods often contain unhealthful trans fats, saturated fats, and far too many calories.

Baked potato and tortilla chips have about half the calories of their fatty counterparts, making them a better choice, though they still have a high GI. Low-fat snack crackers also have fewer calories than high-fat versions, but most brands are made from finely ground, high-GI refined flours. As for fat-free cookies and candies, most kinds contain just as much—or more—sugar than their full-fat counterparts. The fact is low-fat snack foods like pretzels, graham crackers, animal crackers, and jellybeans typically have a glycemic index of over 80! So what should you snack on? Skip the overly processed junk food and snack on real food instead. Here are some ideas for smart snacks. Just be sure to consider your calorie needs:

- Canned peach, pear, or apricot halves filled with a spoonful of soft-curd farmer cheese or cottage cheese
- Celery or leaves of endive stuffed with low-fat tuna or chicken salad
- Celery stuffed with a small amount of peanut butter
- A banana spread with a small amount of peanut butter
- A few whole-grain crackers with some low-fat tuna, chicken, or egg salad
- Hummus with celery sticks or a few whole-grain crackers
- A half sandwich made on low-GI bread
- A cup of soup
- A piece of low-fat string cheese and an apple
- An ounce of low-fat cheese and a few whole-grain crackers
- A hard-boiled omega-3-enriched egg
- A fresh pear, orange, or apple
- A bowl of fresh cherries or berries
- A bowl of fresh or frozen grapes
- A few dried apricots
- A carton of light fruit yogurt
- A glass of low-fat milk (plain or mixed with a sugar-free cocoa mix)
- A smoothie made from low-fat milk, sugar-free instant breakfast, and frozen fruit
- A small handful of mixed nuts, roasted soy nuts, or pumpkinseeds
- A small handful of trail mix
- A bowl of low-fat popcorn
- V•8 or tomato juice

- A refreshing spritzer of fruit juice mixed with club soda
- Fresh cut vegetables—cherry tomatoes, mushrooms, broccoli, cauliflower, red bell peppers, radishes, carrots, celery, etc. (with low-fat dip or dressing if desired)
- An oat bran muffin
- A slice of whole-grain banana bread with a glass of low-fat milk
- A scoop of low-fat ice cream topped with fresh berries
- A frozen 100-percent fruit-juice bar
- A small piece of dark chocolate

Some Cautions About Using the Glycemic Index for Meal Planning

- Remember that calories still count. Just because a food has a low glycemic index does not mean that it can be eaten in unlimited quantities. Even healthful foods like pasta, legumes, and brown rice can cause weight gain if eaten in excess of your calorie needs.

- Just because a food has a low glycemic index does not necessarily mean it is a healthful choice. Sometimes sugary or high-fat foods—such as candy bars, muffins, cookies, cheesecake, and ice cream—have a low glycemic index. These foods should be eaten in moderation.

- Adding fat to a meal lowers its GI because it slows down digestion; however, remember to include fat in your diet only within the bounds of your calorie needs, or you may find yourself gaining unwanted weight.

- Avoid using refined fructose as a sweetener, and limit foods that contain high-fructose corn syrup as the primary sweetener. While fructose has a very low GI, too much can raise blood fats (triglycerides), adding a risk factor for cardiovascular disease. In addition, refined fructose—like other refined sugars—contains no nutrients and adds unneeded calories to your diet.

- As the glycemic index becomes more popular, manufacturers will undoubtedly develop more and more low-GI foods. As with many of the fat-free foods that were developed in the 1990s, many of these low-GI foods will probably contain highly refined and artificial ingredients, too many calories, and too few nutrients. Always beware as new products enter the market, and consider the nutritional qualities of the food before making it a regular part of your diet.

Making the change to a low-GI lifestyle can be both easy and enjoyable. It is primarily a matter of learning about some simple substitutions. And instead of dieting and deprivation, a low-GI lifestyle presents a wide variety of satisfying and delicious meal-planning possibilities. The next chapter expands on this topic by offering a wealth of tips for maintaining your low-GI diet when eating away from home.

5. Dining Defensively in Restaurants

*E*ating low on the glycemic index can be easily accomplished at home, where you control the grocery shopping and meal preparation. But can you keep up your low-GI lifestyle when eating away from home? Absolutely. Many of the suggestions presented in the previous chapter can be applied also to eating in restaurants. And while dining out does present some challenges, many restaurants are making it easier than ever to eat healthfully. Grilled fish and seafood, lean meats and poultry, fresh vegetables, fruits, pasta, and vegetarian dishes can be found in just about any restaurant today. And most chefs are more than happy to modify dishes to suit your nutritional preferences. Many restaurants also have Web sites where you can peruse menus, look up nutrition information, ask questions, and provide feedback. Here are some suggestions for making the most of the menu in any restaurant.

TIPS FOR EATING WELL IN RESTAURANTS

- ◆ Choose restaurants that feature table service instead of an all-you-can-eat food bar or buffet. The sight of a large quantity and variety of food attractively displayed and all for one price encourages overconsumption by even the most disciplined people.

- ◆ Don't go to a restaurant ravenously hungry. If necessary, have a small low-GI snack in the late afternoon before you go out to eat. By taking the edge off your hunger, you'll have more control when ordering.

- ◆ If you must wait at the bar for your table, order mineral water, club soda with lime, tomato juice, V•8 juice, or a Virgin Mary, glass of dry red or white wine, or a wine spritzer (white wine mixed with club soda). Avoid alcoholic beverages made with sweet or creamy mixers.

- ◆ Beware of the breadbasket. Most of the bread served in restaurants is the highly refined, high-GI type. French bread, for instance, has a GI of 95! And it's easy to polish off several pieces of bread and butter (and several hundred calories) before the entrée even arrives.

- ◆ Make smart choices at the salad bar. Start by loading up on fresh vegetables and fruits. For protein, choose low-fat cottage cheese, turkey, steamed seafood, and kidney beans or garbanzo beans. Dress your salad with a light dressing or use just a little olive oil and a splash of vinegar or lemon juice.

- When ordering sandwiches, request whole-grain bread, and use mustard, low-fat mayonnaise, light ranch dressing, or a splash of light Italian dressing as a spread. Be sure to add plenty of lettuce, tomato, and vegetable toppings.

- Ask if tuna and chicken salads and other mayonnaise-based dishes can be made with light mayonnaise. Some restaurants do offer these lighter alternatives.

- Substitute a side salad, cup of soup, sliced tomatoes, steamed vegetables, fresh fruit, pasta salad, or cottage cheese for high-GI accompaniments like fries, baked potatoes, chips, and pretzels.

- At breakfast, ask if you can have omelets, scrambled eggs, and French toast made with a fat-free egg substitute or with more whites and fewer yolks—many restaurants will be happy to do this for you. Have French toast made with whole-wheat bread, and use fresh fruit or applesauce as a topping. Order Canadian bacon or ham instead of regular bacon or sausage. And request unbuttered whole-wheat, rye, or pumpernickel toast instead of buttered white toast.

- Look for menu items that are steamed, broiled, blackened, grilled, roasted, prepared "en papillote" (steamed in parchment paper), stir-fried, stewed, braised, or served "in their own juice." Be sure to order any sauces or dressings on the side so that you can control the amount used.

- Ask if traditional menu items can be prepared with less fat. For instance, many restaurants will prepare stir-fries, pasta, and other dishes with little or no butter or oil. This can easily trim a couple of hundred calories from your meal.

- Be creative when ordering. Consider ordering an à la carte meal of an appetizer, soup, and salad rather than a full-course meal.

- Choose broth-based, vegetable, and bean soups instead of high-fat cream soups.

- If portions are large, take half home or split an entrée with a dinner companion. Note that some restaurants may also offer some of their entrées, salads, and sandwiches in "lighter" or smaller portions for a reduced price.

- If you can't resist dessert, share it with a friend—or with several friends. And remember, the "light" and "low-fat" desserts featured at some restaurants can be very high in carbohydrates and calories if the portions are large, or if they are high in sugar.

Getting Down to Specifics

Each type of restaurant offers its own rewards and challenges. Ethnic restaurants, in particular, present a wide range of delicious possibilities for the discriminating diner. For instance, ethnic specialties like pasta and legumes fit nicely into a low-GI eating plan. Here are some ideas for making the best choices in a wide range of restaurants.

CHINESE

Authentic Chinese food is low in fat and high in nutrients. Traditional dishes feature moderate portions of meat, seafood, poultry, or tofu stir-fried with plenty of vegetables and flavorful sauces. Realize, though, that the Asian-style sticky white rice that accompanies these dishes ranks high on the glycemic index and should be limited. American-style Chinese food tends to be a heavier, fattier version of the traditional cuisine, so it pays to peruse the menu. Here are some of the lighter dishes.

- Broth-based soups like wonton, hot and sour, and egg drop
- Stir-fried combinations of seafood, poultry, lean meat, tofu, and vegetables (Ask for a minimum of oil to be used in preparation.)
- Chop suey and chow mein (served without the fried noodles)
- Noodle dishes like seafood, chicken, or vegetable lo mein (Ask for a minimum of oil to be used in preparation.)
- Steamed fish and vegetable dishes
- Steamed long-grain brown rice (if available)
- Foods cooked in black bean sauce, oyster sauce, hot mustard sauce, and Szechuan sauce
- Fortune cookie (One cookie has only 30 calories and 6 grams of carbohydrate.)

FRENCH

This cuisine, which is often heavy in eggs, butter, cheese, and creamy sauces, can be a difficult one for people who are trying to keep fat within reasonable limits. And French bread ranks exceptionally high on the glycemic index (GI = 95). Fortunately, many French restaurants also serve some lighter Mediterranean-style items, and if you know what to look for, you can actually dine quite healthfully.

- Consommé and broth-based soups
- Broiled, steamed, or poached seafood and poultry (Order sauces to be served on the side.)
- Seafood and poultry cooked *en papillote* (steamed in parchment paper)
- Chicken or fish Provençal (with tomato sauce); chicken or fish cooked with tomato-wine sauces
- Seafood or vegetable stews, such as bouillabaisse and ratatouille
- Chicken, beef, and veal stews with wine or tomato sauces

- Steamed vegetables; salads with vinaigrette dressing on the side
- Poached fruits

GREEK

Roasted lamb and chicken, lemon, yogurt, and herbs like oregano and rosemary are some of the better ingredients featured in this flavorful cuisine. On the other hand, buttery filo-crusted pies, heaps of feta cheese, and pools of olive oil can blow your fat and calorie budgets in a hurry. Choose these items most often:

- Bean and lentil soups; avgolemono (lemon and egg) soup; vegetable soups; fish soups
- Shish kabobs made of roasted lamb or chicken and vegetables
- Baked fish dishes such as Plaki (fish baked with tomatoes, onions, and garlic) and fish baked in grape leaves; baked chicken dishes (Ask the chef to use a minimal amount of butter or oil in baked dishes.)
- Gyro sandwiches made with grilled chicken or lean rotisserie meat
- Greek salads made with just a tablespoon or two of feta cheese and a light vinaigrette dressing
- Fruit compotes; marinated fruits

INDIAN

Here's a cuisine with plenty to offer the low-GI diner. Healthful legumes, chicken, fish, vegetables, and yogurt are featured throughout the menu. Basmati rice is also featured in Indian cuisine, though it is usually white basmati rice. Curry, cumin, coriander, and other flavorful seasonings add exotic and delicious flavors. Indian cooks use ghee (clarified butter) or vegetable oil to prepare dishes like curries, vindaloos, and rice dishes—and some chefs have a heavier hand with the fat than do others. So be sure to request that your food be prepared with a minimum of added fat. If you're eating Indian food, try any of the following:

- Vegetable and dahl (lentil or bean) soups
- Chapati (a whole-wheat tortilla-like bread)
- Raita (a cold side dish made of cucumbers or other vegetables with yogurt sauce)
- Chutney (a spicy accompaniment to meals)
- Vegetable, chicken, or seafood biryanis (basmati rice dishes)
- Vegetable, seafood, and chicken curry dishes (avoid those made with large amounts of coconut or coconut milk)
- Chicken or Shrimp Vindaloo (in a hot and spicy tomato, onion, and curry sauce)
- Tandoori chicken or fish (chicken marinated in yogurt and spices and baked in a clay oven)

- Lamb or chicken kabobs
- Dahls (legume dishes)

ITALIAN

Steer clear of the white Italian bread and the cheese-laden, creamy, and excessively oily dishes; and, instead, go for the pasta, tomato sauces, vegetables, and beans. Many Italian restaurants offer pasta dishes in half portions. Try combining a half portion of pasta with a soup and salad for a filling and satisfying meal. Also, try the following:

- Vegetable or bean-based soups like minestrone and pasta fagioli
- Steamed clams or mussels
- Pasta with tomato-based sauces (like marinara, puttanesca, and arrabbiata); pasta with tomato-seafood sauces like red clam sauce
- Broiled or grilled chicken and fish dishes
- Chicken cacciatore; chicken or veal piccata and marsala (Request that a minimum of oil or butter be used to prepare these dishes.)
- Seafood stews like cioppino
- Thin-crust pizza with lots of vegetable toppings and part-skim mozzarella cheese
- Poached fruits; cappuccino made with low-fat milk

JAPANESE

The Japanese enjoy the greatest longevity in the world, and traditional Japanese cuisine is one reason why. Grilled or stir-fried chicken, seafood, lean beef, and tofu served with plenty of colorful vegetables are featured fare. Teriyaki sauce and ginger are frequently used to add savory flavor to dishes. Realize, however, that the Asian-style sticky white rice that accompanies most dishes ranks very high on the glycemic index and should be limited.

- Miso soup; broth-based soups
- Sashimi (raw, slivered fish, usually served with a dipping sauce), edamame (lightly salted and boiled green soybeans)
- Yakitori (broiled chicken kabobs), teriyaki dishes, "yakimono" (grilled) dishes, sukiyaki (thinly sliced beef and vegetables in a piquant sauce)
- Stir-fried seafood, chicken, lean beef, or tofu and vegetable combinations
- Udon (wheat) noodles, soba (buckwheat) noodles
- Steamed long-grain brown rice (if available)

LOW-GI RESTAURANT ALTERNATIVES TO HIGH-GI RESTAURANT MEALS	
Instead of . . . (High-GI Meal)	Substitute . . . (Lower-GI Alternative)
Breakfast Pancakes made with refined flour topped with butter and syrup Sausage Juice	*Breakfast* French toast (made with fewer yolks and more whites or a fat-free egg substitute and whole-wheat bread) topped with fresh fruit Canadian bacon Skim or low-fat milk
Western omelet Hash browns Buttered white toast Bacon Juice	Western omelet (made with fewer yolks and more whites or a fat-free egg substitute) Unbuttered whole-wheat toast Canadian bacon Fresh fruit cup
Lunch 2 slices thick-crust pizza Bread stick Soda	*Lunch* 2 slices thin-crust pizza Salad with light Italian or olive oil vinaigrette dressing Water or unsweetened tea
Turkey sandwich on Kaiser roll Potato chips Soda	Turkey sandwich on whole-wheat bread Cup of vegetable soup Water or unsweetened tea
Grilled chicken sandwich on a white bun French fries Soda	Grilled chicken salad with light dressing Cup of minestrone soup Water or unsweetened tea
Dinner Steak Baked potato with butter	*Dinner* Steak and vegetable kabob Baked sweet potato

Low-GI Restaurant Alternatives to High-GI Restaurant Meals (cont.)	
Instead of . . . (High-GI Meal)	Substitute . . . (Lower-GI Alternative)
Dinner Bread with butter Salad Sweet tea	*Dinner* Steamed vegetables Salad Unsweetened tea or water
Tortilla chips and salsa Chicken burrito Mexican rice Refried beans Soda	Black-bean soup Chicken burrito Grilled vegetables Salad Unsweetened tea or water
Egg roll Sweet-and-Sour Chicken White rice Soda	Hot-and sour soup Szechuan Chicken Stir-Fried Vegetable Combination Green tea Water

MEXICAN

Much of the food served in Mexican restaurants is high in starch and fat and low in vegetables and fruits, making it easy to get an overdose of carbohydrates and calories. Fortunately, most Tex-Mex restaurants also have a lighter side. Flavorful grilled seafood and chicken entrées, colorful salads, low-fat beans, and grilled vegetables are some of the best-selling items in Tex-Mex restaurants these days. Some restaurants also offer burritos, fajitas, soft tacos, and quesadillas made with whole-wheat tortillas, low-fat cheese, and light sour cream.

When ordering Tex-Mex, you can lighten your glycemic load considerably by skipping the chips that usually precede the meal and replacing the usual rice side dish with some grilled or steamed veggies. Also, try any of the following:

* Black bean soup; ceviche (lime-marinated seafood salad); gazpacho (chilled tomato and cucumber soup)

* Grilled seafood and chicken dishes

- Main-dish salads topped with grilled chicken or seafood and a light dressing (If the salad is served in a fried taco shell, be sure to ask the chef to leave it off.)

- Chicken soft tacos, burritos, chicken and vegetable quesadillas (Limit the cheese and sour cream toppings, and ask if whole-wheat tortillas are available.)

- Chicken enchiladas (request that the tortillas be softened on a dry grill) topped with a red sauce or green chili sauce and a light sprinkling of cheese

- Chicken, shrimp, and vegetable fajitas (Ask that they be cooked in less oil, limit the sour cream and cheese, and ask if whole-wheat tortillas are available.)

- Low-fat bean side dishes; grilled or steamed Mexican vegetables such as zucchini, peppers, corn, and onion medley; fresh fruit

- Salsa, pico de gallo (tomatoes with onions and hot peppers), ranchero sauce, red enchilada sauce, tomatillo sauce, green chili sauce

- Guacamole (limit the amount if you are watching your weight)

- Low-fat sour cream and cheese (if available)

THAI

This flavorful cuisine has much to offer the discriminating diner. Thai dishes typically combine small amounts of meats, seafood, chicken, or tofu with lots of vegetables and spicy curry, chili, and fish sauces. Many Thai dishes are also served with long-grain rice (which has a moderate GI), though it is usually white rice. Lime juice, lemongrass, and basil also add flavor to Thai dishes. Try any of the following:

- Broth-based soups like Tom Yum Gai (chicken with vegetables and Thai seasonings) or Tom Yum Goong (shrimp with vegetables and Thai seasonings)

- Stir-fried combinations of seafood, chicken, tofu, lean meat, and vegetables (Ask for a minimum of oil to be used in preparation.)

- Pad Thai and other stir-fried noodle dishes made with vegetables and seafood, chicken, tofu, or lean meat (Ask for less oil than usual to be used in preparation.)

- Dishes made with basil sauce, lime sauce, chili sauce, and fish sauce

As you can see, a low-GI lifestyle presents plenty of delicious possibilities for those who enjoy the pleasures of dining out. Most restaurants feature a wide variety of menu items that can fit nicely into a healthful low-GI eating plan for every meal of the day. And most chefs are more than willing to prepare menu items and make substitutions to suit your preferences. So there's no reason to sit at home once you know the secrets of eating low on the glycemic index.

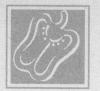

6. Mastering Low-GI Cooking

While many people believe that making the change to a low-GI lifestyle means spending hours in the kitchen learning complicated cooking techniques or perusing specialty stores for exotic and expensive ingredients, nothing could be further from the truth. The fact is, preparing healthful low-GI meals can be both easy and enjoyable. And most of the foods you will need to prepare your meals can be found right in your favorite grocery store.

In this chapter, you will learn about the foods that will get you started on the road to success, along with some tips for using these foods in cooking and meal planning. And, as you will see, once you know the secrets of low-GI cooking, you can also modify many of your favorite recipes to fit your low-GI lifestyle. First, though, let's look at some general tips that can help you survive your next trip to the grocery store.

* Avoid going grocery shopping when you are hungry. This will reduce the likelihood of impulse buying.

* Spend most of your time in the periphery of the store, as this is where the most nutrient-dense, least processed foods tend to be located.

* Peruse the ingredients list before buying packaged foods. This will tell you a product's ingredients in their order of predominance. Limit your use of foods that contain large amounts of hydrogenated vegetable oil, refined grains and flours, sugars, salt, and artificial ingredients.

* Become familiar with the "Nutrition Facts" label on packaged foods. Evaluate the serving size and compare this to what you would call a serving. Then look at the calories, fat, and carbohydrate amounts and see how these amounts fit into your personal nutrition goals. (The tables on pages 19 and 27 can give you an idea of what levels of these nutrients are appropriate for you.)

* Evaluate the fiber content of the food, bearing in mind that most people should aim for *at least* 25 to 35 grams per day. (See page 35 for more on fiber.)

- Look at the sodium content of the food, bearing in mind that a prudent daily intake is 2,400 milligrams or less.

- Look at the sugar content of the food, bearing in mind that most people should aim for an upper limit of 24 to 48 grams (6 to 12 teaspoons) of added refined sugar per day. (See page 19 for more on sugar).

- Be wary, but don't get carried away with counting every calorie, carbohydrate gram, and fat gram that you eat. This is how unhealthy food obsessions are born. Just focus on choosing foods that are wholesome and minimally processed, and eat moderate portions. Otherwise, you might never make it out of the store!

A Health-Minded Tour of the Supermarket

Here are some specific suggestions for choosing and using the foods than can help you lighten your glycemic load, trim fat, and improve your overall health.

DAIRY PRODUCTS

Many people believe that dairy products are taboo on a low-GI eating plan, but the fact is, dairy products like milk, yogurt, and cheese have very low glycemic indexes (less than 35). This is because the sugar in dairy products (lactose) is very slowly released and absorbed by the body. The acidity of cultured dairy products like yogurt and buttermilk also contributes to a low GI by slowing carbohydrate digestion. Plus, these days, it's a simple matter to choose lower-fat and lower-sugar versions of all your favorite dairy products. Here are some products to put in your shopping cart.

Cheese

- Low-fat and nonfat cottage cheese
- Low-fat and nonfat ricotta cheese
- Low-fat and nonfat cream cheese
- Neufchâtel (reduced-fat cream cheese)
- Soft-curd farmer cheese—a soft, slightly crumbly white cheese that is delicious in spreads and fillings or crumbled over a salad
- Reduced-fat and nontat feta cheese
- Parmesan cheese (Although Parmesan contains 8 grams of fat per ounce, a little bit goes a long way, making this an acceptable choice.)
- Reduced-fat and nonfat mozzarella, Cheddar, Monterey Jack, provolone, and Swiss cheeses—

look for brands with no more than 5 grams of fat per ounce (Tip: Reduced-fat cheeses work best in recipes in which you need a cheese that melts well, while nonfat brands work fine atop a salad or in a sandwich.)

- Low-fat string cheese

Milk

- Skim (nonfat) and low-fat (1-percent) milk
- Nonfat and low-fat buttermilk (Tip: If you need a substitute for buttermilk in recipes, you can mix ½ cup of plain yogurt with ½ cup of skim or low-fat milk to make 1 cup of buttermilk substitute.)
- Evaporated skim or low-fat milk—Use as a substitute for cream in pasta dishes and sauces or to lighten your coffee.
- Instant nonfat dry milk powder

Yogurt

- Plain nonfat and low-fat yogurt
- Flavored nonfat and low-fat yogurt—Choose sugar-free or light brands to trim calories by almost half.

Other Dairy Products

- Nonfat and light sour cream
- Low-fat ice cream and frozen yogurt—Watch portions because these products contain sugar.

NONDAIRY ALTERNATIVES

If you choose to avoid dairy products, you'll be glad to know that there are plenty of nondairy options to choose from. Milks made from ingredients like soybeans, brown rice, oats, and almonds are available and can replace cow's milk on cereal and in most recipes. Cheeses, yogurt, and sour cream made from soy-, brown-rice, and nut milks are also widely available. Many of these products can be found in your grocery store, while others are featured in health-food stores. Just be aware that some nondairy products do contain casein, a milk protein that some people need to avoid.

MARGARINE AND BUTTER

Which is better, butter or margarine? Neither should have a prominent place in your diet. Butter is a concentrated source of artery-clogging saturated fat, while margarine often contains equally harmful trans fats (from hydrogenated vegetable oils). If you are watching your weight, you should know that just one tablespoon of either butter or margarine contains 100 calories. Fortunately, reduced-fat and nonfat spreads, with 25- to 95-percent less fat and calories, are also widely available, and some trans-fat-free margarines are available as well. Light butter and margarine can be used for cooking many dishes, but in some cases, a small amount of a full-fat spread works best. The recipes in this book will specify which kind of spread is most appropriate for each recipe. Use the following products in moderation, keeping your health and weight-management goals in mind.

- Light whipped butter
- Light butter
- Light margarine—Look for liquid (nonhydrogenated) canola, soy, or olive oil as the first ingredient.
- Regular margarine—Look for liquid (nonhydrogenated) canola, soy, or olive oil as the first ingredient, and use sparingly if you are watching your weight.

MAYONNAISE AND SALAD DRESSINGS

Some carbohydrate-control books assert that you must use only full-fat mayonnaise and salad dressings because lower-fat versions contain sugar or other carbohydrates. While this may be true, the amount of carbohydrate present in the lower-fat products is usually not enough to worry about, and the calorie savings are considerable. For instance, a tablespoon of nonfat mayonnaise that provides 10 calories and 2 grams of carbohydrate is definitely a better choice than a tablespoon of full-fat mayo with 100 calories and 11 grams of fat!

As for salad dressings, some lower-fat brands contain as much as 10 grams (2½ teaspoons) of sugar per 2-tablespoon serving, while others are practically sugar-free. Read labels and compare calories, sugar, and fat contents of different brands. Then make your decision based on your personal nutrition goals.

What if you don't like the light products? Go ahead and use the full-fat product; just be sure to use it sparingly. If you haven't tried some of the lower-fat products recently, you should give them another try because they are continually improving.

Here are some mayonnaises and salad dressings you can use:

- Nonfat and light mayonnaise
- Regular mayonnaise—Choose brands made with canola, soybean, or olive oil and use sparingly if you are watching your weight.
- Nonfat and low-fat salad dressings—Compare labels for sugar content, and choose accordingly.
- Regular salad dressings—Choose brands made with canola, soybean, or olive oil, and use sparingly if you are watching your weight.

• Vinegars and lemon juice—Because they slow the rate of digestion, acidic ingredients like vinegar and lemon juice should be staples in the low-GI pantry. Adding just 4 teaspoons to a meal can lower its glycemic index by about 30 percent. A wide variety of vinegars are available—including red or white wine, herb flavored, rice, balsamic, and raspberry—to add zing to your homemade salads and dressings. A splash of vinegar or lemon juice can also perk up steamed broccoli, asparagus, greens, and many other vegetables.

OILS

Many people are confused about oils because liquid vegetable oils have long been promoted as being "heart healthy." The reason is, these oils are low in artery-clogging saturated fat and contain no cholesterol. Unfortunately, many people assume that these products are also low in total fat and calories, and therefore may be used liberally. Not so. All oils are pure fat—just one tablespoon of *any* oil has 13.6 grams of fat and 120 calories. So if you are watching your weight, cutting back on oils and other fats is one of the best strategies for trimming calories.

On the other hand, using a little oil in some recipes definitely makes food more palatable, so you needn't completely eliminate this ingredient from your diet. In addition, some oils provide essential fatty acids such as the omega-3 fat alpha-linolenic acid that many people are deficient in. Used judiciously, cooking oils can both enhance flavor and help provide a healthy balance of essential fat. Here are some of the better choices.

Canola Oil

Low in saturated fats and rich in monounsaturated fats, canola oil also contains alpha-linolenic acid, an essential omega-3 fat that is deficient in most people's diets. For these reasons, canola oil should be one of your primary cooking oils. Canola oil has a very mild, bland taste, so it is a good all-purpose oil for cooking and baking when you want no interfering flavors.

Extra-Virgin Olive Oil

Along with canola oil, olive oil should be one of your primary cooking oils. Rich in monounsaturated fat, olive oil also contains phytochemicals that help lower blood cholesterol levels and protect against cancer. Unlike most vegetable oils, which are very bland, olive oil adds its own delicious flavor to foods. Extra-virgin olive oil is the least processed and most flavorful type of olive oil.

Soybean Oil

Most cooking oils that are labeled simply "vegetable oil" are made from soybean oil. Soybean oil is also used as an ingredient in many brands of margarine, mayonnaise, and salad dressing. This oil supplies a fair amount of omega-3 fat, although not as much as canola and walnut oils do. Like canola oil, soybean oil has a bland flavor that works well in dishes where you want no interfering flavors.

Walnut Oil

With a delicate nutty flavor, walnut oil is an excellent choice for baking and salads. Like canola oil, walnut oil contains a substantial amount of the omega-3 fat. Most brands of walnut oil have been only minimally processed and can turn rancid quickly, so once opened, they should be refrigerated.

Nonstick Vegetable Oil Cooking Spray

Available unflavored and in butter, olive oil, and garlic flavors, cooking sprays are pure fat. The advantage to using them is that the amount that comes out during a one-second spray is so small that it adds an insignificant amount of fat to a recipe. Nonstick cooking sprays are very useful to promote the browning of foods and to prevent foods from sticking to pots and pans.

EGGS AND EGG SUBSTITUTES

Everyone knows that eggs are loaded with cholesterol—just one large egg uses up two-thirds of your daily cholesterol budget. One egg also contains close to 5 grams of fat. This may not seem like all that much until you consider that a three-egg omelet contains 15 grams of fat—and that's without counting the cheese filling or the butter used in the skillet! The good news is that it is a simple matter to make dishes with more whites (which are fat- and cholesterol-free) and fewer yolks, or you can use a fat-free egg substitute and enjoy your favorite egg dishes with absolutely no fat or cholesterol at all.

Contrary to what the term *substitute* implies, egg substitutes are made from 99-percent pure egg whites. The remaining 1 percent consists mostly of vegetable thickeners, vitamins, minerals, and yellow coloring—usually beta-carotene or the plant-based coloring agents annatto or turmeric. You will find egg substitutes, like Egg Beaters, in both the refrigerated-foods section and the freezer case of your grocery store.

Realize that although whole eggs are high in cholesterol, most health experts agree that a healthy diet can include four to seven egg yolks per week. Ask your physician or dietitian to make a recommendation for your specific needs.

Finally, some manufacturers are now feeding hens a diet that is enriched with vitamin E and ingredients like flaxseeds, marine algae, and fishmeal. This produces eggs that are nutritionally superior to regular eggs because the yolks are higher in vitamin E and omega-3 fatty acids. When you eat whole eggs, choose these omega-3-enriched products most often.

MEAT, POULTRY, AND SEAFOOD

Including several ounces of protein in a meal will make the meal more filling and satisfying—a real boon to the weight watcher. Be sure to choose lean, well-trimmed meats and skinless poultry to keep saturated fat and calories under control. Realize that processed meats like ham, hot dogs, and luncheon meats are high in sodium and contain artificial ingredients, so use these products less often. Be sure to substitute fish for meat several times a week, and include more of the vegetarian alternatives (listed in the next section) in your diet often. Following are some good meats, poultry, and seafoods to choose:

- Skinless chicken and turkey
- Ground turkey—Look for ground turkey that is at least 93- to 96-percent lean.
- Beef round, eye of round, round tip, top sirloin
- Ground beef—Look for ground beef that is at least 93- to 96-percent lean.
- Pork tenderloin, loin roast, sirloin chops, loin chops
- Ham—Look for ham that is at least 95-percent lean.
- Extra-lean turkey bacon (Tip: For a crisp texture, cook turkey bacon in a microwave oven. Turkey bacon cooked in a skillet will have a chewy texture.)
- Canadian bacon
- Smoked sausage and kielbasa—Look for products that are at least 95- to 97-percent lean.
- Luncheon meats—Look for products that are at least 97-percent lean.
- Fish and shellfish (fresh or plain frozen)—Choose oily fish like salmon often for their healthful omega-3 fatty acids.
- Water-packed canned tuna, salmon, and sardines

VEGETARIAN MEAT ALTERNATIVES

To optimize your health, try to get at least half of your protein from plant sources like the ones listed below. These foods are naturally low in saturated fat, and they contain no cholesterol. In addition, the following foods are loaded with health-promoting phytochemicals that are not present in meats. Some of these foods are rich sources of fiber as well.

- Tofu—Substitute crumbled firm tofu for part or all of the hard-boiled eggs in egg salad; add crumbled firm tofu to scrambled eggs or sprinkle it over a salad as you would cheese. Substitute cubed firm or extra-firm tofu for the meat in stir-fry dishes.
- Tofu hamburger—These mildly seasoned bits of tofu look like cooked ground beef and can substitute for part or all of the ground beef in many recipes. Two cups of tofu hamburger is the equivalent of 1 pound of ground beef.
- Frozen recipe crumbles—Like tofu hamburger, recipe crumbles (like Green Giant's Harvest Burger for Recipes) can substitute for part or all of the ground meat in recipes. Two cups of recipe crumbles are the equivalent of 1 pound of ground beef.

- Texturized vegetable protein (TVP)—Made from defatted soy flour, TVP comes packaged as small nuggets that you rehydrate with water. Substitute the rehydrated product for part or all of the ground meat in recipes. One cup of TVP rehydrated with ⅞ cup of boiling water is the equivalent of 1 pound of ground beef.

- Veggie burgers

- Soy lunchmeats, hot dogs, and sausages—Realize that these products are higher in sodium and may contain artificial ingredients, so use them less often than the other vegetarian alternatives listed. Since they are also diluted with other ingredients, they usually contain fewer beneficial phytochemicals, such as isoflavones, than pure soy foods.

- Legumes (dried beans, peas, and lentils)—Legumes have very low GIs (in the 25 to 45 range) and are rich in cholesterol-lowering soluble fiber as well as a multitude of vitamins and minerals. Stock up on dried kidney, pinto, garbanzo, navy, lima, and black beans as well as lentils, split peas, and black-eyed peas. Canned versions of these products are also excellent ingredients for soups, salads, and other dishes. Draining and rinsing canned beans will remove about 40 percent of the sodium.

BREADS

Bread made from finely ground flours—which are rapidly digested and absorbed—have a very high GI (in the 70 to 90 range). Equally problematic is the fact that the majority of breads sold in grocery stores and bakeries and eaten in restaurants today are made from nutrient-poor refined white flour. However, chosen wisely, the right bread can fit into a low-GI diet and add important nutrients to your diet. What should you look for? Choose breads made with *stone-ground* whole-wheat flour, which is a coarsely ground flour made from whole-grain wheat kernels. Look for coarse, rustic breads that contain intact whole grains, cracked wheat, wheat berries, wheat bran, wheat germ, rolled oats, oat bran, flaxseed, and bits of seeds or nuts. These breads will usually have a GI in the 50 to 60 range. Here are some examples:

- 100-percent stone-ground whole-wheat bread—Look for at least 2 grams of fiber per 1-ounce slice.

- Rye, pumpernickel, oatmeal, oat bran, and multigrain breads made with 100-percent whole-grain ingredients—Look for at least 2 grams of fiber per 1-ounce slice.

- Sourdough bread—The acidity of sourdough bread gives it a lower GI than other breads, even if it is made from white flour. For the most nutrition and fiber, though, choose whole-wheat or rye sourdough breads.

- Burger buns and sandwich rolls—Look for brands made with 100-percent stone-ground whole-wheat flour or a combination of flour and other grains such as oats, oat bran, rolled wheat, and wheat bran. Look for at least 4 grams of fiber per 2-ounce bun.

- Bagels—Look for 100 percent whole-wheat or multigrain bagels. Realize that the big bagels that are commonly available today are the equivalent of four to five slices of bread and can blow your carbohydrate budget in a hurry! Instead, choose small (2- to 3-ounce) bagels or have just half of a large bagel.

- English muffins—Look for whole-wheat or oat-bran English muffins.

- Whole-wheat and oat-bran pita bread—Flatbreads like pita, chapati, and tortillas tend to have a lower GI than soft, airy-textured breads because their starch is not as gelatinized (hydrated with water). The dense structure of flatbreads also resists digestion, contributing to a lower GI.

- Whole-wheat flour tortillas—Use to make wrap-style sandwiches, burritos, quesadillas, and other Tex-Mex favorites. Unleavened breads like tortillas and chapati contain *phytate,* a phytochemical that is naturally present in whole-grains which is associated with a lower GI in breads.

- Chapati—A traditional Indian flatbread made from whole-wheat flour and sometimes chickpea flour. Chapati can be used interchangeably with wheat-flour tortillas in wraps, burritos, and many other recipes.

PASTA

Many people are surprised to discover that in contrast to bread, pasta has a low GI (in the 35 to 50 range). What makes these two wheat products so different? First, pasta is usually made from *semolina* flour, which is more coarsely ground than the flour used to make bread. Second, the starch in cooked pasta is less gelatinized (swollen with water) than the starch in most breads. This makes pasta more resistant to digestive enzymes and slows the rate at which pasta is digested and absorbed. Realize that the longer you cook pasta, the more water it will absorb, and the faster it will be digested. This is why overcooked pasta has a slightly higher GI than does al dente (slightly firm) pasta. Canned pasta products, which are very overcooked, will have the highest GI of all.

Both white and whole-wheat pastas are now widely available in grocery stores, and both have similar GIs. However, since whole-wheat pasta is made from the whole-grain wheat kernel, it provides much more fiber and nutrients than does white pasta, making it a more healthful choice. Try any of the following pastas:

- Dried spaghetti, fettuccine, linguine, and other dried pasta shapes

- Fresh spaghetti, fettuccine, linguine, and other pasta shapes

- Fresh or dried tortellini, ravioli, and other filled pastas—Look for lower-fat varieties.

LEGUMES

With indexes in the 30 to 50 range, legumes are among the lowest-GI foods available. One reason is that these foods are rich in soluble fiber, which slows digestion. Legumes are also rich in protein, vitamins, and minerals, making them excellent substitutes for meat. Canned beans and soft-cooked beans (as in soups) have a higher GI than beans cooked only al dente. However, they are still within the low-to-moderate-GI range, making them a good choice. Some legumes to look for include:

- Black beans
- Black-eyed peas
- Chickpeas
- Kidney beans
- Lentils
- Lima beans
- Navy beans
- Pinto beans
- Soybeans
- Split peas

GRAINS

Grains have been much maligned over the past several years, with many diet gurus advising that they be completely abolished from our diets. However, all grains are not alike. By choosing the *right* grains, you will add fiber and numerous health-protective nutrients to your diet. In fact, studies consistently show that people who eat whole grains substantially reduce their risk for cancer and are about 30-percent less likely to develop heart disease and diabetes than people who eat mostly refined grains. Here are some grains to stock up on.

- Barley—Barley has a light nutty flavor and is delicious in soups, pilafs, and casseroles.
- Buckwheat—Roasted buckwheat kernels, commonly known as *kasha*, are delicious in pilafs and hot breakfast cereals.
- Bulgur wheat—Bulgur, cracked wheat that is precooked and dried, can be prepared in a matter of minutes. Use in pilafs, casseroles, side dishes, salads, and other dishes.
- Couscous—Actually a tiny pasta, couscous cooks in just a couple of minutes. Be sure to choose whole-wheat couscous for the most nutrition.
- Rice—Most of the rice sold in America is the long-grain type, which has a much lower GI than short, sticky Asian rice. For the most nutrition, choose long-grain brown rice, which has all its nutrients and fiber intact. For a real treat, try basmati brown rice, which is revered for its nutty flavor and aroma. Avoid instant rice, which has a higher GI.
- Rice, parboiled—Also known as converted rice, parboiled rice is steamed prior to milling.

This steaming process infuses nutrients from the bran and germ into the kernel's heart and improves its nutritional value compared with regular white rice. The steaming process also inhibits the ability of the rice starch to gelatinize and produces a lower glycemic response. Although parboiled rice has a lower GI than brown rice, brown rice is still the better choice because it has all its fiber and nutrients intact.

- Wheat berries—These whole-grain wheat kernels have a pleasant chewy texture and a nutty flavor. Cooked wheat berries are delicious in salads, casseroles, pilafs, breads, and many other recipes.

- Wild rice—Rich in fiber and nutrients, wild rice has a slightly chewy texture and a delicious nutty flavor. Use wild rice in soups, side dishes, salads, and casseroles.

FLOURS AND BAKING INGREDIENTS

Whether whole-grain or refined, all finely ground flours have a high GI. However, whole-grain flours provide more fiber and nutrients, making them the better choice. When possible, replace part of the flour in recipes with lower-GI alternatives like oats, wheat germ, wheat bran, and flaxmeal.

If you have never used whole-grain products before, a word should be said about storing these foods. Whole grains naturally contain a small amount of polyunsaturated fat, and once cracked open or ground into flour, they can become rancid if stored improperly. Fresh whole-grain flours (and products like wheat germ and cracked grains) will have a light, mildly sweet flavor and aroma, while rancid products will have an unpleasant, slightly bitter flavor and smell. To assure freshness, purchase whole-grain products in a store that has a high turnover rate, and keep them in the refrigerator or freezer after you take them home.

Flaxseeds

These small, nutty-tasting seeds are sometimes referred to as *linseeds*. Flax has long been a popular ingredient with bakers in Europe and Canada, who frequently add the whole seeds or ground flax meal to breads and baked goods. Besides adding flavor and crunch to foods, flaxseeds are loaded with soluble fibers and healthful omega-3 fatty acids. Both flaxseeds and flax meal are widely available in health-food stores. Realize that once ground into meal, flax can turn rancid quickly, so it should be stored in an opaque container in the refrigerator or freezer. Even better, make your own flax meal as you need it, by grinding the whole seeds in a blender or coffee grinder. Flax meal looks similar to wheat bran and can replace 15 to 25 percent of the wheat flour in many baked goods. Flax meal can also be sprinkled over cereals or added to smoothies for a nutrition boost.

Rolled Oats

More than just a breakfast cereal, rolled oats can replace part of the flour in baked goods such as yeast breads, muffins, quick breads, pancakes, waffles, cookies, pie crusts, and crumb toppings. And since oats have a naturally sweet flavor, you can often get by with using less sugar in recipes. Oats can also replace bread crumbs as filler in meatloaf and meatball recipes. Avoid instant oatmeal, which is very thinly cut and has a higher GI than thicker cut oats.

Oat Bran

Not only does oat bran rank low on the glycemic index; it also has a naturally sweet flavor, which reduces the need for sugar, and its soluble fibers reduce the need for fat. All this makes oat bran a superior baking ingredient, which can replace 25 to 50 percent of the flour in muffins, quick breads, pancakes, waffles, cookies, and many other baked goods. Some recipes, such as muffins, can be made with 100-percent oat bran and no flour at all. Look for oat bran in the hot cereal section of your grocery store alongside the oatmeal. The softer products, like Quaker Oat Bran, work best in baked goods.

Rice Bran

The outer layer of the brown rice kernel, rice bran is a rich source of B vitamins, iron, magnesium, vitamin E, and phytochemicals. Rice bran also has a glycemic index of only 19, making it a product worth learning more about. Rice bran can be sprinkled over breakfast cereals, added to smoothies, or used as filler for meatloaf, burgers, and meatballs. This product can also replace 10 to 15 percent of the flour in yeast breads, pancakes, waffles, and cookies and up to a third of the flour in muffins and quick breads. Because rice bran is high in polyunsaturated fat, it can turn rancid quickly if not stored properly. To ensure freshness, purchase rice bran from a store with a high turnover, and store it in the refrigerator or freezer.

Wheat Germ

Wheat germ is the inner part of the wheat kernel. Toasted wheat germ has a nutty flavor and is loaded with vitamin E, trace minerals, and B vitamins. Wheat germ can replace 10 to 15 percent of the flour in muffins, quick breads, pancakes, waffles, cookies, and many other baked goods.

Wheat Bran

The outer part of the wheat kernel, wheat bran is high in fiber, minerals, and phytochemicals. Wheat bran can replace 10 to 15 percent of the flour in yeast breads, pancakes, waffles, and cookies, and up to half of the flour in muffins and quick breads.

Whole-Wheat Flour

Ground from the whole-grain wheat kernel, whole-wheat flour includes the grain's nutrient-rich bran and germ. Nutritionally speaking, whole-wheat flour is far superior to refined white flour. Stone-ground whole-wheat flour, which is a coarsely ground flour, has a lower GI than finely ground whole-wheat flour.

White Whole-Wheat Flour

Made from hard white wheat instead of the hard red wheat used to make regular whole-wheat flour, white whole-wheat flour contains all the nutrients of regular whole-wheat flour but is sweeter and lighter-tasting than its red wheat counterpart. White whole-wheat flour can be used for all your baking needs, including yeast breads.

Whole-Wheat Pastry Flour

Made from soft (low-protein) white whole-wheat flour, whole-wheat pastry flour has a lightly sweet flavor and soft texture that is ideal for making muffins, quick breads, pancakes, cookies, and many other baked goods. This nutritious whole-grain flour can replace 50 to 100 percent of the white flour in any recipe except for yeast bread. Whole-wheat pastry flour is also a nutritious alternative to white flour for thickening gravies. Look for this ingredient in health-food stores, and choose a stone-ground brand for the lowest GI.

BREAKFAST CEREALS

Most ready-to-eat cereals are made from processed grains that have been flaked, popped, puffed, or extruded. This disruption of their natural structure gives cereals a very high glycemic index and leaves us with a very short list of recommended cereals.

One of the most confusing aspects of choosing cereals is that sugary cereals often have a lower GI than cereals made with little or no sugar. How can this be? Sugar has a lower GI than the popped, puffed, or extruded grains that are used to make cereals. Please do not interpret this to mean that the sugary cereals are a better choice. To lower your GI and optimize nutrition, look for minimally processed cereals made from 100 percent whole grains with little or no added sugar. Realize that topping your cereal with milk and some fresh berries or diced peaches will lower the GI of the meal. You can also lighten your glycemic load and boost the staying power of your meal by having a hard-boiled omega-3-enriched egg instead of a side of toast. Here are some of the better cereal choices:

- All Bran

- Bran Buds

- Bran Chex

- Hot cereals made with cracked or thickly cut rolled grains (avoid instant varieties)

- Life

- Müesli

- Nutri-Grain

- Oats, old-fashioned or steel-cut

- Oat bran

- Shredded Wheat

- Shredded Wheat and Bran

- Special K—This is not a 100-percent whole-grain cereal, but its low GI (54) makes it a good substitute for corn flakes and bread crumbs (GI = 70 to 84) in crispy coatings for oven-fried foods.

CANNED GOODS

Although canned foods offer busy cooks convenience, some are definitely better choices than others. For instance, with a few exceptions, most vegetables and fruits are better purchased fresh or frozen. However, if your fresh produce is not really fresh, canned might actually be more nutritious. Here are some canned goods to stock up on:

- Unsweetened applesauce

- Artichoke hearts and bottoms

- Chicken, beef, and vegetable broth and dry bouillons—Look for lower-sodium varieties

- Dill pickles

- Dried beans

- Fruits canned in juice

- Hot peppers

- Olives

- Roasted red bell peppers

- Soups—Choose broth-based, vegetable, bean, and lentil, and low-fat cream soups

- Spaghetti and marinana sauce—Look for brands made with little or no added sugar or fat.

- Tomatoes, stewed tomatoes, tomato sauce, tomato paste
- Tomato juice
- Tuna, salmon, crab, sardines, anchovies
- Vegetable juice cocktail

CONDIMENTS AND SEASONINGS

Condiments such as these can perk up a variety of foods:

- Anchovies and anchovy paste
- Capers
- Curry paste—A flavorful blend of curry spices mixed with canola oil, ground lentils, and other ingredients. Curry paste has a deeper, richer flavor than curry powder. Brands like Patak's curry paste are available in the imported foods section of many grocery stores and in international or Indian markets. If you don't have any curry paste on hand, you can substitute an equal amount of curry powder plus a little salt in recipes.
- *Fines Herbes*—a blend of thyme, oregano, sage, rosemary, marjoram, and basil. This product can be found in the dried spice section of most grocery stores.
- Herbs, spices, and salt-free herb blends
- Horseradish
- Hot sauce
- Jam and preserves—Choose low-sugar and all-fruit types
- Ketchup (in moderation)
- Lemon juice
- Mustard
- Reduced-sodium soy sauce
- Salsa and picante sauce
- Vinegars
- Worcestershire sauce

PRODUCE

Eating generous amounts of vegetables and fruits is at the very heart of a low-GI lifestyle. With a few exceptions—baking potatoes, parsnips, carrots, and watermelon, for instance—the vast majority of produce ranks low to moderate on the glycemic index. In addition, high-GI produce items like carrots are so low in carbohydrate that they do not have a major impact on blood sugar levels in the amounts normally eaten.

In the produce department, potatoes present the biggest threat to a low-GI lifestyle, simply because they make up such a huge percentage of most people's vegetable intake. The best advice is to think of potatoes as a bread substitute instead of a vegetable and to eat them less often. Chapter 4 also presents some lower-GI alternatives to potatoes that will help you with menu planning.

Nuts

Although high in fat, nuts can and should be a regular part of a healthful diet. These tasty morsels supply essential fats and a wide range of phytochemicals, vitamins, and minerals. Nuts also have a very low glycemic index. These qualities put nuts high on the list of healthful foods. In fact, people who eat an ounce of nuts (3 to 4 tablespoons) several times a week are 30- to 50-percent less likely to suffer from heart disease as people who avoid nuts. If you are watching your weight, be aware that a cup of nuts provides about 800 calories, so don't go overboard. However, used moderately, nuts can greatly enhance the joy of eating without blowing your fat or calorie budgets.

Low-GI Cooking Tips

If you know a few tricks of the trade, you can easily lower the glycemic index of many of your favorite recipes and create new dishes that will complement your low-GI lifestyle. Familiarizing yourself with the foods described in the first part of this chapter is the first step toward healthier cooking. The next step is learning which substitutions work best in each particular kind of recipe. The following table presents some tips that will help you master the basics of low-GI cooking.

How to Lower the Glycemic Index of Recipes

Type of Recipe	Tips for Lowering the Glycemic Index
BURGERS, MEATLOAF, MEATBALLS	Substitute rolled oats, oat bran, bulgur wheat, and mashed cooked lentils or legumes for fillers such as bread crumbs and white rice. Incorporate lots of finely chopped vegetables in the burger or loaf mix.
CRUMB COATINGS	Substitute crushed Special K cereal for corn flakes and bread crumbs.
MARINADES	Reduce the amount of sugar in marinades. Add sweetness with fruit juices and fruit juice concentrates instead.
SOUPS	Substitute long-grain or basmati brown rice, wild rice, or barley for white rice. Include legumes, pasta, and generous amounts of vegetables in soup recipes.
PASTA DISHES	Cook the pasta al dente. Do not overcook. Incorporate more vegetables into pasta dishes.
CASSEROLES	Substitute long-grain or basmati brown rice, wild rice, barley, or bulgur wheat for white rice. Incorporate more vegetables and legumes into casseroles.
PILAFS	Substitute long-grain or basmati brown rice, wild rice, barley, bulgur wheat, or whole-wheat couscous for white rice. Incorporate generous amounts of vegetables into pilafs.
STUFFINGS	Use low-GI breads. Add lots of chopped vegetables to the stuffing mixture.
SANDWICHES	Use low-GI breads. Add lots of vegetable toppings.

How to Lower the Glycemic Index of Recipes (CONTINUED)

Type of Recipe	Tips for Lowering the Glycemic Index
FRENCH TOAST	Use low-GI bread. Top with fresh or canned fruit, applesauce, or low-sugar fruit sauces.
PANCAKES, WAFFLES	Replace part of the flour with lower-GI ingredients like oat bran, oats, flax meal, wheat bran, rice bran, or wheat germ. Top with fresh or canned fruit, applesauce, or a low-sugar fruit sauce.
MUFFINS, QUICK BREADS, COOKIES	Replace part of the flour with lower-GI ingredients like oat bran, oats, flax meal, wheat bran, rice bran, or wheat germ. Use fruits, fruit juices, and dried fruits to add sweetness and reduce the need for sugar. Add a little extra cinnamon, nutmeg, orange rind, or vanilla extract to enhance sweetness and reduce the need for sugar.
YEAST BREADS	Use ingredients like stone-ground whole-wheat flour, oats, oat bran, flax meal, wheat germ, wheat bran, rice bran, nuts and seeds, soaked cracked grains, and cooked whole grains. "Doctor up" bread machine mixes by adding ingredients like flax, wheat germ, wheat bran, rice bran, nuts, seeds, and cooked whole or cracked grains.
CUSTARDS, PUDDINGS	Add a little extra cinnamon, nutmeg, orange rind, or vanilla to enhance sweetness and reduce the need for sugar.
CRISPS, COBBLERS, PIES	Prepare recipes with more fruit and less sugar. Substitute oats or oat bran for part of the flour in toppings and crusts.

High-GI Blueberry Muffins (GI = 64)	Low-GI Blueberry Muffins (GI = 50)
2 cups white flour	2 cups oat bran
½ cup sugar	¼ cup sugar
1 tablespoon baking powder	2 teaspoons baking powder
¾ cup milk	¼ teaspoon baking soda
6 tablespoons margarine or butter	½ cup low-fat vanilla yogurt
2 eggs	½ cup orange juice
¾ cup blueberries	½ cup fat-free egg substitute
	2 tablespoons canola oil
	¾ cup blueberries
Nutrition Facts (per muffin)	
Calories: 177	Nutrition Facts (per muffin)
Carbohydrates: 26 g	Calories: 98
Fat: 7 g	Carbohydrates: 18 g
Fiber: 0.7 g	Fat: 3.4 g
	Fiber: 2.7 g

Recipe Makeover

Here is an example of how replacing high-GI ingredients with low-GI ingredients can lower the GI of a recipe, and at the same time, greatly improve its nutritional value. Two adjustments are made that lower the GI of the recipe on the right: Oat bran replaces the high-GI white flour, and vanilla yogurt and orange juice add both moistness and sweetness, reducing the need for sugar. Other adjustments have also been made to the recipe to trim fat. The end result is a muffin with a lower GI, 45-percent fewer calories, half the fat, and almost four times the fiber.

Controlling Fat and Calories

While lowering the glycemic index of recipes makes for a more healthful product, remember that controlling fat and calories is also important for people who are watching their weight. In many recipes, trimming unnecessary fat can slash calories by 25 to 50 percent. Many excellent products are now available that can help you control fat and calories without sacrificing taste. The following table presents some ideas for smart ingredient substitutions and cooking techniques that will help you master lighter cooking.

RECIPE	TIPS FOR TRIMMING FAT
MEATS	Purchase lean cuts (see page 68–69). Trim away any visible fat. Use low-fat cooking methods: bake, broil, grill, stir-fry.
POULTRY	Remove the skin. Use low-fat cooking methods: bake, broil, grill, stir-fry, oven fry.
BURGERS, MEATLOAF, MEATBALLS	Use extra-lean ground meat (93 to 96 percent lean) Replace up to one-third of the ground meat with vegetarian hamburger crumbles, tofu hamburger, or TVP. Add lots of finely chopped mushrooms, onions, bell peppers, and other vegetables to the ground meat mixture.
SOUPS	Use a gravy separator to remove the fat from stocks and broths, or chill the stock or broth and remove the fat that floats to the top. Use leaner meats. Substitute skim or low-fat milk for whole milk. Add 1 to 2 tablespoons of nonfat dry milk powder to each cup of skim or low-fat milk for a richer flavor. Thicken soups with pureed vegetables instead of cream.
SALADS	Substitute lower-fat mayonnaise, sour cream, and dressings for full-fat versions. Use lower-fat meats and cheeses.
SAUCES	Substitute evaporated skim or low-fat milk for cream. Use less butter or margarine, or use a reduced-fat alternative.
CASSEROLES	Use lower-fat cheeses and sour cream. Use leaner meats. Use less butter, margarine, and oil.
OMELETS, FRITTATAS	Substitute fat-free egg substitutes for whole eggs, use fewer yolks and more whites.

continued on next page

Recipe	Tips for Trimming Fat
	Use lower-fat cheeses and meats. Include plenty of vegetable fillings.
Quiches	Substitute evaporated skim or low-fat milk for cream. Use lower-fat cheeses and meats. Substitute fat-free egg substitutes for whole eggs, or use fewer yolks and more whites.
Muffins, quick breads	Substitute applesauce for part of the fat in baked goods. Substitute fat-free egg substitutes or egg whites for whole eggs.
Custards, puddings	Substitute skim or low-fat milk for whole milk. Add 1 to 2 tablespoons of nonfat dry milk powder to each cup of skim or low-fat milk for a richer flavor. Substitute fat-free egg substitutes for whole eggs.

Mastering low-GI cooking is both easy and immensely enjoyable. And if you know the secrets of low-GI cooking, you can easily transform many of your own recipes into low-GI favorites. A wide variety of healthful and delicious foods can star in your low-GI meals, and most of these foods are readily available in your local grocery store. The remainder of this book features over 200 kitchen-tested recipes that put principle into practice and present a wide range of delicious possibilities for every meal of the day and every occasion.

Part II

Low-GI Recipes

About the Nutrition Analysis

The Food Processor Nutrition Analysis software, version 7.5 (ESHA Research), along with product information from manufacturers, was used to calculate the nutrition information for the recipes in this book. For each recipe, information on calories, carbohydrate, protein, fat, cholesterol, dietary fiber, sodium, and calcium content is provided. Nutrients are always given per one serving.

A glycemic index classification of very low (39 or lower), low (40–54), or moderate (55–69), is also assigned to each recipe. Since the GI of every food ingredient is not known and because a variety of factors can affect the GI of individual foods, it would be impossible to assign a specific number on the glycemic index to each recipe with precision. However, there is sufficient knowledge of the GI values of a core group of foods to estimate whether a recipe will provoke a very low, low, moderate, or high glycemic response. Realize that a recipe that contains a small amount of a moderate- or high-GI ingredient may be classified as a low-GI food if it contains a negligible amount of carbohydrate per serving.

Sometimes recipes give you options regarding ingredients. For instance, you might be able to choose between nonfat and reduced-fat cheese, eggs or egg substitute, or sugar-free or regular yogurt. This will help you create dishes that suit your tastes and your nutrition goals. Just bear in mind that the nutrition analysis is based on the first ingredient listed and does not include optional ingredients.

7. Breakfast and Brunch Favorites

*S*tarting your day the low-GI way can go a long way toward lightening your glycemic load. Why? Breakfast foods like processed cereals, refined breads and bagels, toaster pastries, pancakes, and waffles tend to rank very high on the glycemic index. And if you are watching your weight, what you eat for breakfast can make all the difference in your success. By producing a slow and sustained rise in blood sugar, low-GI foods will keep you feeling full and satisfied throughout the morning. On the other hand, a high-GI breakfast can wreak havoc on your blood sugar and set you up for a roller-coaster pattern of overeating that lasts all day long.

This chapter provides a variety of tempting low-GI breakfast and brunch dishes that are worth getting up for. Omelets, frittatas, and quiches are especially filling breakfast foods, due to their high protein content. And as you will see, these dishes can be easily made with a fraction of the usual fat and cholesterol. Frittatas and quiches can be made ahead of time and quickly reheated in a microwave oven for a no-fuss breakfast on a busy morning. Add a bowl of fresh fruit, and you have a super-nutritious meal that will keep you going all morning long. Note that the recipes in this chapter call for fat-free egg substitutes, but feel free to substitute whole eggs (especially omega-3-enriched eggs) within the context of your personal nutrition goals.

Made properly, muffins and quick breads can also be made the low-GI way. Here you will find an assortment of healthful and delicious recipes for muffins and quick breads that can be made ahead, frozen, and thawed in a microwave. Paired with a glass of low-fat milk, any of these would make for a quick and filling breakfast on the run. With a little creativity, even pancakes and French toast can fit into your low-GI eating plan. Healthful whole grains, low-fat dairy products, and light fruit toppings can make all the difference in the glycemic index and nutritional value of these breakfast favorites.

Spinach and Mushroom Omelet

YIELD: 1 SERVING

½ cup sliced fresh mushrooms
Pinch ground black pepper
Pinch dried thyme
½ cup (packed) chopped fresh spinach
½ cup fat-free egg substitute
3 tablespoons shredded nonfat or reduced-fat Swiss, mozzarella, or provolone cheese
1 slice extra-lean turkey bacon, cooked, drained, and crumbled (optional)
Ground paprika

1. Coat an 8-inch nonstick skillet with cooking spray, and preheat over medium heat. Add the mushrooms, pepper, and thyme. Cover and cook, stirring several times, for about 2 minutes, or until the mushrooms are tender and nicely browned. Add the spinach, and cook uncovered for about 30 seconds, stirring frequently, or until the spinach is wilted. Remove the mixture to a small dish, and cover to keep warm.

2. Respray the skillet, and place over medium-low heat. Add the egg substitute, and cook without stirring for about 2 minutes, or until set around the edges.

3. Use a spatula to lift the edges of the omelet, and allow the uncooked egg to flow below the cooked portion. Cook for another minute or two, or until the eggs are almost set.

4. Arrange first the spinach mixture and then the cheese over half of the omelet. Top with the bacon if desired. Fold the other half over the filling, and cook for another minute or two, or until the cheese is melted and the eggs are completely set.

5. Slide the omelet onto a plate, sprinkle with the paprika, and serve hot.

Nutritional Facts

CALORIES: 104   CARBOHYDRATES: 5 G   CHOLESTEROL: 2 MG   FAT: 0.2 G   FIBER: 0.7 G
PROTEIN: 20 G   SODIUM: 395 MG   CALCIUM: 271 MG   GI RATING: VERY LOW

Ham and Swiss Omelet

3 tablespoons diced lean ham or Canadian bacon (about 1 ounce)
½ cup fat-free egg substitute
3 tablespoons shredded nonfat or reduced-fat Swiss cheese
1 tablespoon finely chopped fresh parsley

1. Coat an 8-inch nonstick skillet with cooking spray, and preheat over medium heat. Add the ham or Canadian bacon and cook, stirring frequently, for about 2 minutes, or until the bacon or ham is nicely browned. Remove the meat to a small dish, and cover to keep warm.
2. Respray the skillet, and place over medium-low heat. Add the egg substitute and cook without stirring for about 2 minutes, or until set around the edges.
3. Use a spatula to lift the edges of the omelet, and allow the uncooked egg to flow below the cooked portion. Cook for another minute or two, or until the eggs are almost set.
4. Arrange first the ham or bacon and then the cheese over half of the omelet. Fold the other half over the filling and cook for another minute or two, or until the cheese is melted and the eggs are completely set.
5. Slide the omelet onto a plate, sprinkle with the parsley, and serve hot.

Nutritional Facts

CALORIES: 125 CARBOHYDRATES: 4.6 G CHOLESTEROL: 10 MG FAT: 1 G FIBER: 0.1 G
PROTEIN: 24 G SODIUM: 563 MG CALCIUM: 260 MG GI RATING: VERY LOW

Monterey Crab Omelet

YIELD: 1 SERVING

1 tablespoon chopped red or green bell pepper
1 tablespoon chopped onion
¼ cup cooked crabmeat
½ cup fat-free egg substitute
3 tablespoons shredded nonfat or reduced-fat Monterey Jack cheese (plain or with jalapeño peppers)
Ground paprika

1. Coat an 8-inch nonstick skillet with cooking spray, and preheat over medium heat. Add the bell pepper and onion to the skillet. Cover and cook, stirring frequently, for about 2 minutes, or until the pepper and onion start to soften. Add the crabmeat, and cook uncovered for another minute, or until heated through. Transfer the mixture to a small dish, and cover to keep warm.

2. Respray the skillet, and place over medium-low heat. Add the egg substitute and cook without stirring for about 2 minutes, or until set around the edges.

3. Use a spatula to lift the edges of the omelet, and allow the uncooked egg to flow below the cooked portion. Cook for an additional minute or two, or until the eggs are almost set.

4. Arrange first the crab mixture and then the cheese over half of the omelet. Fold the other half over the filling, and cook for another minute or two, or until the cheese is melted and the eggs are completely set.

5. Slide the omelet onto a plate, sprinkle with some paprika, and serve hot.

Nutritional Facts

CALORIES: 132   CARBOHYDRATES: 5 G   CHOLESTEROL: 24 MG   FAT: 0.4 G   FIBER: 0.4 G
PROTEIN: 25 G   SODIUM: 494 MG   CALCIUM: 275 MG   GI RATING: VERY LOW

Bacon and Tomato Omelet

YIELD: 1 SERVING

1 tablespoon plus 1½ teaspoons sliced scallions, divided
3 tablespoons chopped seeded plum tomatoes
½ cup fat-free egg substitute
1 slice extra-lean turkey bacon, cooked, drained, and crumbled
3 tablespoons shredded nonfat or Monterey Jack cheese (plain or with jalapeño peppers)

1. Coat an 8-inch nonstick skillet with cooking spray, and preheat over medium heat. Add 1 tablespoon of the scallions, cover, and cook for about 1 minute or until the scallions start to soften. Add the tomatoes, cover, and cook for about 30 seconds or until just heated through. Transfer the mixture to a small dish and cover to keep warm.

2. Respray the skillet, and place over medium-low heat. Add the egg substitute, and cook without stirring for about 2 minutes, or until the eggs are set around the edges.

3. Use a spatula to lift the edges of the omelet, and allow the uncooked egg to flow below the cooked portion. Cook for an additional minute or two, or until the eggs are completely set.

4. Arrange the tomato mixture, then the bacon, and finally the cheese over half of the omelet. Fold the other half over the filling, and cook for another minute or two, or until the cheese is melted and the eggs are completely set.

5. Slide the omelet onto a plate, sprinkle with the remaining scallions, and serve hot.

Nutritional Facts

CALORIES: 123   CARBOHYDRATES: 5 G   CHOLESTEROL: 22 MG   FAT: 0.6 G   FIBER: 0.6 G
PROTEIN: 22 G   SODIUM: 516 MG   CALCIUM: 264 MG   GI RATING: VERY LOW

Spring Vegetable Omelet

YIELD: 1 SERVING

⅓ cup 1-inch pieces fresh asparagus
1 tablespoon plus 1½ teaspoons chopped red bell pepper
1 tablespoon plus 1½ teaspoons chopped onion
⅛ teaspoon dried thyme or fines herbes
½ cup fat-free egg substitute
1½ teaspoons grated Parmesan cheese
3 tablespoons shredded nonfat or reduced-fat mozzarella, provolone, or Swiss cheese
2 teaspoons finely chopped fresh parsley or chives

1. Coat an 8-inch nonstick skillet with cooking spray and preheat over medium heat. Add the asparagus, peppers, onions, and herbs to the skillet. Cover and cook, stirring several times, for 2 to 3 minutes, or until the vegetables are crisp-tender (add a little water if the skillet becomes too dry). Remove the mixture to a small dish, and cover to keep warm.

2. Respray the skillet, and place over medium-low heat. Add the egg substitute, and cook without stirring for about 2 minutes, or until set around the edges.

3. Use a spatula to lift the edges of the omelet, and allow the uncooked egg to flow below the cooked portion. Cook for another minute or two, or until the eggs are almost set.

4. Arrange the vegetables over half of the omelet. Sprinkle the vegetables with the Parmesan cheese and then the shredded cheese. Fold the other half over the filling, and cook for another minute or two or until the cheese is melted and the eggs are completely set.

5. Slide the omelet onto a plate, sprinkle with the parsley or chives, and serve hot.

Broccoli Frittata

YIELD: 4 SERVINGS

2 cups fat-free egg substitute
2 tablespoons grated Parmesan cheese
¾ cup chopped fresh mushrooms
1 teaspoon crushed garlic
¼ teaspoon dried thyme
1 package (10 ounces) frozen chopped broccoli, thawed and drained
1 cup shredded nonfat or reduced-fat mozzarella cheese

1. Combine the egg substitute and Parmesan cheese in a medium-sized bowl. Stir to mix well and set aside.
2. Coat a 10-inch nonstick ovenproof skillet with cooking spray and add the mushrooms, garlic, and thyme. Place the skillet over medium heat, cover, and cook for about 2 minutes, stirring several times, or until the mushrooms are tender. Add the broccoli, stir to mix well, and spread the mixture evenly over the bottom of the skillet.
3. Reduce the heat to low, and pour the egg mixture over the vegetables. Cover, and cook without stirring for about 10 minutes, or until the eggs are almost set.
4. Remove the lid from the skillet and wrap the handle in aluminum foil (to ensure that it will not be damaged by the broiler flame). Place the skillet under a preheated broiler, and broil 6 inches from the heat for about 3 minutes, or until the eggs are set but not dry.
5. Sprinkle the mozzarella over the frittata, and broil for an additional minute, or until the cheese has melted. Cut the frittata into wedges, and serve immediately.

Nutritional Facts (per serving)

CALORIES: 140   CARBOHYDRATES: 7 G   CHOLESTEROL: 5 MG   FAT: 1.2 G   FIBER: 2.3 G

PROTEIN: 24 G   SODIUM: 519 MG   CALCIUM: 396 MG   GI RATING: VERY LOW

Ham & Potato Frittata

YIELD: 4 SERVINGS

⅓ cup chopped onion

⅓ cup chopped green bell pepper

¾ cup diced ham (at least 97 percent lean)

1½ cups diced cooked new potatoes

2 cups fat-free egg substitute

1 cup shredded nonfat or reduced-fat Cheddar or Monterey Jack cheese

1. Coat a 10-inch nonstick ovenproof skillet with nonstick cooking spray, and add the onion, bell peppers, and ham. Place the skillet over medium-high heat, cover, and cook, stirring several times, for about 3 minutes or until the onions and peppers start to soften.
2. Add the potatoes to the skillet, and stir to mix. Reduce the heat to medium, cover, and cook for 1 minute or until the mixture is heated through.
3. Reduce the heat to low and pour the egg substitute over the potato mixture. Cover, and cook without stirring for about 10 minutes or until the eggs are almost set.
4. Remove the lid from the skillet and wrap the handle in aluminum foil (to ensure that it will not be damaged by the broiler flame). Place the skillet under a preheated broiler and broil for about 3 minutes or just until the eggs are completely set. Sprinkle the cheese over the top, and broil for another minute or until the cheese is melted.
5. Cut the frittata into wedges, and serve hot.

Nutritional Facts (per serving)

CALORIES: 189 CARBOHYDRATES: 18 G CHOLESTEROL: 9 MG FAT: 0.9 G FIBER: 1.7 G
PROTEIN: 26 G SODIUM: 627 MG CALCIUM: 322 MG GI RATING: MODERATE

Breakfast Burritos

YIELD: 4 SERVINGS

¾ cup diced ham (at least 97 percent lean)

1½ cups fat-free egg substitute

½ cup shredded nonfat or reduced-fat Monterey Jack cheese
    (plain or with jalapeño peppers)

4 whole-wheat flour tortillas (8-inch rounds)
Picante sauce (optional)

1. Coat a large nonstick skillet with cooking spray and preheat over medium-high heat. Add the ham, cover, and cook, stirring once or twice, for about 2 minutes or until the ham is heated through and begins to brown.
2. Reduce the heat to medium-low, and pour the egg substitute over the ham. Cook without stirring for 3 to 4 minutes or until the eggs are partially set. Stirring gently to scramble, continue to cook for another minute or two or until the eggs are almost set.
3. Sprinkle the cheese over the eggs, and cook, stirring gently, for another minute or until the eggs are cooked but not dry, and the cheese is melted.
4. While the eggs are cooking, warm the tortillas according to the manufacturer's directions.
5. Arrange the warm tortillas on a flat surface. Place a quarter of the egg mixture along the right side of each tortilla, stopping 1½ inches from the bottom. Top the eggs with some of the picante sauce if desired.
6. Fold the bottom edge of each tortilla up about 1 inch. (This fold will prevent the filling from falling out.) Then, beginning at the right edge, roll each tortilla up jellyroll style. (See below.) Serve hot.

Nutritional Facts (per serving)

CALORIES: 230 CARBOHYDRATES: 25 G CHOLESTEROL: 8 MG FAT: 3.7 G FIBER: 2 G
PROTEIN: 21 G SODIUM: 727 MG CALCIUM: 125 MG GI RATING: MODERATE

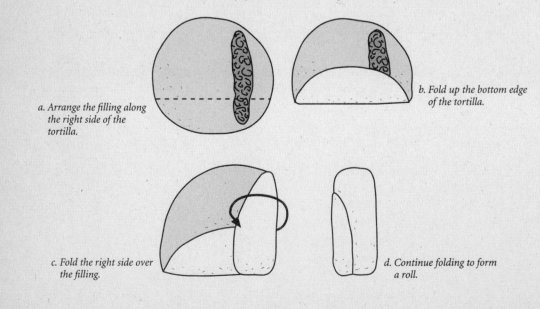

a. Arrange the filling along the right side of the tortilla.

b. Fold up the bottom edge of the tortilla.

c. Fold the right side over the filling.

d. Continue folding to form a roll.

Ham & Asparagus Quiche

For variety, substitute cooked crabmeat for the ham.

YIELD: 6 SERVINGS

Crust
1½ cups cooked brown rice
2 tablespoons grated Parmesan cheese
1 tablespoon fat-free egg substitute

Filling
1¼ cups shredded nonfat or reduced-fat Swiss or mozzarella cheese
¾ cup diced ham (at least 97 percent lean)
¾ cup ¾-inch pieces fresh asparagus
Pinch ground nutmeg
1 cup fat-free egg substitute
1 cup evaporated skim or low-fat milk
1 large plum tomato, thinly sliced
2 tablespoons grated Parmesan cheese

1. To make the crust, combine the rice, Parmesan cheese, and egg substitute in a medium bowl, and stir to mix well. Coat a 9-inch deep-dish pie pan with nonstick cooking spray, and pat the mixture evenly over the bottom and up the sides of the pan, forming an even crust. Set aside.
2. For the filling, combine the cheese, ham, asparagus, and nutmeg in a medium bowl and toss to mix well. Add the egg substitute and evaporated milk, and stir to mix well. Pour the egg mixture into the rice crust.
3. Arrange the tomato slices on the top of the quiche, and then sprinkle with Parmesan cheese. Bake at 350° F for about 45 minutes or just until a sharp knife inserted near the center of the quiche comes out clean, and the top is nicely browned. Remove the dish from the oven, and let sit for 15 minutes before cutting into wedges and serving.

Nutritional Facts (per serving)
CALORIES: 190 CARBOHYDRATES: 20 G CHOLESTEROL: 12 MG FAT: 2.4 G FIBER: 1.4 G
PROTEIN: 22 G SODIUM: 582 MG CALCIUM: 412 MG GI RATING: LOW

Quiche Lorraine

Filling
1 medium yellow onion, cut into very thin wedges (about 1 cup)
1 tablespoon dry sherry
1¼ cups shredded nonfat or reduced-fat Swiss cheese
1 tablespoon unbleached flour
Pinch ground nutmeg
5 slices extra-lean turkey bacon, cooked and crumbled
1 cup fat-free egg substitute
1½ cups evaporated skim or low-fat milk
2 tablespoons grated Parmesan cheese

Crust
1½ cups cooked brown rice
2 tablespoons grated Parmesan cheese
1 tablespoon fat-free egg substitute

1. Coat a small nonstick skillet with cooking spray, and add the onions and sherry. Place the skillet over medium heat, cover, and cook for several minutes, stirring occasionally until the onions are tender. Add a little water if the skillet becomes too dry, but only enough to prevent scorching. Remove the skillet from the heat, and set aside to cool slightly.

2. To make the crust, combine the rice, Parmesan cheese, and egg substitute in a medium bowl, and stir to mix well. Coat a 9-inch deep-dish pie pan with nonstick cooking spray, and pat the mixture evenly over the bottom and up the sides of the pan, forming an even crust. Set aside.

3. For the filling, combine the Swiss cheese, flour, and nutmeg in a medium bowl, and toss to mix well. Add the bacon and cooked onions and toss again. Add the egg substitute and evaporated milk to the cheese mixture and stir to mix well. Pour the filling into the crust, and sprinkle the Parmesan cheese over the top.

4. Bake at 350° F for about 45 minutes, or until a sharp knife inserted near the center of the quiche comes out clean and the top is nicely browned. Remove the dish from the oven, and let sit for 15 minutes before cutting into wedges and serving.

Nutritional Facts (per serving)

CALORIES: 202 CARBOHYDRATES: 21 G CHOLESTEROL: 24 MG FAT: 2.3 G FIBER: 1.4 G
PROTEIN: 20 G SODIUM: 581 MG CALCIUM: 440 MG GI RATING: LOW

Light Eggs Benedict

Eggs
5 large eggs
5 slices (1 ounce each) Canadian bacon or ham (at least 97 percent lean)
5 whole-wheat or oat-bran English muffin halves, toasted
Ground paprika

Sauce
½ teaspoon dry mustard
Pinch ground white pepper
1 tablespoon water
1 cup plain nonfat or low-fat yogurt
3 tablespoons fat-free egg substitute
2 tablespoons reduced-fat margarine or light butter
1½ teaspoons lemon juice

1. Coat a large nonstick skillet with cooking spray and preheat over medium-high heat. Add the Canadian bacon or ham to the skillet and cook for about 1 minute on each side or until lightly browned and heated through. Remove the skillet from the heat, cover, and set aside to keep warm.

2. To poach the eggs, fill a large nonstick skillet with 3 inches of water and bring the water to a boil over high heat. Reduce the heat to low to keep the water gently simmering. Break one of the eggs into a custard cup. Holding the cup close to the water's surface, slip the egg into the water. Add the remaining eggs to the skillet in the same manner, spacing them evenly apart. Cover the skillet, and cook for 3 to 5 minutes or until the whites are completely set and the yolks thickened.

3. While the eggs are cooking, make the sauce. Put the mustard, pepper, and water in a 1-quart glass bowl and stir with a wire whisk to mix well. Whisk in the yogurt and the egg substitute. Add the margarine or butter to the yogurt mixture. (There is no need to melt the margarine or butter first.)

4. Place the bowl containing the yogurt mixture in a microwave oven and microwave at high power for 1½ minutes, then whisk to mix well. Microwave for an additional 1½ to 2 minutes, whisking every 30 seconds, until the mixture is thickened. (Note that the mixture may seem curdled when you first stir it, but it will become smooth as you keep whisking.) Remove the mixture from the microwave oven, and whisk in the lemon juice.

5. To assemble the dish, place one English muffin half on each of 5 serving plates. Top each muffin half with 1 slice of Canadian bacon and 1 egg. Spoon ¼ cup of sauce over each serving, and sprinkle with some of the paprika. Serve hot.

Nutritional Facts (per serving)

CALORIES: 222 CARBOHYDRATES: 19 G CHOLESTEROL: 220 MG FAT: 8.5 G FIBER: 2.3 G
PROTEIN: 18 G SODIUM: 634 MG CALCIUM: 215 MG GI RATING: MODERATE

Variations

To make **Seafood Eggs Benedict,** substitute 1 cup of cooked crabmeat or shrimp (or ½ cup of each) for the Canadian bacon or ham.

Nutritional Facts (per serving)

CALORIES: 217 CARBOHYDRATES: 18 G CHOLESTEROL: 231 MG FAT: 8.1 G
FIBER: 2.3 G PROTEIN: 18 G SODIUM: 454 MG CALCIUM: 229 MG
GI RATING: MODERATE

To make **Eggs Benedict Florentine,** place 1½ cups sliced mushrooms, ¼ teaspoon dried thyme, and ⅛ teaspoon each salt and pepper in a large nonstick skillet. Cover and cook over medium heat for about 3 minutes or until the mushrooms begin to brown and release their juices. Add 3 cups coarsely chopped fresh spinach, and cook for a minute or two or until the spinach is wilted. Substitute the spinach mixture for the Canadian bacon.

Nutritional Facts (per serving)

CALORIES: 201 CARBOHYDRATES: 19 G CHOLESTEROL: 213 MG FAT: 7.9 G
FIBER: 3 G PROTEIN: 14 G SODIUM: 380 MG CALCIUM: 234 MG
GI RATING: MODERATE

Bacon, Egg, and Cheese Breakfast Sandwich

YIELD: 1 SERVING

1 slice (½ ounce) Canadian bacon (at least 97 percent lean)
¼ cup plus 2 tablespoons fat-free egg substitute
1 slice (¾ ounce) nonfat or reduced-fat Cheddar cheese
1 whole-wheat or oat-bran English muffin

1. Coat a medium-sized skillet with nonstick cooking spray, and preheat over medium-high heat. Add the Canadian bacon and cook for about 1 minute on each side or until nicely browned. Remove the bacon from the skillet, and set aside to keep warm.
2. Respray the skillet and reduce the heat under the skillet to medium. Pour in the egg substitute and cook without stirring for a minute or two, or until the eggs are set around the edges. Use a spatula to lift the edges of the eggs, and allow the uncooked egg to flow underneath the cooked portion. Cook for another minute or until the eggs are almost set.
3. Using a spatula, fold the eggs in half, then fold in half again (so it will fit on the bread). Place the Canadian bacon on top of the eggs, and top with the cheese. Reduce the heat to low, cover, and cook for another minute or until the cheese begins to melt.
4. Transfer the eggs, bacon, and cheese to the lower half of the English muffin, cover with the top half, and serve hot.

Nutritional Facts (per serving)
CALORIES: 224   CARBOHYDRATES: 29 G   CHOLESTEROL: 6 MG   FAT: 1.8 G   FIBER: 4.4 G
PROTEIN: 23 G   SODIUM: 841 MG   CALCIUM: 395 MG   GI RATING: MODERATE

Morning Müesli

YIELD: 8 CUPS

4 cups old-fashioned oats
1¼ cups whole-bran cereal (like All Bran or Bran Buds)
¾ cup chopped almonds, walnuts, hazelnuts, or pecans
1 cup chopped dried apricots or dried pitted sweet cherries
1 cup dark or golden raisins

1. Place all the ingredients in a large bowl and stir to mix well. Transfer to an airtight container, and store for up to 1 month.
2. To serve, place ½ cup of the müesli in an individual serving bowl. Add ¾ skim or low-fat milk or plain or vanilla yogurt. Stir, and let sit for 5 minutes before serving.

Nutritional Facts (per ½-cup serving, cereal only)
CALORIES: 168 CARBOHYDRATES: 28 G CHOLESTEROL: 0 MG FAT: 3.9 G FIBER: 5.9 G
PROTEIN: 5.6 G SODIUM: 65 MG CALCIUM: 54 MG GI RATING: LOW

Nutritional Facts (per ½-cup serving with skim milk)
CALORIES: 232 CARBOHYDRATES: 37 G CHOLESTEROL: 3 MG FAT: 4.2 G FIBER: 5.9 G
PROTEIN: 11.9 G SODIUM: 160 MG CALCIUM: 280 MG GI RATING: LOW

Sunrise Smoothie

Have this nutritious smoothie for a quick breakfast or a filling snack anytime.

YIELD: 1 SERVING

¾ cup nonfat or low-fat vanilla yogurt (sugar-free or regular)
1 cup fresh or frozen fruit (use strawberries, blueberries, raspberries, blackberries, dark sweet cherries, diced peaches, or any combination)
¼ cup orange juice
2 ice cubes
1 heaping tablespoon flax meal, oat bran, rice bran, or toasted wheat germ (optional)

1. Place all the ingredients in a blender, and blend until smooth.
2. Pour into a 16-ounce glass and serve immediately.

Nutritional Facts
CALORIES: 182 CARBOHYDRATES: 35 G CHOLESTEROL: 4 MG FAT: 0.7 G FIBER: 3.4 G
PROTEIN: 10 G SODIUM: 139 MG CALCIUM: 327 MG GI RATING: VERY LOW

Buttermilk—Oat-Bran Pancakes

YIELD: 12 PANCAKES

1 cup oat bran
½ cup whole-wheat pastry flour
2 teaspoons baking powder
2 teaspoons sugar
1¾ cups nonfat or low-fat buttermilk
¼ cup fat-free egg substitute or 2 egg whites, lightly beaten

1. Combine the oat bran, flour, baking powder, and sugar in a medium-sized bowl, and stir to mix well. Add the buttermilk and the egg substitute or egg whites, and stir with a wire whisk to mix well.
2. Coat a large griddle or nonstick skillet with cooking spray, and preheat over medium heat until a drop of water sizzles when it hits the heated surface. (If using an electric griddle, heat the griddle according to manufacturer's directions.)
3. For each pancake, pour ¼ cup of the batter onto the griddle or skillet and spread into a 4-inch circle. Cook for about 1½ minutes, or until the top is bubbly and the edges are dry. Turn and cook for an additional minute or until the second side is golden brown.
4. As the pancakes are done, place them on a serving plate, and keep warm in a 200° F preheated oven.
5. Serve hot, topped with Summer Berry Sauce (page 103), Cinnamon-Apple Topping (page 104), or fresh fruit, and a dollop of vanilla yogurt.

Nutritional Facts (per pancake)
CALORIES: 56 CARBOHYDRATES: 11 G CHOLESTEROL: 1 MG FAT: 0.9 G FIBER: 1.8 G
PROTEIN: 3.9 G SODIUM: 41 MG CALCIUM: 42 MG GI RATING: LOW

Breakfast Crepes with Summer Berry Sauce

YIELD: 4 SERVINGS

½ cup whole-wheat pastry flour
½ cup oat bran
1½ teaspoons baking powder
¾ cup skim or low-fat milk

¾ cup fat-free egg substitute

¼ cup plus 2 tablespoons applesauce

1½ cups nonfat or low-fat cottage or ricotta cheese or soft-curd farmer cheese,
brought to room temperature

1 cup Summer Berry Sauce (page 103) or Cinnamon-Apple Topping (page 104)

3 tablespoons chopped walnuts or pecans (optional)

1. Place the flour, oat bran, and baking powder in a medium-sized bowl and stir to mix well. Add the milk, egg substitute, and applesauce, and stir with a wire whisk to mix well. (The batter will be thin.)

2. Coat a large griddle or nonstick skillet with cooking spray, and preheat over medium heat until a drop of water sizzles when it hits the heated surface. (If using an electric griddle, heat the griddle according to manufacturer's directions.)

3. For each crepe, pour ¼ cup plus 1 tablespoon of the batter onto the griddle or skillet. (Tilt the pan so that the batter spreads out to form a 7-inch circle.) Cook for about 1½ minutes or until the top is bubbly and the edges are dry. Turn and cook for an additional 30 seconds or until the second side is golden brown. Repeat until all the batter is used up, respraying the griddle or skillet between crepes.

4. As the crepes are done, roll them up, place on a serving plate, and keep warm in a 200° F preheated oven.

5. To assemble, unroll a crepe, and spread 3 tablespoons of cheese along one side. Reroll the crepe to enclose the filling, and place on a serving plate. Repeat with the remaining ingredients to make 8 filled crepes. Place 2 crepes on each of 4 serving plates and top each serving with ¼ cup of the topping and a sprinkling of nuts if desired. Serve hot.

Nutritional Facts (per serving)

CALORIES: 233 CARBOHYDRATES: 33 G CHOLESTEROL: 8 MG FAT: 1.8 G FIBER: 6.2 G
PROTEIN: 22 G SODIUM: 562 MG CALCIUM: 155 MG GI RATING: LOW

Variation: Breakfast Crepes with Bananas and Pecans

Instead of the Summer Berry Topping, top each serving with ¼ cup sliced bananas, 1 tablespoon maple syrup or honey, and 2 teaspoons of chopped pecans.

Nutritional Facts (per serving)

CALORIES: 308 CARBOHYDRATES: 44 G CHOLESTEROL: 8 MG FAT: 4.8 G
FIBER: 5.2 G PROTEIN: 22 G SODIUM: 378 MG CALCIUM: 161 MG
GI RATING: MODERATE

Sourdough French Toast

For variety, substitute a firm oat-bran, or multigrain, bread for the sourdough bread.

YIELD: 8 SLICES

1 cup fat-free egg substitute
⅔ cup evaporated skim or low-fat milk
1 tablespoon frozen (thawed) orange or apple juice concentrate
¼ teaspoon ground cinnamon
8 slices sourdough bread (preferably whole-wheat sourdough bread)
Butter-flavored nonstick cooking spray

1. Combine the egg substitute, evaporated milk, juice concentrate, and cinnamon in a shallow bowl, and stir with a wire whisk to mix well. Dip the bread slices in the egg mixture, turning to allow both sides to soak up some of the mixture.
2. Coat a large nonstick skillet or griddle with the butter-flavored spray and preheat over medium heat. Lay the bread slices in the skillet and cook for 1½ minutes or until the bottoms are nicely browned. Spray the tops of the bread slices lightly with more cooking spray, turn, and cook for an additional minute, or until both sides are nicely browned. Serve hot topped with Summer Berry Sauce (below) or Cinnamon-Apple Topping (page 104).

Nutritional Facts (per slice)
CALORIES: 103 CARBOHYDRATES: 16 G CHOLESTEROL: 1 MG FAT: 1 G FIBER: 2 G
PROTEIN: 6.9 G SODIUM: 239 MG CALCIUM: 91 MG GI RATING: LOW

Summer Berry Sauce

YIELD: ABOUT 2 CUPS

¼ cup white grape or orange juice
2 teaspoons cornstarch
3½ cups mixed fresh or frozen berries (such as sliced strawberries, blueberries, blackberries, and raspberries)
2 to 3 tablespoons sugar or honey

1. Combine 1 tablespoon of the juice and all the cornstarch in a small bowl. Stir to dissolve the cornstarch, and set aside.
2. Combine the berries, the remaining juice, and the sugar or honey in a 2-quart pot. Stir to mix well, cover, and bring to a boil over medium-high heat. Reduce the heat to medium-low and cook, stirring occasionally, for an additional 5 minutes or until the fruit is soft.
3. Stir the cornstarch mixture and add about half of it to the pot. Cook, stirring constantly, for another minute or two or until the mixture is thickened and bubbly. If the mixture seems too thin, add a little more of the cornstarch mixture to thicken the sauce to the desired consistency. Serve warm over pancakes, French toast, or waffles; or use as a topping for ice cream.

Nutritional Facts (per ¼-cup serving)

CALORIES: 44   CARBOHYDRATES: 11 G   CHOLESTEROL: 0 MG   FAT: 0.3 G   FIBER: 2.3 G
PROTEIN: 0.5 G   SODIUM: 2 MG   CALCIUM: 10 MG   GI RATING: LOW

Cinnamon-Apple Topping

YIELD: 2 CUPS

½ cup plus 2 tablespoons apple juice
2 teaspoons cornstarch
2–3 tablespoons light brown sugar
¼ teaspoon ground cinnamon
Pinch salt
3½ cups thinly sliced peeled apples (about 4 medium)

1. Place 1 tablespoon of the apple juice and all the cornstarch in a small bowl, stir to mix well, and set aside.
2. Place the light brown sugar, cinnamon, and salt in a 2-quart pot, and stir to mix well. Add the remaining apple juice, and stir to mix well.
3. Add the apples to the pot, and bring to a boil over medium-high heat. Reduce the heat to medium-low, cover, and simmer, stirring occasionally, for about 5 minutes or until the apples are tender.
4. Stir the cornstarch mixture and add it to the pot. Cook and stir for another minute or two or until thickened and bubbly. Serve warm over pancakes, French toast, or waffles, or use as a topping for ice cream.

CALORIES: 52 CARBOHYDRATES: 13 G CHOLESTEROL: 0 MG FAT: 0.2 G FIBER: 1 G

PROTEIN: 0.1 G SODIUM: 19 MG CALCIUM: 6 MG GI RATING: LOW

Blueberry Oat-Bran Muffins

YIELD: 12 MUFFINS

2 cups oat bran
¼ cup sugar
2 teaspoons baking powder
¼ teaspoon baking soda
½ cup nonfat or low-fat vanilla yogurt
½ cup orange juice
½ cup fat-free egg substitute; or 2 large eggs plus 1 egg white, lightly beaten
2 tablespoons canola or walnut oil
¾ cup fresh or frozen (unthawed) blueberries

1. Combine the oat bran, sugar, baking powder, and baking soda in a large bowl, and stir to mix well.
2. Combine the yogurt, orange juice, egg substitute or eggs, and oil in a small bowl and stir to mix well. Add the yogurt mixture to the oat-bran mixture and stir to mix well. Fold in the blueberries.
3. Coat the bottoms only of muffin cups with nonstick cooking spray, and fill ¾ full with the batter. Bake at 350° F for about 16 minutes or just until a wooden toothpick inserted in the center of a muffin comes out clean.
4. Remove the muffin tin from the oven and allow it to sit for 5 minutes before removing the muffins. Serve warm or at room temperature. Refrigerate or freeze any leftovers not eaten within 24 hours.

Nutritional Facts (per muffin)

CALORIES: 98 CARBOHYDRATES: 18 G CHOLESTEROL: 0 MG FAT: 3.4 G FIBER: 2.7 G

PROTEIN: 4.5 G SODIUM: 132 MG CALCIUM: 80 MG GI RATING: LOW

Apple Oat-Bran Muffins

YIELD: 12 MUFFINS

2 cups oat bran

2 teaspoons baking powder

¼ teaspoon baking soda

1 teaspoon ground cinnamon

¼ cup dark brown sugar

½ cup nonfat or low-fat vanilla yogurt

½ cup apple juice

½ cup fat-free egg substitute; or 2 large eggs plus 1 egg white, lightly beaten

2 tablespoons canola or walnut oil

1 cup finely chopped peeled apples (about 1 medium-large)

½ cup chopped walnuts, pecans, dried cranberries, or dark raisins (optional)

1. Combine the oat bran, baking powder, baking soda, and cinnamon in a large bowl and stir to mix well. Add the brown sugar, and stir to mix well. Use the back of a wooden spoon to press out any lumps in the brown sugar.

2. Put the yogurt, apple juice, egg substitute or eggs, and oil in a small bowl, and stir to mix well. Add the yogurt mixture to the oat-bran mixture and stir to mix well. Fold in the apples and, if desired, the nuts or dried fruit.

3. Coat the bottoms only of muffin cups with nonstick cooking spray, and fill ¾ full with the batter. Bake at 350° F for about 16 minutes or just until a wooden toothpick inserted in the center of a muffin comes out clean.

4. Remove the muffin tin from the oven and allow it to sit for 5 minutes before removing the muffins. Serve warm or at room temperature. Refrigerate or freeze any leftovers not eaten within 24 hours.

Nutritional Facts (per muffin)

CALORIES: 100 CARBOHYDRATES: 19 G CHOLESTEROL: 0 MG FAT: 3.4 G FIBER: 2.6 G
PROTEIN: 4.4 G SODIUM: 133 MG CALCIUM: 83 MG GI RATING: LOW

Muffins and quick breads make great quick breakfasts or satisfying snacks anytime. And these treats are easy to freeze, so you can always have a supply on hand. To freeze for later use, cool the muffins or bread to room temperature. Slice the bread into individual servings. Wrap the muffins or individual bread slices in plastic wrap, place the wrapped muffins or bread slices in a freezer bag, and freeze for up to 3 weeks. Remove individual servings from the freezer bag as you need them, and thaw at room temperature. Or remove the plastic wrap and heat the muffin or bread slice at medium-low power for 1 minute in a microwave oven, or until thawed and warmed through.

Cranberry-Applesauce Bread

For variety, substitute mashed very ripe bananas for the applesauce

YIELD: 16 SLICES

1¼ cups whole-wheat pastry flour
1 cup oat bran; or ½ cup oat bran plus ½ cup flax meal
⅓ cup sugar
1 tablespoon baking powder
½ teaspoon ground nutmeg
⅛ teaspoon salt
1¼ cups applesauce
½ cup fat-free egg substitute; or 2 eggs plus 1 egg white, lightly beaten
¼ cup canola oil
1½ teaspoons vanilla extract
½ cup dried sweetened cranberries, cherries, or blueberries
½ cup chopped walnuts or pecans (optional)

1. Put the flour, oat bran, sugar, baking powder, nutmeg, and salt in a large bowl and stir to mix well. Put the applesauce, egg substitute or eggs, oil, and vanilla extract in a medium-sized bowl and stir to mix well. Add the applesauce mixture to the flour mixture and stir to mix well. Fold in the berries or cherries and, if desired, the nuts.

2. Coat an 8-by-4-inch pan with nonstick cooking spray. Spread the batter evenly in the pan and bake at 350° F for about 50 minutes or just until a wooden toothpick inserted in the center of the loaf comes out clean. Be careful not to overbake.

3. Remove the bread from the oven and let sit for 15 minutes. Invert the loaf onto a wire rack, turn right side up, and cool to room temperature before slicing and serving. Refrigerate or freeze any leftovers not eaten within 24 hours.

Nutritional Facts (per slice)

CALORIES: 122 CARBOHYDRATES: 21 G CHOLESTEROL: 0 MG FAT: 3.9 G FIBER: 2.8 G
PROTEIN: 3.3 G SODIUM: 78 MG CALCIUM: 9 MG GI RATING: MODERATE

Fruit & Bran Bread

YIELD: 16 SLICES

15-ounce can pears in juice
¼ cup canola oil
¼ cup plus 2 tablespoons fat-free egg substitute; or 2 eggs lightly beaten
1 teaspoon vanilla extract
1⅓ cups whole-wheat pastry flour
⅔ cup oat bran
⅔ cup wheat bran
⅓ cup sugar
1 tablespoon baking powder
½ teaspoon ground cinnamon
⅛ teaspoon salt
⅔ cup chopped pitted prunes or dried apricots
⅓ cup chopped walnuts or pecans (optional)

1. Drain the pears, reserving the juice. Place the pears and about half of the juice in a blender and blend until smooth. Transfer the pears to a 2-cup measure and add enough of the remaining juice to bring the volume up to 1⅓ cups. Add the oil, eggs or egg substitute, and vanilla extract to the puréed pears and stir to mix well. Set aside.

2. Put the flour, oat bran, wheat bran, sugar, baking powder, cinnamon, and salt in a large bowl and stir to mix well. Add the pear mixture to the flour mixture and stir to mix well. Fold in the prunes or apricots and, if desired, the nuts.

3. Coat an 8-by-4-inch pan with nonstick cooking spray. Spread the batter evenly in the pan, and bake at 350° F for about 45 minutes or just until a wooden toothpick inserted in the center of the loaf comes out clean. Be careful not to overbake.

4. Remove the bread from the oven and let sit for 15 minutes. Invert the loaf onto a wire rack, turn right side up, and cool to room temperature before slicing and serving. Refrigerate or freeze any leftovers not eaten within 24 hours.

Nutritional Facts (per slice)

CALORIES: 128   CARBOHYDRATES: 23 G   CHOLESTEROL: 0 MG   FAT: 4 G   FIBER: 2.7 G
PROTEIN: 3.2 G   SODIUM: 75 MG   CALCIUM: 11 MG   GI RATING: LOW

Mandarin-Blueberry Bread

YIELD: 16 SLICES

1 cup plus 2 tablespoons whole-wheat pastry flour
¾ cup oat bran
½ cup wheat bran
⅓ cup sugar
1 tablespoon baking powder
⅛ teaspoon salt
11-ounce can mandarin oranges in juice or light syrup, undrained
½ cup fat-free egg substitute; or 2 large eggs plus 1 egg white, lightly beaten
¼ cup canola oil
1½ teaspoons vanilla extract
½ cup dried blueberries, cranberries, or cherries
½ cup chopped toasted pecans (optional)

1. Place the flour, oat bran, wheat bran, sugar, baking powder, and salt in a large bowl and stir to mix well. Using a wooden spoon, crush the oranges into bits. Place the undrained oranges, egg substitute or eggs, oil, and vanilla extract in a medium-sized bowl, and stir to mix well. Add the orange mixture to the flour mixture and stir to mix well. Fold in the berries or cherries and, if desired, the pecans.

2. Coat an 8-by-4-inch pan with nonstick cooking spray. Spread the batter evenly in the pan, and bake at 350° F for about 50 minutes or just until a wooden toothpick inserted in the center of the loaf comes out clean. Be careful not to overbake.

3. Remove the bread from the oven, and let sit for 15 minutes. Invert the loaf onto a wire rack, turn right side up, and cool to room temperature before slicing and serving. Refrigerate or freeze any leftovers not eaten within 24 hours.

Nutritional Facts (per slice)

CALORIES: 119   CARBOHYDRATES: 20 G   CHOLESTEROL: 0 MG   FAT: 3.9 G   FIBER: 2.9 G
PROTEIN: 3 G   SODIUM: 78 MG   CALCIUM: 8 MG   GI RATING: MODERATE

8. Hors D'Oeuvres with a Difference

f *or most of us, party foods spell fun, festivity—and an overdose of fat, calories, and high-GI carbs. Crackers, chips, snack mixes, and other party staples top the list of high-GI foods, while creamy dips and high-fat finger foods can make special occasions a real obstacle for anyone who's trying to watch fat and calories.*

Fortunately, adopting a healthy low-GI lifestyle does not mean giving up party foods. Ingredients like low-fat cheeses, ultralean lunchmeats, low-fat sour cream and mayonnaise, and wholesome whole-grain breads can substantially lighten up your celebrations and get-togethers. This chapter uses these ingredients plus plenty of fresh vegetables and fruits to create a variety of hot and cold hors d'oeuvres, both plain and fancy. So whether you are looking for some mini shish kabobs to start your next cookout, a creamy dip to accompany a fresh vegetable tray, or a platter of festive finger sandwiches, this chapter offers plenty of ideas for light and healthy fare that is so delicious no one will guess that they're also good for you.

Spicy Shrimp Skewers

YIELD: 16 APPETIZERS

1 pound cleaned raw shrimp
1½–2 tablespoons Ragin' Cajun Rub (page 175)
1 tablespoon extra-virgin olive oil
16 six-inch skewers

1. Place the shrimp in a large bowl, sprinkle with the rub, and drizzle with the olive oil. Toss to mix well, and set aside for 15 to 30 minutes.
2. Thread about 4 shrimp onto each skewer as follows: Bend each shrimp almost in half, so that the large end nearly touches the smaller tail end. Insert the skewer just above the tail so that it passes through the shrimp twice. (If you are using wooden skewers, soak them in water for 20 minutes before using, to prevent burning.)

3. Grill the skewers over medium coals for about 6 minutes, turning occasionally, or until the shrimp turn pink and are cooked through. (Alternatively, broil the skewers under a preheated broiler for about 6 minutes, turning occasionally.)

Nutritional Facts (per appetizer)
CALORIES: 28 CARBOHYDRATES: 0.2 G CHOLESTEROL: 40 MG FAT: 1.2 G FIBER: 0 G
PROTEIN: 4.4 G SODIUM: 60 MG CALCIUM: 21 MG GI rating: VERY LOW

Peanutty Chicken Skewers

YIELD: 24 APPETIZERS

Marinade
½ cup plus 2 tablespoons orange or pineapple juice
3 tablespoons peanut butter
3 tablespoons reduced-sodium soy sauce
1 tablespoon light brown sugar
1½ teaspoons ground ginger
2 teaspoons crushed garlic

1¼ pounds boneless skinless chicken breast
48 one-inch pieces scallion
48 pieces red bell pepper (½ inch by 1 inch)
24 six-inch skewers

1. Rinse the chicken with cool water, and pat it dry with paper towels. Cut the chicken into thin strips (about ¼ inch), and place the strips in a shallow nonmetal container.
2. Place all the marinade ingredients in a blender, and process until smooth. Remove ⅓ cup of the marinade, transfer to a covered container, and refrigerate until ready to cook the skewers.
3. Pour the remaining marinade over the chicken strips and toss to mix well. Cover and refrigerate for 6 to 24 hours.
4. Loosely weave 2 scallion pieces, 2 bell pepper pieces, and a 6-inch strip of the chicken onto each skewer. (If you are using wooden skewers, soak them in water for 20 minutes before using, to prevent burning.)
5. Coat a large broiler pan with nonstick cooking spray, and arrange the skewers on the pan. Broil for about 8 minutes, turning occasionally or until the chicken is nicely browned and no longer

pink inside. Baste with the reserved marinade during the last 3 minutes of cooking. (Alternatively, grill the skewers over medium coals for about 8 minutes, turning occasionally.) Place the skewers on a serving platter, and serve hot.

Nutritional Facts (per appetizer)

CALORIES: 37 CARBOHYDRATES: 1.5 G CHOLESTEROL: 14 MG FAT: 0.8 G FIBER: 0.3 G
PROTEIN: 6 G SODIUM: 56 MG CALCIUM: 7 MG GI RATING: VERY LOW

Steak on a Stick

YIELD: 28 APPETIZERS

1¼ pounds well-trimmed beef top sirloin steak
2–3 tablespoons Zesty Herb Rub (page 175)
1 tablespoon extra-virgin olive oil
56 medium-small fresh mushrooms
28 six-inch skewers
Olive oil nonstick cooking spray

1. Rinse the meat with cool water and pat it dry with paper towels. Slice the meat into thin strips (about ¼ inch), and place the strips in a shallow nonmetal container.
2. Sprinkle the rub over the steak strips and toss to mix well. Drizzle the olive oil over the steak strips and toss again. Set aside for 15 to 30 minutes, or for more intense flavor cover and refrigerate for up to 24 hours.
3. Thread one mushroom onto each skewer. Then loosely thread a 3- to 4-inch steak strip onto the skewers followed by another mushroom. (If you are using wooden skewers, soak them in water for 20 minutes before using, to prevent burning.)
4. Coat a large broiler pan with nonstick cooking spray and arrange the skewers on the pan. Spray the skewers lightly with the olive oil cooking spray and broil for about 8 minutes, turning occasionally, or until the skewers are nicely browned and the steak is done. (Alternatively, grill the skewers over medium coals for about 8 minutes.) Place the skewers on a serving platter, and serve hot.

Nutritional Facts (per appetizer)

CALORIES: 41 CARBOHYDRATES: 2 G CHOLESTEROL: 12 MG FAT: 1.6 G FIBER: 0.6 G
PROTEIN: 5.1 G SODIUM: 38 MG CALCIUM: 4 MG GI RATING: VERY LOW

Spinach and Cheese Roll-Ups

YIELD: 30 APPETIZERS

1 tablespoon plus 1 teaspoon chopped sun-dried tomatoes
1 tablespoon plus 1 teaspoon water
8-ounce block nonfat or reduced-fat cream cheese, softened to room temperature
1 teaspoon crushed garlic
10-ounce package frozen chopped spinach, thawed and squeezed dry
½ cup chopped black olives
3 flour tortillas (10-inch rounds) warmed to room temperature

1. Place the tomatoes and water in a small microwave-safe dish and microwave for about 30 seconds or until the water comes to a boil. Remove the dish from the microwave and set aside for 10 minutes or until the water has been absorbed and the tomatoes are softened.
2. Place the cream cheese and garlic in a large bowl and stir to mix well. Finely chop the tomatoes and add them to the cheese mixture along with the spinach and olives. Stir to mix well.
3. Spread each tortilla with ⅓ of the cheese mixture, extending the mixture all the way to the top and bottom edges, but only to within 1 inch of the sides.
4. Starting at the bottom, roll each tortilla up tightly. Cut a 1¼-inch piece off each end, and discard. Slice the remainder of each tortilla into ten ¾-inch pieces. Arrange the rolls on a platter, and serve immediately. Or leave the rolls uncut, wrap in plastic wrap, and refrigerate for up to 8 hours before slicing and serving.

Nutritional Facts (per appetizer)
CALORIES: 23 CARBOHYDRATES: 3.4 G CHOLESTEROL: 0 MG FAT: 0.3 G FIBER: 0.6 G
PROTEIN: 1.8 G SODIUM: 72 MG CALCIUM: 34 MG GI RATING: MODERATE

Gorgonzola Party Pizzas

YIELD: 24 APPETIZERS

4 pieces whole-wheat or oat-bran pita bread or flatbread (6-inch rounds)

Toppings
1 cup finely chopped plum tomatoes (about 3 medium)
1 cup shredded reduced-fat mozzarella cheese

⅓ cup crumbled Gorgonzola or blue cheese
¼ cup sliced scallions
¾ teaspoon dried Italian seasoning

1. Spread a quarter of the tomatoes over each piece of pita bread or flatbread crust to within ¼ inch of the edges. Sprinkle first the mozzarella and then the Gorgonzola over the tomatoes. Sprinkle with the scallions, and then the Italian seasoning.
2. Arrange the pizzas on a large baking sheet and bake at 400° F for about 10 minutes, or until the cheese is melted and the pizzas are just beginning to brown. Transfer the pizzas to a cutting board, and cut each one into 6 wedges. Serve hot.

Nutritional Facts (per appetizer)

CALORIES: 40 CARBOHYDRATES: 6 G CHOLESTEROL: 4 MG FAT: 1.2 G FIBER: 0.8 G
PROTEIN: 2.9 G SODIUM: 102 MG CALCIUM: 35 MG GI RATING: MODERATE

Righteous Roll-Ups

YIELD: 28 APPETIZERS

4 flour tortillas (10-inch rounds), warmed to room temperature
1 cup Veggie–Cream Cheese Spread (page 000)
6 ounces thinly sliced roasted turkey breast
4 ounces thinly sliced nonfat or reduced-fat Swiss cheese
12 thin rings red bell pepper
1⅓ cups alfalfa or spicy sprouts or 24 tender fresh spinach leaves

1. Spread each tortilla with ¼ cup of the cheese spread, extending it all the way to the outer edges. Lay a quarter of the turkey over the *bottom half only* of each tortilla, leaving a 1-inch margin on each outer edge. Arrange a quarter of the cheese and 3 bell pepper rings over the turkey. Finally, spread a quarter of the sprouts or spinach leaves over the bell pepper layer.
2. Starting at the bottom, roll each tortilla up tightly. Cut a 1¼-inch piece off each end, and discard. Slice the remainder of each tortilla into seven 1-inch pieces. Arrange the rolls on a platter, and serve immediately. Or wrap the rolls in plastic wrap, and refrigerate for up to 3 hours before slicing and serving.

Nutritional Facts (per appetizer)

CALORIES: 40 CARBOHYDRATES: 4 G CHOLESTEROL: 6 MG FAT: 0.4 G FIBER: 0.4 G
PROTEIN: 4.5 G SODIUM: 89 MG CALCIUM: 79 MG GI RATING: MODERATE

Ham & Asparagus Tarts

YIELD: 24 APPETIZERS

4 ounces thinly sliced ham, cut into thin strips
4 thin slices onion, separated into rings
1½ cups ¾-inch pieces fresh asparagus
4 pieces whole-wheat or oat-bran pita bread or flatbread (6-inch rounds)
8 ounces soft-curd farmer cheese or soft goat cheese
2 tablespoons grated Parmesan cheese
Olive oil nonstick cooking spray

1. Coat a large nonstick skillet with the olive oil cooking spray. Add the ham, onion, and aspara-gus and cook, stirring frequently, for several minutes or until the asparagus is crisp-tender and the ham is beginning to brown. Place a lid over the skillet periodically if the skillet becomes too dry. (The steam released during cooking will moisten the skillet.)

2. Place the pita rounds on a flat surface and spread each with a quarter of the farmer or goat cheese. Top the cheese on each pita with a quarter of the asparagus mixture, then sprinkle 1½ teaspoons of the Parmesan cheese over each tart. Spray the top of each tart lightly with the cooking spray.

3. Place the tarts on a baking sheet and bake at 400° F for about 10 minutes or until the cheese is melted and the tarts are just beginning to brown. Transfer the tarts to a cutting board, and cut each one into 6 wedges. Serve hot.

Nutritional Facts (per appetizer)

CALORIES: 47 CARBOHYDRATES: 6 G CHOLESTEROL: 5 MG FAT: 1.2 G FIBER: 0.9 G
PROTEIN: 3.8 G SODIUM: 142 MG CALCIUM: 28 MG GI RATING: MODERATE

Mediterranean White Bean Dip

YIELD: 1¼ CUPS

15-ounce can white beans, rinsed and drained
1 tablespoon plus 1 teaspoon lemon juice
1–2 tablespoons extra-virgin olive oil

1½ teaspoons crushed garlic
¼ teaspoon dried oregano
⅛ teaspoon ground black pepper
2 tablespoons finely chopped black olives
2 tablespoons finely chopped fresh parsley

1. Place all the ingredients except the olives and parsley in a food processor and process until smooth. Add a few teaspoons of water if the mixture seems too thick.
2. Spread the bean mixture in a small shallow dish. Combine the olives and parsley in a small bowl, toss to mix well, and sprinkle over the bean dip. Serve immediately with wedges of whole-grain pita bread, whole-grain crackers, leaves of Belgian endive, celery sticks, and carrot sticks. Or cover and refrigerate until ready to serve, but let the spread come to room temperature before serving.

Nutritional Facts (per tablespoon)

CALORIES: 26 CARBOHYDRATES: 3.6 G CHOLESTEROL: 0 MG FAT: 0.9 G FIBER: 1.4 G
PROTEIN: 1.2 G SODIUM: 39 MG CALCIUM: 11 MG GI RATING: LOW

Garden Hummus

YIELD: 2 CUPS

16-ounce can garbanzo beans (chickpeas), rinsed and drained
¼ cup toasted sesame tahini (sesame butter)
¼ cup plain nonfat or low-fat yogurt
2 tablespoons lemon juice
1½ teaspoons crushed garlic
¼ teaspoon ground cumin
¼ cup chopped carrots
3 tablespoons chopped fresh parsley
2 tablespoons sliced scallions

1. Combine the garbanzo beans, tahini, yogurt, lemon juice, garlic, and cumin in a food processor and process until smooth. Add a little more yogurt if the mixture seems too thick. Add the carrots and process until the carrots are finely chopped. Add the parsley and scallions and process until finely chopped.

2. Serve immediately with wedges of whole-grain pita bread, whole-grain crackers, celery sticks, and carrot sticks. Or cover and refrigerate until ready to serve, but let the spread come to room temperature before serving.

Nutritional Facts (per tablespoon)

CALORIES: 28   CARBOHYDRATES: 3.2 G   CHOLESTEROL: 0 MG   FAT: 1.2 G   FIBER: 0.9 G
PROTEIN: 1.3 G   SODIUM: 26 MG   CALCIUM: 17 MG   GI RATING: LOW

Roasted Red Pepper Dip

YIELD: 1 CUP

¾ cup nonfat or light mayonnaise
½ cup chopped drained roasted red peppers (about 3½ ounces)
1 teaspoon crushed garlic
¼ teaspoon dried oregano
¼ teaspoon ground black pepper

1. Combine all the ingredients in a blender or mini food processor and process until smooth.
2. Cover and chill for at least 2 hours before serving. Serve with an assortment of fresh-cut vegetables and rolled-up slices of roasted turkey breast and lean roast beef.

Nutritional Facts (per tablespoon)

CALORIES: 9   CARBOHYDRATES: 1.8 G   CHOLESTEROL: 0 MG   FAT: 0 G   FIBER: 0 G
PROTEIN: 0.1 G   SODIUM: 101 MG   CALCIUM: 1 MG   GI RATING: LOW

Creamy Herb Dip

YIELD: 1¼ CUPS

¾ cup nonfat or light mayonnaise
½ cup nonfat or light sour cream
1 teaspoon crushed garlic
1 tablespoon finely chopped fresh parsley or 1 teaspoon dried parsley
1 tablespoon finely chopped fresh chives or 1 teaspoon dried chives

¾ teaspoon finely chopped fresh dill or ¼ teaspoon dried dill
¼ teaspoon ground black pepper

1. Combine all the ingredients in a small bowl and stir to mix well.
2. Transfer the mixture to a covered container and refrigerate for several hours before serving. Serve with an assortment of fresh-cut vegetables and rolled-up slices of roasted turkey breast and lean roast beef.

Nutritional Facts (per tablespoon)

CALORIES: 12 CARBOHYDRATES: 2 G CHOLESTEROL: 0 MG FAT: 0 G FIBER: 0 G
PROTEIN: 0.4 G SODIUM: 67 MG CALCIUM: 8 MG GI RATING: LOW

Chutney-Cheese Spread

YIELD: 1 CUP

8-ounce block nonfat or reduced-fat cream cheese, softened to room temperature
3 tablespoons mango chutney

1. Put the cream cheese in a medium-sized bowl, and beat with an electric mixer until smooth. Beat in the chutney.
2. Serve immediately, or transfer the dip to a covered container and refrigerate until ready to serve. Serve with wedges of whole-grain pita bread, whole-grain crackers, celery sticks, apple wedges, and rolled-up slices of thinly shaved turkey breast.

Nutritional Facts (per tablespoon)

CALORIES: 18 CARBOHYDRATES: 2.1 G CHOLESTEROL: 1 MG FAT: 0 G FIBER: 0.1 G
PROTEIN: 2.2 G SODIUM: 75 MG CALCIUM: 44 MG GI RATING: LOW

Veggie–Cream Cheese Spread

YIELD: 1¼ CUPS

8-ounce block nonfat or reduced-fat cream cheese, softened to room temperature
1 teaspoon crushed garlic

3 tablespoons finely chopped scallions
3 tablespoons finely chopped green bell pepper
3 tablespoons grated carrots

1. Combine the cream cheese and garlic in a medium-sized bowl and beat with an electric mixer until smooth. Stir in the remaining ingredients. Transfer the dip to a covered container and refrigerate for at least 2 hours before serving.
2. Serve with whole-grain crackers and fresh-cut vegetables or use as a filling for finger sandwiches.

Nutritional Facts (per tablespoon)
CALORIES: 12 CARBOHYDRATES: 0.8 G CHOLESTEROL: 1 MG FAT: 0 G FIBER: 0.1 G
PROTEIN: 1.8 G SODIUM: 55 MG CALCIUM: 35 MG GI RATING: VERY LOW

Tasty Tuna Spread

For variety, substitute ¾ cup flaked smoked salmon for the tuna.

YIELD: 2 CUPS

8-ounce block nonfat or reduced-fat cream cheese
¼ cup nonfat or light sour cream or mayonnaise
6-ounce can albacore tuna, drained
¼ cup finely chopped scallions
¼ cup finely chopped celery
¼ cup finely chopped black olives

1. Place the cream cheese and the sour cream or mayonnaise in a medium bowl and beat with an electric mixer until smooth. Stir in the remaining ingredients.
2. Transfer to a covered container and refrigerate for at least 1 hour. Serve with whole-grain crackers. Or use as a filling for celery sticks, hollowed-out cherry tomatoes, or finger sandwiches.

Nutritional Facts (per tablespoon)
CALORIES: 15 CARBOHYDRATES: 1 G CHOLESTEROL: 2 MG FAT: 0.2 G FIBER: 0.1 G
PROTEIN: 2.2 G SODIUM: 58 MG CALCIUM: 23 MG GI RATING: VERY LOW

Creamy Seafood Spread

YIELD: 1½ CUPS

8-ounce block nonfat or reduced-fat cream cheese, softened to room temperature
2 tablespoons chili sauce or cocktail sauce
1 cup flaked cooked crabmeat or diced cooked shrimp
3 tablespoons finely chopped scallions

1. Put the cream cheese and chili sauce in a medium-sized bowl and beat with an electric mixer until smooth. Stir in the crabmeat or shrimp.
2. Spread the mixture evenly into a 2-cup serving dish. Cover and refrigerate for at least 1 hour. Sprinkle the scallions over the spread just before serving. Serve with whole-grain crackers and celery sticks.

Nutritional Facts (per tablespoon)
   CALORIES: 16   CARBOHYDRATES: 1 G   CHOLESTEROL: 4 MG   FAT: 0.1 G   FIBER: 0 G
   PROTEIN: 2.6 G   SODIUM: 83 MG   CALCIUM: 32 MG   GI RATING: LOW

Baked Crab and Artichoke Dip

YIELD: 3 CUPS

14½-ounce can artichoke hearts, drained and finely chopped
1½ cups finely flaked cooked crabmeat; or 2 cans (6 ounces each) crabmeat, drained
1 cup nonfat or light mayonnaise
2 teaspoons Dijon mustard
½ teaspoon crushed garlic
⅛ teaspoon ground white pepper
½ cup grated Parmesan cheese

1. Combine all the ingredients except 2 tablespoons of the Parmesan cheese in a medium-sized bowl and stir to mix well. Coat a 1-quart casserole dish with nonstick cooking spray, and spread the mixture evenly in the dish. Sprinkle the remaining Parmesan cheese over the top.

2. Cover the dish with aluminum foil and bake at 350° F for 25 minutes. Remove the foil and bake for an additional 10 minutes or until the top is lightly browned. Serve hot with whole-grain crackers or wedges of whole-grain pita bread.

Nutritional Facts (per tablespoon)

CALORIES: 14 CARBOHYDRATES: 1.3 G CHOLESTEROL: 4 MG FAT: 0.4 G FIBER: 0.3 G
PROTEIN: 1.4 G SODIUM: 74 MG CALCIUM: 19 MG GI RATING: LOW

Spinach and Mushroom Quesadillas

YIELD: 32 APPETIZERS

2½ cups sliced fresh mushrooms
2 teaspoons crushed garlic
½ teaspoon dried thyme
5 cups (moderately packed) fresh coarsely chopped spinach leaves
8 flour tortillas (8-inch rounds), warmed to room temperature
2 cups shredded nonfat or reduced-fat mozzarella, provolone, or Swiss cheese
Olive oil nonstick cooking spray

1. Coat a large nonstick skillet with the olive oil cooking spray, and preheat over medium-high heat. Add the mushrooms, garlic, and thyme and cook, stirring frequently, until the mushrooms release their juices and are nicely browned. Periodically place a lid on the skillet if mixture begins to dry out. (The steam released during cooking will moisten the skillet.) Add the spinach to the skillet and cook, stirring frequently, for a minute or two or until the spinach is wilted. Remove the skillet from the heat and set aside.

2. Lay a tortilla out on a flat surface, and spread ⅛ of the spinach mixture over the bottom half of the tortilla, then sprinkle with ¼ cup of the cheese. Fold the top half of the tortilla over to enclose the filling. Repeat with the remaining ingredients to make 8 filled tortillas.

3. Coat 2 large baking sheets with nonstick cooking spray, and lay the folded tortillas on the sheets. Spray the tops lightly with the cooking spray. Bake at 425° F for 5 minutes, turn the quesadillas with a spatula, and bake for 4 minutes more or until lightly browned and the cheese is melted.

4. Place each quesadilla on a cutting board and cut into 4 wedges. Serve hot.

Nutritional Facts (per appetizer)

CALORIES: 45 CARBOHYDRATES: 6 G CHOLESTEROL: 0 MG FAT: 0.8 G FIBER: 0.7 G
PROTEIN: 2.8 G SODIUM: 105 MG CALCIUM: 52 MG GI RATING: MODERATE

Crab-Stuffed Mushrooms

YIELD: 24 APPETIZERS

24 medium–large fresh mushrooms (about 1 pound)
⅓ cup finely chopped red bell pepper
⅓ cup finely chopped green bell pepper
¼ cup finely chopped onion
1 teaspoon dried thyme
½ teaspoon ground black pepper
¼ cup chicken broth
1 cup finely flaked cooked crabmeat (about 5 ounces)
2 cups multigrain or sourdough bread crumbs*
¼ cup grated Parmesan cheese
Butter-flavored nonstick cooking spray

1. Remove the stems from the mushrooms and finely chop enough of the stems to yield ¾ cup. Coat a large nonstick skillet with the butter-flavored cooking spray, and preheat over medium heat. Add the chopped mushroom stems, red and green bell peppers, onions, thyme, black pepper, and 1 tablespoon of the broth. Cover and cook, stirring frequently, for about 3 minutes or until the vegetables are tender. Add a little more broth during cooking if the skillet becomes too dry.

2. Remove the skillet from the heat and set aside for a few minutes to cool slightly. Add the crabmeat to the skillet mixture and toss to mix well. Add the bread crumbs and Parmesan cheese and toss to mix well. Slowly add the remaining broth while tossing gently to mix well. The mixture should be moist but not wet and should hold together loosely when gently pressed. Toss in a little more broth if needed.

3. Coat a 9-by-13-inch pan with the cooking spray. Place about 1 tablespoonful of the stuffing in each mushroom cap, pressing the stuffing gently to make it hold together, and arrange the mushrooms in the pan. Spray the tops of the mushrooms lightly with cooking spray.

4. Cover the pan with aluminum foil, and bake at 400° F for 12 minutes. Remove the foil and bake for about 5 minutes more or until the mushrooms are tender and the stuffing is lightly browned. Serve hot.

To make the bread crumbs, tear about 3 slices of firm multigrain or sourdough bread into chunks. Place in a food processor or blender, and process into crumbs.

Nutritional Facts (per appetizer)

CALORIES: 24   CARBOHYDRATES: 3 G   CHOLESTEROL: 4 MG   FAT: 0.6 G   FIBER: 0.6 G
PROTEIN: 2.4 G   SODIUM: 57 MG   CALCIUM: 22 MG   GI RATING: LOW

Sausage-Stuffed Mushrooms

YIELD: 24 APPETIZERS

24 medium–large fresh mushrooms (about 1 pound)
8 ounces ground turkey breakfast or Italian sausage
¼ cup finely chopped onion
½ teaspoon dried thyme
⅛ teaspoon ground black pepper
¼ cup chicken broth
2 cups multigrain or sourdough bread crumbs*
Butter-flavored nonstick cooking spray

1. Remove the stems from the mushrooms and finely chop enough of the stems to yield 1 cup. Set aside.
2. Coat a large nonstick skillet with the butter-flavored cooking spray, and preheat over medium heat. Add the sausage and cook, stirring to finely crumble, until the meat is no longer pink. Add the chopped mushroom stems, onions, thyme, black pepper, and 1 tablespoon of the broth. Cover and cook, stirring frequently, for about 3 minutes or until the vegetables are tender. Add a little more broth during cooking if the skillet becomes too dry.
3. Remove the skillet from the heat and set aside for a few minutes to cool slightly. Add the bread crumbs to the skillet mixture and toss gently to mix well. Slowly add the remaining broth to the skillet mixture, while tossing gently to mix well. The mixture should be moist but not wet and should hold together when gently pressed. Toss in a little more broth if needed.
4. Coat a 9-by-13-inch pan with the cooking spray. Place about 1 tablespoonful of the stuffing in each mushroom cap, pressing the stuffing gently to make it hold together, and arrange the mushrooms in the pan. Spray the tops of the mushrooms lightly with the butter-flavored cooking spray.

*To make the bread crumbs, tear about 3 slices of firm multigrain or sourdough bread into chunks. Place in a food processor or blender and process into crumbs.

5. Cover the pan with aluminum foil, and bake at 400° F for 12 minutes. Remove the foil and bake for about 5 minutes more or until the mushrooms are tender and the stuffing is lightly browned. Serve hot.

Nutritional Facts (per appetizer)

CALORIES: 27 CARBOHYDRATES: 3 G CHOLESTEROL: 6 MG FAT: 0.6 G FIBER: 0.5 G
PROTEIN: 3 G SODIUM: 53 MG CALCIUM: 4 MG GI RATING: LOW

Crab-Stuffed Cucumbers

YIELD: 14 APPETIZERS

¾ cup finely flaked cooked crabmeat or 1 6-ounce can crabmeat, drained
2 tablespoons finely chopped red bell pepper
2 tablespoons finely chopped scallions
3 tablespoons nonfat or light mayonnaise
¼ teaspoon dried dill
Pinch ground white pepper
2 medium cucumbers

1. Combine the crabmeat, red bell pepper, and scallions in a small bowl and toss to mix well. Add the mayonnaise, dill, and white pepper, and stir to mix well. Transfer the mixture to a covered container and refrigerate for at least 1 hour or until well chilled.
2. To assemble the appetizers, peel the cucumbers and cut them into ¾-inch-thick slices. Using a melon-baller or a small spoon, scoop out the seeds, leaving a ¼-inch-thick shell covering the bottom of the slice. Fill each cucumber cup with a tablespoon of the crab mixture. Arrange the appetizers on a serving platter and serve immediately.

Nutritional Facts (per appetizer)

CALORIES: 14 CARBOHYDRATES: 2.5 G CHOLESTEROL: 5 MG FAT: 0.1 G FIBER: 0.3 G
PROTEIN: 1.7 G SODIUM: 47 MG CALCIUM: 9 MG GI RATING: VERY LOW

Need More Ideas?

When creating appetizers and snacks, don't limit yourself to the recipes in this chapter. Here are some other ideas for healthy and delicious finger foods that will keep you eating low on the glycemic index.

* Hollow out cherry tomatoes, and fill with Orzo Shrimp Salad (page 162). Or fill with Spicy Egg Salad (page 161), and top with a sprinkling of ground paprika

* Cut 2-inch lengths of celery, and stuff with Almond-Dill Chicken Salad (page 158), Tasty Tuna Spread (page 120), or Spicy Egg Salad (page 161).

* Lay leaves of Belgian endive on a serving platter with the hollow sides up so that they form shallow containers. Fill each leaf with a tablespoon of Tasty Tuna Spread (page 120), Cashew Crunch Turkey Salad (page 159), West Coast Crab Salad (page 160), Spicy Egg Salad (page 161), or Orzo Shrimp Salad (page 162).

* Serve Country Chicken Salad (page 157), Almond-Dill Chicken Salad (page 158), Cashew Crunch Turkey Salad (page 159), West Coast Crab Salad (page 160), or Spicy Egg Salad (page 161) with an assortment of whole-grain crackers. Or use them as a filling for finger sandwiches made with firm multigrain or pumpernickel bread.

* Thread cherry tomatoes, mushrooms, zucchini, scallions, pitted black olives, and cubes of low-fat cheese onto 6-inch skewers. Serve with Creamy Herb Dip (page 118) or Roasted Red Pepper Dip (page 118)

* Thread balls or cubes of fresh melon, whole fresh strawberries, grapes, and pineapple chunks onto 6-inch skewers.

* Serve an assortment of fresh fruits on a platter with low-fat vanilla yogurt for dipping.

9. Heartwarming Soups

There's nothing quite as warming and comforting as a steaming bowl of homemade soup. And soups that feature ingredients like lean meats, poultry, seafood, whole grains, beans, pasta, and garden vegetables are a natural for low-GI living.

Perhaps the most versatile of foods, a cup of soup is the perfect low-GI accompaniment to a sandwich or main-course salad. And a bowl of hearty soup needs only a fresh garden salad and a piece of crusty whole-grain bread to make a satisfying lunch or light supper. And even when you take the time to make soups from scratch, you'll find that soups are perfect for a busy lifestyle. Most soups can be prepared ahead of time and refrigerated or frozen until needed. In fact, many soups taste even better when refrigerated overnight, allowing the flavors to marry and blend.

Watching your weight? A big bowl of soup may be just what the doctor ordered. Because soup has a high water content, you get a big portion for relatively few calories. This makes soup exceptionally filling and satisfying.

This chapter combines wholesome ingredients to produce a variety of delectable low-GI soups that are bursting with flavor and brimming with important nutrients. So take out your kettle and get ready to make soups a healthful part of your menus.

Chicken & Wild Rice Soup

🌿 For variety, substitute brown rice or barley for the wild rice.

YIELD: 8 CUPS

2 skinless bone-in chicken breast halves (about 1 pound)
7 cups water or unsalted chicken broth
1 tablespoon plus 1 teaspoon instant chicken bouillon granules

2 cups sliced fresh mushrooms
1 cup chopped onion
1 cup sliced celery (include the leaves)
¾ cup wild rice
2 teaspoons crushed garlic
¾ teaspoon dried thyme
¾ teaspoon dried rosemary
⅛ teaspoon ground white pepper

1. Coat a 4-quart pot with nonstick cooking spray and preheat over medium-high heat. Add the chicken breasts and cook for a couple of minutes on each side or until the chicken is nicely browned.
2. Add all the remaining ingredients to the pot, and bring to a boil over high heat. Reduce the heat to low, cover, and simmer for 25 minutes or until the chicken is tender and thoroughly cooked. Remove the chicken from the pot and set aside. Cook the soup for an additional 30 minutes or until the rice is tender.
3. Pull the chicken meat from the bones, and tear it into bite-sized pieces. Add the chicken to the soup, and simmer for an additional minute or two. Serve hot.

Nutritional Facts (per 1-cup serving)
CALORIES: 121 CARBOHYDRATES: 15 G CHOLESTEROL: 27 MG FAT: 1 G FIBER: 1.9 G
PROTEIN: 14 G SODIUM: 365 MG CALCIUM: 19 MG GI RATING: LOW

Creole Chicken Soup

YIELD: 8 CUPS

2 bone-in skinless chicken breast halves (about 1 pound)
4½ cups water or unsalted chicken broth
14½-ounce can stewed tomatoes, undrained and crushed
1 cup chopped onion
1 cup sliced fresh mushrooms
¾ cup sliced celery (include the leaves)
½ cup uncooked brown rice
1 tablespoon instant chicken bouillon granules
2 teaspoons crushed garlic
1½–2 teaspoons Cajun seasoning

1½ teaspoons dried thyme
1 cup fresh or frozen whole kernel corn
1 cup fresh or frozen sliced okra

1. Coat a 4-quart pot with nonstick cooking spray and preheat over medium-high heat. Add the chicken breasts and cook for a couple of minutes on each side or until the chicken is nicely browned.
2. Add the water or broth, tomatoes, onions, mushrooms, celery, rice, bouillon granules, garlic, Cajun seasoning, and thyme to the pot with the chicken, and bring the mixture to a boil. Reduce the heat to low, cover, and simmer for 25 minutes or until the chicken is tender and thoroughly cooked.
3. Remove the chicken from the pot and set aside. Cook the soup for an additional 20 minutes or until the rice is almost tender.
4. Add the corn and okra to the soup and cook for 10 minutes or until the okra, corn, and rice are tender. Pull the chicken meat from the bones and tear it into bite-sized pieces. Add the chicken to the soup and simmer for an additional minute or two. Serve hot.

Nutritional Facts (per 1-cup serving)
CALORIES: 145 CARBOHYDRATES: 20 G CHOLESTEROL: 24 MG FAT: 1.3 G FIBER: 2.8 G PROTEIN: 13 G SODIUM: 446 MG CALCIUM: 45 MG GI RATING: LOW

Manhattan Clam Chowder

YIELD: 7 SERVINGS

2 cans chopped clams (6 ounces each)
1 cup vegetable juice cocktail (like V•8)
14½-ounce can stewed tomatoes, undrained and crushed
1½ cups diced new potatoes
1¼ cups sliced fresh mushrooms
¾ cup sliced celery (include the leaves)
¾ cup chopped onion
½ cup diced carrots
1 teaspoon dried thyme
1 teaspoon dried parsley
¼ teaspoon ground black pepper
1 tablespoon extra-virgin olive oil

1. Drain the clams, reserving the juice, and set aside. Pour the clam juice into a 2-cup measure, and add enough water to bring the volume to 1½ cups.

2. Pour the clam juice mixture into a 3-quart pot and add the remaining ingredients except the clams and olive oil. Bring the mixture to a boil over high heat, then reduce the heat to low. Cover and simmer for 30 minutes or until the vegetables are tender and the flavors are well blended. Add the olive oil and clams to the soup and simmer for another minute or two or until the mixture is heated through. Serve hot.

Nutritional Facts (per 1-cup serving)

CALORIES: 87 CARBOHYDRATES: 15 G CHOLESTEROL: 1 MG FAT: 2.1 G FIBER: 2.2 G
PROTEIN: 2.1 G SODIUM: 330 MG CALCIUM: 45 MG GI RATING: LOW

Sicilian Meatball Soup

YIELD: 10 CUPS

Meatballs
1 pound 95-percent lean ground beef
2 teaspoons dried parsley
1 teaspoon instant beef bouillon granules
¾ teaspoon dried Italian seasoning
¼ teaspoon ground black pepper
3 tablespoons fat-free egg substitute
¼ cup orzo pasta, uncooked

Soup
6 cups water
1 tablespoon instant beef bouillon granules
1 teaspoon dried Italian seasoning
2 teaspoons crushed garlic
1 cup chopped onion (about 1 medium)
1 cup diced carrots (about 2 medium)
14½-ounce can Italian-style stewed tomatoes, undrained
½ cup orzo pasta
2 medium-small zucchini squash, halved lengthwise and sliced ½ inch thick (to make 1½ cups)
1 cup (packed) chopped fresh spinach

1. To make the meatballs, combine all the meatball ingredients except the orzo and mix well. Add the uncooked orzo, and mix again. Shape the meat mixture into 1-inch balls and set aside.
2. Combine the water, bouillon granules, Italian seasoning, garlic, onions, and carrots in a 4-quart pot and bring to a boil over high heat. Reduce the heat to low, cover, and simmer for 5 minutes or until the carrots start to soften.
3. Place the undrained tomatoes in a blender, and purée until smooth. Add the puréed tomatoes to the simmering broth mixture and increase the heat slightly to return the mixture to a simmer.
4. Add the meatballs, a few at a time, to the simmering soup. Cover and simmer over low heat for 20 minutes. Add the orzo and increase the heat to medium. Cook covered for about 10 minutes or until the orzo is almost done. (Stir occasionally to prevent the orzo from sticking to the bottom of the pot.) Add the zucchini and cook for 3 minutes more or until the zucchini is tender and the orzo is done. Add the spinach and cook for another minute or just until the spinach wilts. Serve hot.

Nutritional Facts (per 1-cup serving)

CALORIES: 136 CARBOHYDRATES: 15 G CHOLESTEROL: 24 MG FAT: 2.3 G FIBER: 1.7 G
PROTEIN: 12.1 G SODIUM: 391 MG CALCIUM: 30 MG GI RATING: LOW

Country Beef & Cabbage Soup

YIELD: 7 CUPS

12 ounces 95-percent lean ground beef
2 cups beef broth
14½-ounce can stewed tomatoes, undrained and crushed
1 cup chopped onion
1 teaspoon dried thyme
1 bay leaf
⅛ teaspoon ground black pepper
4 cups coarsely chopped cabbage (about ½ medium head)
15-ounce can red kidney beans, rinsed and drained

1. Coat a 4-quart pot with nonstick cooking spray and add the ground beef. Place the pot over medium heat and cook, stirring to crumble, until the meat is no longer pink. Add the remaining ingredients except the cabbage and kidney beans, and bring to a boil over high heat. Reduce the heat to low, cover, and simmer for 15 minutes.

2. Add the cabbage and kidney beans to the pot and raise the heat to bring the mixture to a boil. Reduce the heat to low, cover, and simmer for an additional 15 to 20 minutes or until the cabbage is tender and the flavors are well blended. Remove the bay leaf, and serve hot.

Nutritional Facts (per 1-cup serving)

CALORIES: 162 CARBOHYDRATES: 20 G CHOLESTEROL: 20 MG FAT: 2.6 G FIBER: 7 G
PROTEIN: 15 G SODIUM: 353 MG CALCIUM: 43 MG GI RATING: VERY LOW

Zippy Vegetable-Beef Soup

YIELD: 10 CUPS

1 pound 95-percent lean ground beef
6 cups water
14½-ounce can stewed tomatoes, undrained and crushed
1 medium yellow onion, cut into thin wedges
1 medium carrot, peeled and diced
1 tablespoon plus 1 teaspoon instant beef bouillon granules
1½ teaspoons chili powder
¾ teaspoon dried thyme
½ teaspoon dried oregano
1 cup fresh or frozen whole kernel corn
1 cup 1-inch pieces fresh green beans
1½ cups coarsely chopped cabbage
3 ounces wagon-wheel pasta (about 1 cup)

1. Coat a 5-quart pot with nonstick cooking spray and add the ground beef. Place the pot over medium heat and cook, stirring to crumble, until the meat is no longer pink. Add the water, tomatoes, onion, carrot, bouillon granules, chili powder, thyme, and oregano and bring to a boil over high heat. Reduce the heat to low, cover, and simmer for 15 minutes.
2. Add the corn and green beans to the pot and return the mixture to a boil. Reduce the heat to low, cover, and simmer for 10 minutes.
3. Add the cabbage and pasta and cook for about 10 minutes more or until the pasta is al dente. (Be careful not to overcook, as the pasta will continue to soften as long as it remains in the hot broth.) Serve hot.

Nutritional Facts (per 1-cup serving)

CALORIES: 134 CARBOHYDRATES: 16 G CHOLESTEROL: 24 MG FAT: 2.4 G FIBER: 2 G
PROTEIN: 12 G SODIUM: 127 MG CALCIUM: 32 MG GI RATING: VERY LOW

Zesty Chili

YIELD: 8 CUPS

½ teaspoon whole cumin seed
1 pound 95-percent lean ground beef
14½-ounce can Mexican-style stewed tomatoes, undrained and crushed
1½ cups vegetable juice cocktail (like V•8)
1 cup chopped onion
4-ounce can chopped green chilies
2 tablespoons chili powder
1½ teaspoons crushed garlic
½ teaspoon dried oregano
¼ teaspoon ground cinnamon
2 cans (15 ounces each) red kidney beans or black beans, drained
1 cup shredded nonfat or reduced-fat Monterey Jack or Cheddar cheese (optional)
½ cup sliced scallions (optional)

1. Place the cumin seeds in a 4-quart nonstick pot (do not coat the pot with cooking spray or oil) and place the pot over medium heat. Cook, stirring frequently, for 30 to 60 seconds or until the cumin smells toasted and fragrant. Pour the seeds into a small dish and set aside.

2. Coat the pot with nonstick cooking spray, add the ground beef, and place over medium heat. Cook, stirring to crumble, until the meat is no longer pink. Drain off and discard any excess fat.

3. Add the cumin, tomatoes, vegetable juice, onions, chilies, chili powder, garlic, oregano, and cinnamon to the pot and bring the mixture to a boil. Reduce the heat to low, cover, and simmer for 20 minutes.

4. Add the beans to the pot. Cover and simmer for 15 minutes or until the onions are soft and the flavors are well blended. Serve hot, topping each serving with 2 tablespoons of the cheese and a tablespoon of the scallions, if desired.

Nutritional Facts (per 1-cup serving)

CALORIES: 232 CARBOHYDRATES: 30 G CHOLESTEROL: 30 MG FAT: 3.5 G FIBER: 11 G
PROTEIN: 20 G SODIUM: 355 MG CALCIUM: 63 GI RATING: VERY LOW

Very Veggie Chili

YIELD: 7 CUPS

14½-ounce can unsalted stewed tomatoes, undrained and crushed
15-ounce can tomato sauce
1 medium onion, chopped
2–3 tablespoons chili powder
1½ teaspoons crushed garlic
1 teaspoon ground cumin
¾ teaspoon dried oregano
2 cans (15 ounces each) red kidney beans, drained
1½ cups fresh or frozen whole kernel corn
1½ cups diced zucchini (about 1 medium)
¾ cup plus 2 tablespoons nonfat or reduced-fat Cheddar or Monterey Jack cheese

1. Place the tomatoes, tomato sauce, onions, chili powder, garlic, cumin, and oregano in a 3-quart pot, and bring the mixture to a boil over medium-high heat. Reduce the heat to low, cover, and simmer for 12 minutes.
2. Add the beans, corn, and zucchini and raise the heat under the pot to return the mixture to a boil. Reduce the heat to low, cover, and simmer for about 10 minutes more, or until the vegetables are tender and the flavors are well blended.
3. Serve hot, topping each serving with 2 tablespoons of the cheese.

Nutritional Facts (per 1-cup serving)

CALORIES: 234 CARBOHYDRATES: 43 G CHOLESTEROL: 1 MG FAT: 1.4 G FIBER: 13 G
PROTEIN: 14 G SODIUM: 510 MG CALCIUM: 140 MG GI RATING: VERY LOW

Tortellini & Spinach Soup

For variety, substitute 1½ cups of diced roasted chicken for the beans.

YIELD: 8 CUPS

5 cups no-added-salt chicken broth or water
2½ teaspoons instant chicken bouillon granules

1 cup chopped onion

½ cup chopped carrot

2 teaspoons crushed garlic

⅛ teaspoon ground white pepper

9 ounces refrigerated cheese tortellini (about 3 cups)

15-ounce can navy or white beans, rinsed and drained

3 cups (packed) chopped fresh spinach

1. Place the broth or water, bouillon granules, onion, carrot, garlic, and white pepper in a 4-quart pot, and bring to a boil over high heat. Reduce the heat to low, cover, and simmer for 15 minutes or until the vegetables are soft.

2. Remove the pot from the heat and, using a slotted spoon, transfer the vegetables to a blender. Pour about 1 cup of the broth into the blender. Carefully blend the mixture at low speed, leaving the lid slightly ajar (to allow steam to escape) until the vegetables are puréed. Pour the blended vegetable mixture back into the pot.

3. Return the pot to the heat and bring to a boil. Add the tortellini and the beans and let the mixture return to a boil. Reduce the heat to medium, cover, and cook for about 4 minutes or until the tortellini are almost done. Add the spinach and cook, stirring frequently, for a minute or two or until the tortellini are just done and the spinach is wilted. (Be careful not to overcook, as the tortellini will continue to soften as long as it remains in the hot broth.) Serve hot.

Nutritional Facts (per 1-cup serving)

CALORIES: 179 CARBOHYDRATES: 26 G CHOLESTEROL: 14 MG FAT: 3.1 G FIBER: 5.2 G
PROTEIN: 12 G SODIUM: 496 MG CALCIUM: 116 MG GI RATING: LOW

Barley-Vegetable Soup

YIELD: 8 CUPS

5 cups water or unsalted beef broth

14½-ounce can stewed tomatoes, undrained and crushed

1 cup chopped onion

1 cup sliced fresh mushrooms

½ cup sliced celery (include the leaves)

½ cup hulled or pearl barley

1 tablespoon instant beef bouillon granules

1 teaspoon dried thyme

¼ teaspoon ground black pepper
1 cup diced carrots
1 cup 1-inch pieces fresh green beans
1 cup fresh or frozen whole kernel corn

1. Put the water or broth, undrained tomatoes, onion, mushrooms, celery, barley, bouillon granules, thyme, and black pepper in a 4-quart pot and bring to a boil over high heat. Reduce the heat to low, cover, and simmer for 40 minutes.
2. Add the carrots and green beans to the pot and simmer for an additional 10 minutes. Add the corn and simmer for 5 minutes more or until the barley and all the vegetables are tender. Serve hot.

Nutritional Facts (per 1-cup serving)
CALORIES: 101 CARBOHYDRATES: 22 G CHOLESTEROL: 0 MG FAT: 0.8 G FIBER: 4.7 G
PROTEIN: 3.2 G SODIUM: 369 MG CALCIUM: 39 MG GI RATING: VERY LOW

Creamy Mushroom & Wild Rice Soup

YIELD: 5 CUPS

3½ cups water
1 tablespoon instant chicken bouillon granules
4 cups sliced fresh mushrooms
¾ cup chopped onion
½ cup uncooked wild rice
¼ teaspoon dried thyme
¼ teaspoon dried rosemary
⅛ teaspoon ground white pepper
12-ounce can evaporated skim or low-fat milk
3 tablespoons whole-wheat pastry flour or unbleached flour
2 tablespoons dry sherry
⅓ cup sliced scallions (garnish)

1. Place the water, bouillon granules, mushrooms, onion, wild rice, thyme, rosemary, and white pepper in a 3-quart pot and bring to a boil over high heat. Reduce the heat to low, cover, and simmer for about 1 hour or until the rice is tender.

2. Place ½ cup of the milk and all the flour in a jar with a tight-fitting lid and shake until smooth. Set aside.

3. Add the remaining milk to the pot, increase the heat to medium, and let the mixture come to a boil. Slowly pour in the flour mixture while stirring constantly. Cook and stir for a minute or two or until the mixture comes to a boil and thickens slightly.

4. Stir sherry into the soup and serve immediately, topping each serving with some of the scallions.

Nutritional Facts (per 1-cup serving)

CALORIES: 164 CARBOHYDRATES: 30 G CHOLESTEROL: 2 MG FAT: 0.6 G FIBER: 2.9 G
PROTEIN: 9.7 G SODIUM: 468 MG CALCIUM: 212 MG GI RATING: LOW

Savory Lentil Soup

YIELD: 9 SERVINGS

1½ cups brown lentils
1½ cups diced ham (at least 96-percent lean); or 1 large, meaty ham bone
1 cup chopped celery (include the leaves)
1 cup chopped onion
¾ cup diced carrot
1 teaspoon instant chicken bouillon granules
2 teaspoons crushed garlic
1½ teaspoons dried thyme
1 bay leaf
¼ teaspoon ground black pepper
5 cups water
14½-ounce can stewed tomatoes, undrained and crushed

1. Put the lentils in a wire strainer and rinse with cool water. Combine the lentils and the remaining ingredients except the tomatoes in a 4-quart pot and bring to a boil over high heat.

2. Reduce the heat to low, cover, and simmer for 40 minutes. If using a ham bone, remove it from the pot and set aside to cool slightly. Add the undrained tomatoes to the soup and cook for an additional 20 minutes or until the lentils are soft and the liquid is thick.

3. Cut the meat from the ham bone and add it to the soup. Cook for another minute or two to heat through. Serve hot.

Nutritional Facts (per 1-cup serving)

CALORIES: 167 CARBOHYDRATES: 25 G CHOLESTEROL: 7 MG FAT: 1.5 G FIBER: 11 G

PROTEIN: 14 G SODIUM: 421 MG CALCIUM: 42 MG GI RATING: VERY LOW

Tuscan Lentil Soup

YIELD: 8 SERVINGS

¾ cup brown lentils
¼ cup plus 2 tablespoons brown rice
1½ cups coarsely chopped fresh mushrooms
1 cup chopped celery (include the leaves)
1 cup chopped onion
1 tablespoon instant beef bouillon granules
2 teaspoons crushed garlic
1½ teaspoons dried Italian seasoning
¼ teaspoon ground black pepper
5 cups water
14½-ounce can stewed tomatoes, crushed, undrained
3 cups (packed) chopped fresh spinach
1–2 tablespoons extra-virgin olive oil
¼ cup grated Parmesan cheese (optional)

1. Put the lentils in a wire strainer and rinse with cool water. Combine the lentils, rice, mushrooms, celery, onions, bouillon granules, garlic, Italian seasoning, black pepper, and water in a 4-quart pot, and bring to a boil over high heat.
2. Reduce the heat to low, cover, and simmer for 40 minutes. Add the undrained tomatoes and cook for an additional 20 minutes or until the lentils are soft and the liquid is thick. Add the spinach and olive oil and cook for another minute or two or until the spinach is wilted. Serve hot, topping each serving with some of the Parmesan cheese if desired.

Nutritional Facts (per 1-cup serving)

CALORIES: 140 CARBOHYDRATES: 23 G CHOLESTEROL: 0 MG FAT: 2.2 G FIBER: 7.4 G

PROTEIN: 6.9 G SODIUM: 371 MG CALCIUM: 50 MG GI RATING: VERY LOW

Split Pea & Sausage Soup

1½ cups dried green split peas
6 cups water
1¼ cups diced smoked sausage or kielbasa (at least 97 percent lean)
1 cup diced new potatoes
¾ cup diced carrots
¾ cup chopped onion
¾ cup sliced celery (include the leaves)
2 teaspoons instant chicken bouillon granules
1½ teaspoons crushed garlic
1½ teaspoons dried sage
¾ teaspoon dried thyme
¼ teaspoon ground black pepper

1. Place the peas in a wire strainer and rinse with cool water. Combine the peas and the remaining ingredients in a 4-quart pot and bring to a boil over high heat.
2. Reduce the heat to low, cover, and simmer for about 1 hour or until the peas are soft and the liquid is thick. Serve hot.

Nutritional Facts (per 1-cup serving)
CALORIES: 178 CARBOHYDRATES: 29 G CHOLESTEROL: 8 MG FAT: 1.1 G FIBER: 9.8 G
PROTEIN: 12.5 G SODIUM: 409 MG CALCIUM: 35 MG GI RATING: VERY LOW

Split Pea & Barley Soup

YIELD: 7 SERVINGS

1 cup dried green split peas
6 cups water
1 cup diced carrots
1 cup chopped onion
1 cup sliced celery (include the leaves)

¼ cup plus 2 tablespoons hulled or pearled barley

1 tablespoon plus 1 teaspoon instant chicken bouillon granules

2 teaspoons crushed garlic

1 teaspoon dried thyme

¾ teaspoon dried marjoram

1 bay leaf

¼ teaspoon ground black pepper

1. Put the peas in a wire strainer and rinse with cool water. Combine the peas and the remaining ingredients in a 4-quart pot and bring to a boil over high heat.
2. Reduce the heat to low, cover, and simmer for 1 hour or until the barley is tender, the peas are soft, and the liquid is thick. Add a little more water if the mixture seems too thick. Serve hot.

Nutritional Facts (per 1-cup serving)

CALORIES: 153 CARBOHYDRATES: 32 G CHOLESTEROL: 0 MG FAT: 0.6 G FIBER: 9.5 G
PROTEIN: 9 G SODIUM: 390 MG CALCIUM: 34 MG GI RATING: VERY LOW

Quick Chicken Chili

YIELD: 6 SERVINGS

2 cans (15 ounces each) navy or Great Northern beans, drained

1¼ cups unsalted chicken broth

½ cup chopped onion

4-ounce can chopped green chilies

1½ teaspoons ground cumin

1 teaspoon crushed garlic

¼ teaspoon dried oregano

⅛ teaspoon ground white pepper

2 cups cooked shredded chicken breast

½ cup shredded nonfat or reduced-fat Monterey Jack cheese

½ cup nonfat or light sour cream

1. Combine the beans, broth, onion, chilies, cumin, garlic, oregano, and white pepper in a 2½-quart pot and bring to a boil over high heat. Cover and simmer for 10 minutes. Remove about ½ cup of the beans to a small dish, mash with a fork, and return the mashed beans to the pot.
2. Add the chicken to the pot and raise the heat under the pot to bring the mixture to a boil. Re-

duce the heat to low, cover, and simmer for an additional 5 minutes. Serve hot, topping each serving with some of the cheese and sour cream.

Nutritional Facts (per 1-cup serving)
CALORIES: 249 CARBOHYDRATES: 28 G CHOLESTEROL: 41 MG FAT: 2 G FIBER: 6.2 G
PROTEIN: 27 G SODIUM: 373 MG CALCIUM: 156 MG GI RATING: VERY LOW

Bueno Black Bean Soup

YIELD: 8 SERVINGS

2½ cups black beans
6½ cups water
1 tablespoon plus 1 teaspoon instant ham or chicken bouillon granules
1½ cups finely chopped onion (about 1 large)
1 cup finely chopped green bell pepper (about 1 medium)
½ cup bottled salsa
1 tablespoon crushed garlic
1 tablespoon chili powder
2 teaspoons ground cumin
1½ teaspoons dried oregano
½ cup nonfat or light sour cream
½ cup finely chopped green bell pepper
½ cup finely chopped red onion

1. Rinse the beans well and place in a 4-quart pot. Cover the beans with several inches of water and discard any beans that float to the top. Soak the beans for at least 4 hours or for as long as twelve hours. (If soaking the beans for more than 4 hours, place the bowl or pot in the refrigerator.)
2. Discard the soaking water and return the beans to the pot. Add the 6½ cups of water and the bouillon granules and bring to a boil over high heat. Reduce the heat to low, cover, and simmer, stirring occasionally, for 1½ hours or until the beans are tender. Add a little water during cooking, if needed, to keep the beans barely covered with water.
3. Add the onions, bell peppers, salsa, garlic, chili powder, cumin, and oregano, and cook for 30 minutes more or until the beans are easily mashed with a fork and the liquid is thick.
4. Remove 2 cups of the soup and purée in a blender until smooth. Return the puréed soup to the pot and stir to mix well. Cover and simmer for 5 minutes more. Add a little water if the mixture is too thick.

5. Serve hot, topping each serving with a tablespoon each of sour cream, green peppers, and onions. If desired, serve over brown rice.

Nutritional Facts (per 1-cup serving)

CALORIES: 222 CARBOHYDRATES: 40 G CHOLESTEROL: 0 MG FAT: 1 G FIBER: 13.2 G

PROTEIN: 13.7 G SODIUM: 384 MG CALCIUM: 107 MG GI RATING: LOW

Southwestern Pinto Bean Soup

YIELD: 9 SERVINGS

2 cups dried pinto beans

5½ cups water

1 cup chopped onion

1 tablespoon plus 1 teaspoon instant chicken bouillon granules

1 pound bone-in skinless chicken breast halves (about 2 large) or extra-lean pork chops (about 3 medium)

2 teaspoons crushed garlic

1 tablespoon chili powder

1 teaspoon ground cumin

14½-ounce can Mexican-style stewed tomatoes, crushed, undrained

½ cup sliced scallions or finely chopped fresh cilantro

1. Rinse the beans well and place in a 4-quart pot. Cover the beans with several inches of water and discard any beans that float to the top. Soak the beans for at least 4 hours or for as long as twelve hours. (If soaking the beans for more than 4 hours, place the bowl or pot in the refrigerator.)

2. Discard the soaking water and return the beans to the pot. Add the 5½ cups of water, onions, and the bouillon granules, and bring to a boil over high heat. Reduce the heat to low, cover, and simmer, stirring occasionally, for 50 minutes.

3. Add the chicken or pork chops, garlic, chili powder, and cumin to the pot, and cook for 30 minutes more or until the chicken or pork chops are tender and the meat pulls easily away from the bones. Remove the chicken or pork chops to a cutting board, and set aside to cool slightly. Add the undrained tomatoes to the soup, and cook for an additional 30 minutes, or until the beans are soft and the liquid is thick.

4. Remove the meat from the bones and tear into shreds or cut into bite-sized pieces. Add the chicken or pork to the pot and raise the heat slightly to return the mixture to a boil. Reduce the

heat to low, cover, and simmer, stirring occasionally, for 5 minutes or until the flavors are well blended. Serve hot, topping each serving with some of the scallions or cilantro.

Nutritional Facts (per 1-cup serving)

CALORIES: 228   CARBOHYDRATES: 32 G   CHOLESTEROL: 30 MG   FAT: 1.9 G   FIBER: 10 G
PROTEIN: 20 G   SODIUM: 402 MG   CALCIUM: 76 MG   GI RATING: LOW

Italian Garden Soup

YIELD: 10 SERVINGS

6 cups water
1 medium onion, cut into thin wedges
1 cup sliced fresh mushrooms
¾ cup diced carrots (about 1½ medium)
1 tablespoon instant vegetable or beef bouillon granules
2 teaspoons crushed garlic
1 teaspoon dried Italian seasoning
⅛ teaspoon ground black pepper
14½-ounce can Italian-style stewed tomatoes, undrained
4 ounces fusilli pasta (about 1⅓ cups) or macaroni (about 1 cup)
15-ounce can red kidney beans, garbanzo beans (chickpeas), or navy beans, rinsed
    and drained
1 medium zucchini squash, halved lengthwise and sliced ½-inch thick (to make 1 cup)
¾ cup frozen green peas, thawed
2 cups (packed) chopped fresh spinach
1 tablespoon extra-virgin olive oil
⅓ cup grated Parmesan cheese

1. Combine the water, onion, mushrooms, carrots, bouillon granules, garlic, Italian seasoning, and black pepper in a 4-quart pot. Place the undrained tomatoes in a blender, blend until smooth, and add to the pot. Bring the mixture to a boil over high heat. Reduce the heat to low, cover, and simmer for 25 minutes.
2. Add the pasta and beans to the soup and raise the heat to return the mixture to a boil. Reduce the heat to medium and cook covered for about 8 minutes, stirring occasionally, or until the pasta is almost al dente.

3. Add the zucchini and peas to the pot, and cook for an additional 2 minutes or until the zucchini is tender and the pasta is al dente. Add the spinach and olive oil to the soup and cook for another minute or just until the spinach wilts. Serve hot, topping each serving with some of the Parmesan cheese.

Nutritional Facts (per 1-cup serving)

CALORIES: 152 CARBOHYDRATES: 24 G CHOLESTEROL: 2 MG FAT: 2.9 G FIBER: 5.5 G PROTEIN: 7.3 G SODIUM: 362 MG CALCIUM: 77 MG GI RATING: VERY LOW

Country Bean Soup

YIELD: 7 SERVINGS

1¼ cups navy or white beans
5 cups water
1 cup chopped onion
½ cup sliced celery (include the leaves)
2 teaspoons ham or chicken bouillon granules
¼ teaspoon ground black pepper
1½ cups diced ham (at least 97-percent lean)
1½ cups small new potatoes, cut into ¾-inch chunks
¾ cup diced carrots
1½ cups (packed) chopped fresh spinach

1. Rinse the beans well and place in a 4-quart pot. Cover the beans with several inches of water and discard any beans that float to the top. Soak the beans for at least 4 hours, or for as long as 12 hours. (If soaking the beans for more than 4 hours, place the bowl or pot in the refrigerator.)
2. Discard the soaking water and return the beans to the pot. Add the 5 cups of water, onions, celery, bouillon granules, and black pepper, and bring to a boil over high heat. Reduce the heat to low, cover, and simmer, stirring occasionally, for 1 hour.
3. Add the ham, potatoes, and carrots to the pot, and cook for 45 minutes more or until the beans are soft and the liquid is thick. Add a little more water during cooking if necessary. Add the spinach and cook for an additional 2 minutes, or until the spinach wilts. Serve hot.

Nutritional Facts (per 1-cup serving)

CALORIES: 218 CARBOHYDRATES: 38 G CHOLESTEROL: 8 MG FAT: 1.5 G FIBER: 11.5 G PROTEIN: 15 G SODIUM: 514 MG CALCIUM: 88 MG GI RATING: LOW

10. Salads for All Seasons

Salads play an important role in any healthful cuisine, and low-GI cooking is no exception. Besides being packed with essential nutrients, antioxidants, and phytochemicals, salad ingredients such as leafy greens and nonstarchy vegetables do not have a significant impact on blood sugar and should be thought of as "free foods." Other salad ingredients like pasta, legumes, and many fruits rank low on the glycemic index as well.

Besides being super-nutritious and GI-friendly, salads are among the most versatile of dishes. Depending on their ingredients, they can be a protein-packed entrée or a refreshing side dish. Because most salads can be made ahead of time, they are great for entertaining. And because they are portable, they are as much at home at picnics and potluck suppers as they are on your own dining room table.

If you are watching your weight, though, beware. Despite the salad's reputation as being "diet" food, many are anything but. Salads made with high-fat meats and cheeses and drenched in oily or full-fat mayonnaise dressings are definitely not what the doctor ordered. Rest assured that the recipes in this chapter will keep you eating low on the glycemic index without busting your fat or calorie budgets. Ingredients like lean meats, low-fat cheeses, and light mayonnaise, sour cream, and dressings are combined with crisp vegetables, ripe fruits, satisfying pastas, and nutritious whole grains and legumes to create a variety of sensational salads that are sure to make any meal special.

Greek Grilled Shrimp Salad

YIELD: 4 SERVINGS

1 pound peeled and deveined raw shrimp
1½–2 tablespoons Zesty Herb Rub (page 175)
1 tablespoon extra-virgin olive oil

6–8 12-inch skewers
10 cups torn romaine lettuce
1 cup chopped canned artichoke hearts, drained
1 cucumber, peeled, halved lengthwise, and sliced
12 cherry tomatoes, halved
1 cup garbanzo beans (chickpeas), rinsed and drained
½ cup sliced black olives
½ cup crumbled nonfat or reduced-fat feta cheese
½ cup sliced scallions
¾ cup bottled nonfat or light red wine vinaigrette or balsamic vinaigrette salad dressing

1. Rinse the shrimp with cool water, pat dry with paper towels, and put them in a large bowl. Sprinkle the rub over the shrimp, drizzle with the olive oil, and toss to mix well. Set aside for 15 to 30 minutes.
2. Thread the shrimp loosely onto skewers as follows: Bend each shrimp almost in half, so that the large end nearly touches the smaller tail end. Insert the skewer just above the tail so that it passes through the shrimp twice.
3. Broil the shrimp skewers, turning occasionally, for about 6 minutes or until the shrimp turn pink and are cooked through. (Alternatively, grill the skewers over medium coals for about 5 minutes, turning occasionally.)
4. To assemble the salads, arrange a quarter of the lettuce over the bottom of each of 4 plates. Arrange a quarter of the artichoke hearts, cucumber, tomatoes, garbanzo beans, and olives over the outer edges of the lettuce on each plate. Remove the shrimp from the skewers and place a quarter of the shrimp over the center of each salad. Top each salad with some of the feta cheese and scallions and serve immediately, accompanied by the dressing.

Nutritional Facts (per serving)

CALORIES: 288 CARBOHYDRATES: 30 G CHOLESTEROL: 172 MG FAT: 7.7 G FIBER: 10 G
PROTEIN: 29 G SODIUM: 1,252 MG CALCIUM: 216 MG GI RATING: VERY LOW

Jerk Chicken Salad

YIELD: 4 SERVINGS

4 boneless, skinless chicken breast halves (4 ounces each)
1–2 tablespoons Jamaican Jerk Rub (page 176)
Nonstick olive oil cooking spray
10 cups torn romaine lettuce or mixed salad greens
½ cup diagonally sliced celery
1 medium carrot, shredded with a potato peeler
4 thin slices red onion, separated into rings
8 thin rings green bell pepper
½ cup shredded nonfat or reduced-fat Monterey Jack or Cheddar cheese
¼ cup dark raisins
¼ cup chopped toasted sliced almonds (page 78) or chopped roasted peanuts
¾ cup Yogurt Ranch Dressing (page 174) or bottled nonfat or light ranch or bal-
  samic vinaigrette salad dressing

1. Rinse the chicken and pat dry with paper towels. Using your fingers, rub both sides of the chicken breasts with some of the rub, and set aside for 15 to 30 minutes. Or for more intense flavor, cover and refrigerate for up to 24 hours.

2. Coat a broiler pan with the cooking spray, and place the chicken on the pan. Spray the tops of the chicken lightly with the cooking spray, and broil 6 inches under a preheated broiler, turning occasionally, for 12 to 15 minutes or until the meat is nicely browned and no longer pink inside. (Alternatively, grill the chicken in the same manner over medium coals.) Remove the chicken to a cutting board, let sit for 5 minutes, then slice thinly across the grain. Set aside. (Note: The chicken can be cooked the day before, refrigerated, and sliced just before assembling the salads.)

3. To serve, toss the lettuce with the celery and carrots, and arrange a quarter of the mixture over the bottom of each of 4 plates. Arrange some of the onion and green pepper rings over the lettuce on each plate, and sprinkle each salad with 2 tablespoons of the cheese and a tablespoon each of raisins and nuts. Arrange a sliced chicken breast over the top. Serve immediately, accompanied by some of the dressing.

Nutritional Facts (per serving)

CALORIES: 286 CARBOHYDRATES: 23 G CHOLESTEROL: 67 MG FAT: 5 G FIBER: 5.2 G
PROTEIN: 36 G SODIUM: 580 MG CALCIUM: 231 MG GI RATING: LOW

Asian Chicken Salad

YIELD: 4 SERVINGS

4 boneless skinless chicken breast halves (4 ounces each)
10 cups torn romaine lettuce or mixed salad greens
8-ounce can sliced water chestnuts, drained
4 thin slices red onion, separated into rings
10-ounce can mandarin oranges, drained
⅓ cup diced red bell pepper
¼ cup chopped honey-roasted peanuts or cashews (optional)
¾ cup Sesame-Ginger Dressing (page 172)

Marinade
½ cup orange juice
3 tablespoons reduced-sodium soy sauce
2 tablespoons dark brown sugar
2 teaspoons toasted-sesame (dark) oil
1 teaspoon crushed garlic
¾ teaspoon ground ginger

1. To make the marinade, combine all the marinade ingredients in a small bowl and stir to mix well. Remove 3 tablespoons of the marinade, transfer to a covered container, and place in the re-frigerator. Place the chicken in a shallow nonmetal container, and pour the remaining marinade over the chicken, lifting the chicken to allow the marinade to flow underneath. Cover and re-frigerate for 6 to 24 hours.

2. Coat a broiler pan with nonstick cooking spray. Remove the chicken from the marinade (discard the marinade) and place the chicken on the pan. Broil 6 inches under a preheated broiler, turning occasionally, for 12 to 15 minutes or until the meat is nicely browned and no longer pink inside. Baste the chicken with the reserved marinade several times during the last five minutes of cooking. (Alternatively, grill the chicken in the same manner over medium coals.) Remove the chicken to a cutting board, let sit for 5 minutes to cool, then slice thinly across the grain. Set aside. (Note: The chicken can be cooked the day before, refrigerated, and sliced just before assembling the salads.)

3. To serve, spread a quarter of the lettuce over the bottom of each of 4 plates. Arrange some of the drained water chestnuts and onion rings over the lettuce on each plate. Arrange a sliced chicken breast over the lettuce, and arrange some of the drained mandarin oranges and diced red bell peppers around the edge of the plate. Sprinkle some of the peanuts or cashews over the top of each salad if desired. Serve immediately, accompanied by some of the dressing.

Nutritional Facts (per serving)

CALORIES: 356 CARBOHYDRATES: 35 G CHOLESTEROL: 66 MG FAT: 9.4 G FIBER: 8 G
PROTEIN: 32 G SODIUM: 738 MG CALCIUM: 111 MG GI RATING: LOW

Grilled Chicken Caesar Salad

For variety, substitute fresh tuna or salmon steaks for the chicken.

YIELD: 4 SERVINGS

Dressing
1 tablespoon lemon juice
1 teaspoon crushed garlic
¾ teaspoon anchovy paste
½ cup nonfat or light mayonnaise
2 tablespoons fat-free egg substitute
3 tablespoons grated Parmesan cheese
¼ teaspoon coarsely ground black pepper

Salad
4 boneless, skinless chicken breast halves (4 ounces each)
1–2 tablespoons Zesty Herb Rub (page 175)
12 cups torn romaine lettuce

3 tablespoons grated Parmesan cheese
1⅓ cups ready-made sourdough croutons

1. To make the dressing, combine the lemon juice, garlic, and anchovy paste in a small bowl and stir until smooth. Add the remaining dressing ingredients and stir to mix well. Cover the dressing, and refrigerate for at least 1 hour.

2. Rinse the chicken and pat dry with paper towels. Using your fingers, rub both sides of each piece of chicken with some of the rub, and if you have time, set aside for 15 to 30 minutes. Or for more intense flavor, cover, and refrigerate for up to 24 hours.

3. Coat a broiler pan with nonstick cooking spray and place the chicken on the pan. Spray the tops of the chicken lightly with cooking spray, and broil 6 inches under a preheated broiler, turning occasionally, for 12 to 15 minutes or until the meat is nicely browned and no longer pink inside. Remove the chicken to a cutting board, let sit for 5 minutes to cool, then slice thinly across the grain. Set aside. (Note: The chicken can be cooked the day before, refrigerated, and sliced just before assembling the salads.)

4. Place the lettuce in a large bowl. Add the dressing, and toss to mix well. Add the Parmesan cheese, and toss again. To assemble the salads, arrange a quarter of the lettuce mixture over the bottoms of each of 4 plates. Sprinkle a quarter of the croutons over the lettuce on each plate. Arrange a sliced chicken breast over each salad. Serve immediately.

Nutritional Facts (per serving)

CALORIES: 308 CARBOHYDRATES: 23 G CHOLESTEROL: 74 MG FAT: 5.9 G FIBER: 3.3 G PROTEIN: 37 G SODIUM: 697 MG CALCIUM: 224 MG GI RATING: MODERATE

Citrus Grilled Chicken Salad

YIELD: 4 SERVINGS

4 boneless, skinless chicken breast halves (4 ounces each)
10 cups mixed baby salad greens
¾ cup diagonally sliced celery
10-ounce can mandarin oranges packed in juice, drained
4 thin slices red onion, separated into rings
½ cup crumbled nonfat or reduced-fat feta cheese; or ½ cup crumbled blue cheese
¼ cup chopped walnuts
¾ cup bottled nonfat or light balsamic, red wine, or raspberry vinaigrette salad dressing

Rub

1 tablespoon plus 1 teaspoon frozen (thawed) orange juice concentrate
1 tablespoon dried rosemary or fines herbes
1 tablespoon Dijon mustard
1 teaspoon lemon pepper
½ teaspoon garlic powder

1. To make the rub, combine all the rub ingredients in a small bowl and stir to mix well.
2. Rinse the chicken and pat dry with paper towels. Brush both sides of each piece of chicken with some of the rub and set aside for 15 to 30 minutes. Or for more intense flavor, transfer the chicken to a covered container and refrigerate for up to 24 hours before cooking.
3. Coat a broiler pan with nonstick cooking spray and place the chicken on the pan. Broil 6 inches under a preheated broiler, turning occasionally, for 12 to15 minutes or until the meat is nicely browned and no longer pink inside. (Alternatively, grill the chicken in the same manner over medium coals.) Remove the chicken to a cutting board, let sit for 5 minutes, then slice thinly across the grain. Set aside. (Note: The chicken can be cooked the day before, refrigerated, and sliced just before assembling the salads.)
4. To serve, spread a quarter of the lettuce over the bottom of each of 4 plates. Arrange some of the celery, oranges, and onion rings over the lettuce on each plate. Arrange a sliced chicken breast over the lettuce, and sprinkle each salad with some of the cheese and walnuts. Serve immediately, accompanied by some of the dressing.

Nutritional Facts (per serving)

CALORIES: 301 CARBOHYDRATES: 29 G CHOLESTEROL: 63 MG FAT: 7.5 G FIBER: 5.1 G
PROTEIN: 32 G SODIUM: 801 MG CALCIUM: 149 MG GI RATING: LOW

Cajun Grilled Tuna Salad

YIELD: 4 SERVINGS

4 fresh tuna steaks (about 4 ounces each)
1–2 tablespoons Ragin' Cajun Rub (page 175)
Nonstick olive oil cooking spray
10 cups torn romaine lettuce or mixed salad greens
1 cup sliced fresh mushrooms
2 plum tomatoes, thinly sliced
4 thin slices of red onion, separated into rings

¾ cup shredded nonfat or reduced-fat Cheddar cheese

1 cup ready-made sourdough croutons

¾ cup Yogurt Ranch Dressing (page 174), Sun-Dried Tomato Dressing (page 173),
  Parmesan Peppercorn Dressing (page 172), or bottled nonfat or light ranch
  dressing or sun-dried tomato vinaigrette

1. Rinse the tuna and pat dry with paper towels. Using your fingers, rub both sides of each piece of tuna with some of the rub. Set aside for 15 to 30 minutes. Or for more intense flavor, cover, and refrigerate for up to 24 hours.

2. Coat a broiler pan with nonstick cooking spray, and arrange the tuna steaks on the pan. Spray the tops of the tuna lightly with the cooking spray and cook over medium coals, turning occasionally, or broil 6 inches under a preheated broiler for 10 minutes or until the meat is nicely browned and no longer pink inside. Remove the tuna steaks to a cutting board, let sit for 5 minutes, then slice thinly across the grain. Set aside.

3. To serve, toss the lettuce with the mushrooms and tomatoes and arrange a quarter of the mixture over the bottom of each of 4 plates. Arrange some of the onion rings over the lettuce on each plate. Arrange a sliced tuna steak over the lettuce and sprinkle with some of the cheese and croutons. Serve immediately, accompanied by some of the dressing.

Nutritional Facts (per serving)

CALORIES: 290 CARBOHYDRATES: 24 G CHOLESTEROL: 53 MG FAT: 3 G FIBER: 4 G
PROTEIN: 40 G SODIUM: 749 MG CALCIUM: 295 MG GI RATING: LOW

Variation: Cajun Grilled Shrimp Salad

Place 1 pound of cleaned raw shrimp in a large bowl, add the rub, and toss to mix well. Thread the shrimp loosely onto 6 to 8 12-inch skewers. (If you use wooden skewers rather than metal, soak them in water for at least 20 minutes to prevent burning.) Spray the shrimp lightly with cooking spray and grill or broil for about 3 minutes on each side, or until the shrimp turn pink and are cooked through. Prepare the salad as directed, substituting the shrimp for the fish steaks.

Nutritional Facts (per serving)

CALORIES: 249 CARBOHYDRATES: 24 G CHOLESTEROL: 163 MG FAT: 2.8 G
FIBER: 4 G PROTEIN: 30 G SODIUM: 893 MG CALCIUM: 309 MG GI RATING: LOW

Roasted Vegetable Salad

Roasted Vegetable Mixture

8 ounces sliced baby Portabella mushrooms or
    12 large fresh mushrooms, sliced ½-inch thick
20 fresh asparagus spears
4 (½-inch thick) slices red or Spanish onion
1 large red bell pepper, cut into ½-inch-thick strips
1 teaspoon dried thyme or fines herbes
¼ teaspoon ground black pepper
¼ teaspoon salt (optional)
Nonstick olive oil cooking spray

Salad

8 cups torn romaine lettuce or mixed salad greens
2 cups diced roasted or grilled chicken breast or 1⅓ cups canned (drained)
    garbanzo beans (chickpeas)
¼ cup sliced black olives
¾ cup crumbled nonfat or reduced-fat feta cheese
1 cup ready-made sourdough croutons
½ cup bottled nonfat or light balsamic vinaigrette salad dressing

1. To prepare the roasted vegetable mixture, coat 2 large baking sheets with nonstick cooking spray. Arrange the mushrooms in a single layer on one of the sheets, and the asparagus, onions, and red bell pepper strips in a single layer on the second sheet. Sprinkle the vegetables with the herbs, black pepper, and, if desired, the salt. Spray the tops of the vegetables lightly with the olive oil cooking spray.

2. Bake at 450° F for 10 minutes or until the asparagus are tender. Transfer the asparagus to a cutting board and set aside. Using a spatula, turn the remaining vegetables over and bake for an additional 5 to 10 minutes or until tender and nicely browned. Remove the vegetables from the oven and allow them to cool to room temperature.

3. When the vegetables have cooled, cut the asparagus into 1½-inch pieces and separate the onion slices into rings. Place all the vegetables in a medium-sized bowl and toss to mix well. (Note that you can prepare the vegetable mixture the day before and refrigerate until ready to assemble the salad.)

4. To assemble the salads, arrange 2 cups of salad greens over the bottom of each of 4 large serving plates. Top the greens on each plate with a fourth of the roasted vegetable mixture, chicken or garbanzo beans, olives, feta cheese, and croutons. Serve immediately, accompanied by the dressing.

Nutritional Facts (per serving)

CALORIES: 291 CARBOHYDRATES: 29 G CHOLESTEROL: 62 MG FAT: 6 G FIBER: 6 G
PROTEIN: 35 G SODIUM: 956 MG CALCIUM: 182 MG GI RATING: LOW

Mediterranean Chicken and Pasta Salad

YIELD: 4 SERVINGS

¼ cup chopped sun-dried tomatoes (not packed in oil)
¼ cup water
4 ounces bow tie pasta (about 2 cups) or rigatoni pasta (about 3 cups)
1½ cups diced roasted or grilled chicken breast (about 8 ounces)
1 cup chopped canned (drained) artichoke hearts
¼ cup sliced black olives
¼ cup sliced scallions
½ cup plus 2 tablespoons bottled nonfat or light Italian or red-wine vinaigrette salad dressing
8 cups torn romaine lettuce
¼ cup chopped walnuts (optional)
¼ cup grated Parmesan cheese

1. Combine the dried tomatoes and water in a small pot and bring to a boil over high heat. Reduce the heat to low, cover, and simmer for 2 minutes or until the tomatoes are soft and the liquid is absorbed. Set aside to cool to room temperature.
2. Cook the pasta al dente according to package directions. Drain, rinse with cool water, and drain again.
3. Put the cooked pasta in a medium-sized bowl. Add the tomatoes, chicken, artichoke hearts, olives, and scallions, and toss to mix well. Pour ¼ cup of the dressing over the pasta mixture, and toss to mix well. Cover the pasta mixture and refrigerate for at least 2 hours.
4. When ready to serve, place the romaine in a large bowl and add the pasta mixture, the remaining dressing, and, if desired, the walnuts. Toss to mix well. Sprinkle the Parmesan cheese over the salad, and toss again. Serve immediately.

Herbed Turkey and Pasta Salad

YIELD: 5 SERVINGS

Salad

8 ounces tricolor rotini pasta (about 3 cups)

1⅓ cups 1-inch pieces fresh asparagus or small broccoli florets

⅔ cup diagonally sliced carrots

1 cup diced cooked turkey breast

1 cup diced nonfat or reduced-fat mozzarella or Swiss cheese

⅓ cup sliced black olives

¼ cup sliced scallions

Dressing

¼ cup plus 2 tablespoons nonfat or light mayonnaise

¼ cup nonfat or light sour cream

1 tablespoon Dijon mustard

2 tablespoons orange juice

1½ teaspoons fines herbes or ½ teaspoon each dried parsley, thyme, and rosemary

⅛ teaspoon ground white pepper

1. Cook the pasta until almost al dente according to package directions. Add the asparagus or broccoli and the carrots to the pot, and cook for another 30 to 60 seconds or until the asparagus or broccoli turns bright green and is crisp-tender and the pasta is al dente. Drain, rinse with cold water, and drain again. Transfer the mixture to a large bowl, and toss in the turkey, cheese, olives, and scallions.

2. In a small bowl, combine all the dressing ingredients, and stir to mix well. Pour the dressing over the salad, and toss gently to mix well.

3. Cover the salad and chill for at least 2 hours before serving. Toss in a little more mayonnaise just before serving if the salad seems too dry. Serve over a bed of fresh salad greens if desired.

Nutritional Facts (per 1⅔-cup serving)

CALORIES: 297   CARBOHYDRATES: 44 G   CHOLESTEROL: 25 MG   FAT: 2.3 G   FIBER: 2.7 G

PROTEIN: 23 G   SODIUM: 484 MG   CALCIUM: 239 MG   GI RATING: LOW

Mediterranean Tuna Salad

YIELD: 5 SERVINGS

8 ounces rigatoni pasta (about 3 cups)
15-ounce can small white beans or navy beans, rinsed and drained
⅓ cup chopped red onion
⅓ cup thinly sliced celery
½ cup sliced black olives
¼ teaspoon dried oregano
½ cup bottled nonfat or light Italian or red-wine vinaigrette salad dressing
12-ounce can albacore tuna in water, drained
10 cups mixed salad greens or torn romaine lettuce
½ cup crumbled nonfat or reduced-fat feta cheese

1. Cook the pasta al dente according to package directions. Drain, rinse with cool water, and drain again.
2. Put the pasta in a large bowl. Add the beans, onion, celery, olives, and oregano, and toss to mix well. Add the dressing and toss to mix well, then add the drained tuna, and toss again lightly. Cover the salad and chill for at least 2 hours. Toss in a little more dressing if the salad seems too dry.
3. To assemble the salads, place 2 cups of the salad greens on each of 5 plates. Top the lettuce on each plate with 1½ cups of the pasta mixture and sprinkle some of the feta cheese over each salad. Serve immediately.

Nutritional Facts (per serving)

CALORIES: 392 CARBOHYDRATES: 58 G CHOLESTEROL: 21 MG FAT: 3.3 G FIBER: 7.6 G
PROTEIN: 33 G SODIUM: 829 MG CALCIUM: 161 MG GI RATING: LOW

Shanghai Chicken Salad

YIELD: 5 SERVINGS

8 ounces udon noodles* or fettuccine
1½ cups fresh snow peas or 1-inch pieces of asparagus
2 cups cooked, shredded chicken breast
¾ cup matchstick-sized pieces of red bell pepper
½ cup sliced scallions
8-ounce can water chestnuts, drained and coarsely chopped; or 8-ounce can
   bamboo shoots, drained
½ cup plus 2 tablespoons Sesame-Ginger Dressing (page 172)

1. Cook the noodles until almost al dente according to package directions. Add the snow peas or asparagus to the pot and cook for another minute or until the snow peas or asparagus turn bright green and are crisp-tender and the pasta is al dente.
2. Drain the pasta and vegetables, rinse with cold water, and drain again. Transfer the mixture to a large bowl and toss in the chicken, red bell pepper, scallions, and water chestnuts or bamboo shoots. Pour the dressing over the salad, and toss gently to mix well.
3. Cover the salad and chill for at least 2 hours before serving. Toss in a little more dressing just before serving if the salad seems too dry. Serve over a bed of fresh salad greens if desired.

Nutritional Facts (per 1⅔-cup serving)
   CALORIES: 316 CARBOHYDRATES: 36 G CHOLESTEROL: 48 MG FAT: 6.6 G FIBER: 4.3 G
   PROTEIN: 23 G SODIUM: 637 MG CALCIUM: 44 MG GI RATING: LOW

Country Chicken Salad

YIELD: 4 SERVINGS

1½ cups diced cooked chicken or turkey breast (about 8 ounces); or 12-ounce can
   chicken or turkey breast, drained
¾ cup peeled diced Granny Smith apples (about 1 medium)

*A long, thick wheat noodle, similar to fettuccine, that is used in Asian cooking. Udon noodles are available in Asian markets and many grocery stores.

¼ cup plus 2 tablespoons finely chopped celery
¼ cup chopped toasted pecans (page 78)
¼ cup nonfat or light mayonnaise
3 tablespoons nonfat or light sour cream
Pinch ground white pepper

1. Place the chicken, apples, celery, and pecans in a large bowl and toss to mix well. Put the mayonnaise, sour cream, and white pepper in a small bowl and stir to mix well. Add the mayonnaise mixture to the chicken mixture and toss to mix well. Stir in a little more mayonnaise if the mixture seems too dry.
2. Cover the salad and chill for at least 2 hours before serving. Use as a sandwich filling, serve over a bed of fresh salad greens, or use to fill a cantaloupe half.

Nutritional Facts (per ¾-cup serving)

CALORIES: 160 CARBOHYDRATES: 6 G CHOLESTEROL: 45 MG FAT: 6.9 G FIBER: 0.8 G
PROTEIN: 18 G SODIUM: 162 MG CALCIUM: 28 MG GI RATING: VERY LOW

Almond-Dill Chicken Salad

YIELD: 6 SERVINGS

2 cups diced cooked chicken or turkey breast (about 10 ounces); or 3 6-ounce cans
  chicken or turkey breast, drained
8-ounce can water chestnuts, drained and coarsely chopped
½ cup thinly sliced celery
½ cup sliced toasted almonds (page 78)
¼ cup sliced scallions
⅓ cup nonfat or light mayonnaise
¼ cup nonfat or light sour cream
1 tablespoon finely chopped fresh dill weed or 1 teaspoon dried
⅛ teaspoon ground white pepper

1. Place the chicken, water chestnuts, celery, almonds, and scallions in a large bowl and toss to mix well. Put the mayonnaise, sour cream, dill, and white pepper in a small bowl and stir to mix well. Add the mayonnaise mixture to the chicken mixture and toss to mix well. Stir in a little more mayonnaise if the mixture seems too dry.

2. Cover the salad and chill for at least 2 hours before serving. Use as a sandwich filling, serve over a bed of fresh salad greens, or use to fill a cantaloupe or avocado half.

Nutritional Facts (per ¾-cup serving)

CALORIES: 164 CARBOHYDRATES: 10 G CHOLESTEROL: 40 MG FAT: 5.8 G FIBER: 2 G
PROTEIN: 17 G SODIUM: 150 MG CALCIUM: 48 MG GI RATING: VERY LOW

Cashew Crunch Turkey Salad

YIELD: 4 SERVINGS

1½ cups diced cooked turkey or chicken breast (about 8 ounces); or 12-ounce can
   turkey or chicken breast, drained
¾ cup chopped celery
¼ cup plus 2 tablespoons chopped roasted cashews
¼ cup thinly sliced scallions
¼ cup finely chopped red bell pepper
¼ cup nonfat or light mayonnaise
3 tablespoons nonfat or light sour cream
Pinch ground white pepper

1. Place the turkey, celery, cashews, scallions, and bell peppers in a large bowl and toss to mix well. Put the mayonnaise, sour cream, and white pepper in a small bowl and stir to mix well. Add the mayonnaise mixture to the turkey mixture and toss to mix well. Stir in a little more mayonnaise if the mixture seems too dry.
2. Cover the salad and chill for at least 2 hours before serving. Use as a sandwich filling, serve over a bed of fresh salad greens, or use to fill a cantaloupe half.

Nutritional Facts (per ¾-cup serving)

CALORIES: 176 CARBOHYDRATES: 9 G CHOLESTEROL: 47 MG FAT: 6.3 G FIBER: 1.2 G
PROTEIN: 20 G SODIUM: 240 MG CALCIUM: 40 MG GI RATING: VERY LOW

Big Sur Turkey Salad

For variety, add ½ to 1 teaspoon curry paste to the dressing.

1½ cups shredded or diced cooked turkey breast (about 8 ounces);
    or 12-ounce can turkey breast, drained
¾ cup seedless red grapes
½ cup finely chopped celery
¼ cup chopped almonds or walnuts (optional)
¼ cup nonfat or light mayonnaise
3 tablespoons nonfat or light sour cream
Pinch ground white pepper

1. Place the turkey, grapes, celery, and, if desired, the nuts in a large bowl and toss to mix well. Put the mayonnaise, sour cream, and white pepper in a small bowl and stir to mix well. Add the mayonnaise mixture to the turkey mixture and toss to mix well. Stir in a little more mayonnaise if the mixture seems too dry.
2. Cover the salad, and chill for at least 2 hours before serving. Use as a sandwich filling, serve over a bed of fresh salad greens, or serve in a cantaloupe half.

Nutritional Facts (per ¾-cup serving)
CALORIES: 121 CARBOHYDRATES: 9 G CHOLESTEROL: 43 MG FAT: 0.9 G FIBER: 0.7 G
PROTEIN: 18 G SODIUM: 171 MG CALCIUM: 24 MG GI RATING: LOW

West Coast Crab Salad

YIELD: 4 SERVINGS

2¼ cups cooked crabmeat; or 3 cans (6 ounces each) crabmeat, drained
¾ cup chopped canned artichoke hearts, drained
½ cup frozen green peas, thawed
3 tablespoons chopped onion
⅓ cup nonfat or light mayonnaise
3 tablespoons nonfat or light sour cream

⅛ teaspoon dried thyme
Pinch ground white pepper

1. Place the crabmeat, artichoke hearts, peas, and onions in a large bowl and toss to mix well. Put the mayonnaise, sour cream, thyme, and white pepper in a small bowl and stir to mix well. Add the mayonnaise mixture to the crab mixture and toss to mix well. Stir in a little more mayonnaise if the mixture seems too dry.
2. Cover the salad and chill for at least 2 hours before serving. Use as a sandwich filling, serve over a bed of fresh salad greens, or use to fill an avocado half.

Nutritional Facts (per ¾-cup serving)
CALORIES: 132 CARBOHYDRATES: 12 G CHOLESTEROL: 50 MG FAT: 1 G FIBER: 2.8 G
PROTEIN: 17 G SODIUM: 441 MG CALCIUM: 75 MG GI RATING: LOW

Spicy Egg Salad

To maximize nutrition, be sure to use omega-3-enriched eggs in this salad.

YIELD: 4 SERVINGS

6 hard-boiled eggs
½ cup finely chopped celery
1 tablespoon finely chopped fresh chives; or 1 teaspoon dried chives
1½ teaspoons finely chopped fresh dill; or ½ teaspoon dried dill
¼ cup nonfat or light mayonnaise
2 tablespoons spicy mustard
⅛ teaspoon ground white pepper

1. Chop the eggs and place in a medium-sized bowl. Add the celery, chives, and dill, and toss to mix well. Add the mayonnaise, mustard, and white pepper to the egg mixture and stir to mix well. Add a little more mayonnaise if the mixture seems too dry.
2. Cover the salad and chill for at least 2 hours before serving. Use as a sandwich filling or serve with whole-grain crackers.

Nutritional Facts (per ½-cup serving)
CALORIES: 123 CARBOHYDRATES: 3 G CHOLESTEROL: 322 MG FAT: 7.1 G FIBER: 0.5 G
PROTEIN: 9.5 G SODIUM: 313 MG CALCIUM: 43 MG GI RATING: VERY LOW

Variation

To make **Traditional Egg Salad,** substitute 2 tablespoons of chopped dill or sweet pickles for the chives and dill.

Nutritional Facts (per ½-cup serving)

CALORIES: 123 CARBOHYDRATES: 3 G CHOLESTEROL: 322 MG FAT: 7.1 G
FIBER: 0.5 G PROTEIN: 9.5 G SODIUM: 375 MG CALCIUM: 43 MG
GI RATING: VERY LOW

Orzo Shrimp Salad

For variety, substitute salmon or crabmeat for the shrimp.

YIELD: 4 SERVINGS

1 cup orzo pasta (about 7 ounces)
1½ cups cooked peeled and deveined shrimp (about 8 ounces)
¼ cup finely chopped scallions
¼ cup finely chopped celery
1½–2 tablespoons finely chopped fresh dill; or 1½–2 teaspoons dried dill

Dressing
½ cup nonfat or light mayonnaise
2 teaspoons lemon juice
Pinch ground white pepper

1. Cook the orzo according to package directions, drain, rinse with cool water, and drain again. Put the orzo in a large bowl, add the shrimp, scallions, celery, and dill, and toss to mix well.
2. Combine the dressing ingredients in a small bowl and stir to mix well. Add the dressing to the orzo mixture and toss to mix well.
3. Cover the salad and refrigerate for at least 2 hours before serving. Stir in a little more mayonnaise if the mixture seems too dry. Serve on a bed of mixed salad greens if desired.

Nutritional Facts (per 1⅛-cup serving)

CALORIES: 264 CARBOHYDRATES: 42 G CHOLESTEROL: 110 MG FAT: 1.4 G FIBER: 1.5 G
PROTEIN: 18 G SODIUM: 348 MG CALCIUM: 43 MG GI RATING: LOW

Crunchy Layered Salad

YIELD: 8 SERVINGS

10 cups shredded romaine lettuce (about 1 medium head)
8-ounce can sliced water chestnuts, drained
1 cup frozen green peas
1 cup thinly sliced celery
1 cup sliced scallions
1 cup shredded nonfat or reduced-fat mozzarella or Swiss cheese
1½ cups nonfat or light mayonnaise
¾ cup chopped seeded plum tomato (about 3 medium)
2 hard-boiled eggs, chopped

1. Place the lettuce in a 4-quart glass bowl and layer the water chestnuts, peas, celery, scallions, and cheese over the top.
2. Spread the mayonnaise in an even layer over the top of the salad, extending it all the way to the edges.
3. Cover the bowl with plastic wrap and chill for several hours or overnight. Just before serving, sprinkle the tomatoes and eggs over the top of the salad, toss to mix well, and serve immediately.

Nutritional Facts (per 1½-cup serving)
CALORIES: 120 CARBOHYDRATES: 16 G CHOLESTEROL: 54 MG FAT: 1.7 G FIBER: 4.2 G
PROTEIN: 8.8 G SODIUM: 482 MG CALCIUM: 169 MG GI RATING: LOW

Apple-Crunch Coleslaw

YIELD: 8 SERVINGS

1¼ pounds cabbage (about 1 small head)
1 medium-small carrot, peeled and shredded with a potato peeler (about ¾ cup)
1 large Gala or Red Delicious apple, unpeeled and diced
½ cup dark raisins
¼ cup plus 2 tablespoons roasted salted sunflower seeds
¾ cup plus 2 tablespoons nonfat or light mayonnaise

1. Remove the outer leaves from the cabbage and cut the cabbage lengthwise into 2-inch wedges. Cut away the core from each wedge then cut each wedge into very thin slices so that you have coarsely shredded cabbage. Measure the cabbage. There should be 6 cups. Adjust the amount if necessary.
2. Place the cabbage in a large bowl. Add the carrots, apple, raisins, and sunflower seeds and toss to mix well. Add the mayonnaise and toss to mix well.
3. Cover the salad and chill for at least 2 hours before serving.

Nutritional Facts (per ¾-cup serving)

CALORIES: 116 CARBOHYDRATES: 19 G CHOLESTEROL: 0 MG FAT: 3.9 G FIBER: 3.3 G
PROTEIN: 2.6 G SODIUM: 236 MG CALCIUM: 37 MG GI RATING: LOW

Greek Tabbouleh

YIELD: 8 SERVINGS

Salad
3 cups prepared bulgur wheat
1¼ cups peeled, seeded, chopped cucumber (about 1 large)
1¼ cups chopped seeded plum tomato (about 4 medium)
½ cup chopped red onion
½ cup chopped fresh parsley
½ cup crumbled nonfat or reduced-fat feta cheese
⅓ cup chopped black olives

Dressing
3 tablespoons lemon juice
2 tablespoons extra-virgin olive oil
¼ teaspoon salt
¼ teaspoon ground black pepper

1. Combine the bulgur wheat, cucumber, tomatoes, onions, parsley, feta cheese, and olives in a large bowl, and toss to mix well.
2. Combine all the dressing ingredients in a small bowl, and stir to mix well. Pour the dressing over the salad and toss to mix well. Cover the salad and chill for at least 2 hours before serving.

CALORIES: 115 CARBOHYDRATES: 16 G CHOLESTEROL: 0 MG FAT: 4.3 G FIBER: 4 G
PROTEIN: 4.4 G SODIUM: 221 MG CALCIUM: 51 MG GI RATING: LOW

Spinach and Pear Salad

YIELD: 4 SERVINGS

6 cups fresh spinach leaves
2 fresh ripe pears, peeled and sliced
¼ cup plus 2 tablespoons crumbled nonfat or reduced-fat feta cheese
¼ cup chopped toasted pecans (page 78)
¼ cup plus 2 tablespoons bottled nonfat or light balsamic vinaigrette salad dressing

1. Divide the spinach among 4 salad plates, and top the spinach on each plate with a quarter of the pear slices.
2. Sprinkle each salad with 1½ tablespoons of the feta cheese and a tablespoon of the pecans. Serve immediately accompanied by the dressing.

Nutritional Facts (per serving)

CALORIES: 125 CARBOHYDRATES: 17 G CHOLESTEROL: 1 MG FAT: 5.5 G FIBER: 3.8 G
PROTEIN: 4.6 G SODIUM: 434 MG CALCIUM: 99 MG GI RATING: VERY LOW

Orange-Avocado Salad

YIELD: 4 SERVINGS

8 cups mixed salad greens or fresh spinach leaves
1 cup chilled fresh orange sections
1 small avocado, peeled and sliced
4 slices red onion, separated into rings
½ cup bottled nonfat or light balsamic vinaigrette salad dressing
¼ cup crumbled blue cheese, optional

1. Place 2 cups of lettuce or spinach on each of 4 salad plates. Top the greens on each plate with a quarter of the orange sections, a quarter of the avocado slices, and a quarter of the onion rings.

2. Drizzle two tablespoons of the dressing over the top of each salad and sprinkle each salad with some of the blue cheese if desired. Serve immediately.

Nutritional Facts (per serving)

CALORIES: 116 CARBOHYDRATES: 15 G CHOLESTEROL: 0 MG FAT: 6.4 G FIBER: 5.1 G
PROTEIN: 3 G SODIUM: 311 MG CALCIUM: 67 MG GI RATING: VERY LOW

Glorious Greens

YIELD: 4 SERVINGS

8 cups mixed baby salad greens
½ cup crumbled nonfat or reduced-fat feta cheese
¼ cup nonfat or light red-wine or balsamic vinaigrette salad dressing
¾ cup ready-made sourdough croutons (optional)

1. Put the salad greens and the feta cheese in a large bowl and toss to mix well. Pour the dressing over the salad and toss again.
2. Serve immediately, topping each serving with some of the croutons if desired.

Nutritional Facts (per 2-cup serving)

CALORIES: 56 CARBOHYDRATES: 10 G CHOLESTEROL: 1 MG FAT: 0.4 G FIBER: 2 G
PROTEIN: 5.2 G SODIUM: 434 MG CALCIUM: 117 MG GI RATING: VERY LOW

Balsamic Three Bean Salad

For variety, substitute a light raspberry vinaigrette dressing for the balsamic vinaigrette.

YIELD: 8 SERVINGS

2 cans (1 pound each) cut green beans, drained
15-ounce can garbanzo beans (chickpeas), rinsed and drained
15-ounce can red kidney beans, rinsed and drained
¾ cup bottled nonfat or light balsamic vinaigrette salad dressing

1. Combine all the ingredients in a large bowl and toss to mix well.
2. Cover the salad and refrigerate for at least 3 hours before serving.

Nutritional Facts (per ¾-cup serving)

CALORIES: 128   CARBOHYDRATES: 23 G   CHOLESTEROL: 0 MG   FAT: 1.2 G   FIBER: 7.9 G

PROTEIN: 7.3 G   SODIUM: 224 MG   CALCIUM: 25 MG   GI RATING: VERY LOW

Broccoli-Peanut Salad

YIELD: 10 SERVINGS

Salad
1 head fresh broccoli (about 1¼ pounds)
½ cup chopped red onion
½ cup dark raisins
½ cup chopped roasted salted peanuts

Dressing
½ cup nonfat or light mayonnaise
½ cup nonfat or light sour cream
1 tablespoon honey
Pinch ground ginger
Pinch ground white pepper

1. Peel the tough outer skin from the broccoli stalk and discard. Chop the stalks into ½-inch pieces and cut the tops into small florets. (There should be about 6 cups of broccoli florets and stems.)
2. Combine the broccoli, onions, raisins, and peanuts in a large bowl and toss to mix well.
3. Combine the dressing ingredients in a small bowl and stir to mix well. Add the dressing to the broccoli mixture and toss to mix well.
4. Cover the salad and refrigerate for several hours or overnight before serving.

Nutritional Facts (per ⅔-cup serving)

CALORIES: 108   CARBOHYDRATES: 15 G   CHOLESTEROL: 0 MG   FAT: 3.7 G   FIBER: 2.9 G

PROTEIN: 4.5 G   SODIUM: 139 MG   CALCIUM: 509 MG   GI RATING: LOW

Springtime Asparagus Salad

YIELD: 6 SERVINGS

1 pound fresh asparagus spears
½ cup bottled nonfat or light red-wine vinaigrette or balsamic vinaigrette salad
  dressing
2 medium plum tomatoes, thinly sliced
4 thin slices of red onion, separated into rings
¼ cup crumbled nonfat or reduced-fat feta cheese
2 tablespoons chopped walnuts or toasted pecans

1. Rinse the asparagus spears with cool water and snap off the tough stem ends. Bring a large pot of water to a boil over high heat, add the asparagus spears, and cook for 2 to 3 minutes or until the spears are just crisp-tender. Drain the spears, then plunge them into a large bowl of ice water to stop the cooking process. Drain again and arrange the spears in a single layer on a large serving platter.
2. Drizzle the asparagus with half of the salad dressing. Arrange the tomato slices over the asparagus spears, and top with the onion rings. Drizzle the remaining dressing over the onion layer.
3. Cover the salad and refrigerate for 1 to 3 hours. Sprinkle the feta cheese and the nuts over the salad and serve immediately.

Nutritional Facts (per serving)

CALORIES: 64 CARBOHYDRATES: 10 G CHOLESTEROL: 0 MG FAT: 1.8 G FIBER: 2.1 G
PROTEIN: 3.4 G SODIUM: 268 MG CALCIUM: 31 MG GI RATING: VERY LOW

Tortellini Salad

YIELD: 7 SERVINGS

9-ounce package refrigerated cheese tortellini
1½ cups small broccoli florets
1½ cups sliced fresh mushrooms
1½ cups chopped canned artichoke hearts, drained
¾ cup matchstick-sized pieces red bell pepper

½ cup nonfat or light bottled Italian or red-wine vinaigrette salad dressing
½ teaspoon dried oregano or Italian seasoning
⅓ cup crumbled nonfat or reduced-fat feta cheese or 3 tablespoons grated Parmesan cheese (optional)

1. Cook the tortellini al dente according to package directions. One minute before the pasta is done, add the broccoli and mushrooms and cook for an additional minute or until the broccoli turns bright green and is crisp-tender and the pasta is al dente. Drain the pasta and vegetables, rinse with cool water, and drain again.
2. Put the pasta mixture in a large bowl, add the artichoke hearts, red bell peppers, dressing, oregano, and toss to mix well. If desired, add the feta or Parmesan cheese, and toss again.
3. Cover the salad and refrigerate for at least 2 hours before serving.

Nutritional Facts (per 1-cup serving)

CALORIES: 150 CARBOHYDRATES: 25 G CHOLESTEROL: 15 MG FAT: 3.4 G FIBER: 4.1 G
PROTEIN: 7 G SODIUM: 353 MG CALCIUM: 93 MG GI RATING: LOW

Simple Pear Salad

YIELD: 6 SERVINGS

2 cans (15 ounces each) pear halves packed in juice
6 leaves Boston or Bibb lettuce
½ cup nonfat or light sour cream
3 tablespoons shredded nonfat or reduced-fat Cheddar cheese
2 tablespoons chopped toasted pecans

1. Refrigerate the cans of pears for at least 2 hours before assembling the salad.
2. Place 1 lettuce leaf on each of 6 small salad plates.
3. Drain the pears and arrange 2 small pear halves over the lettuce leaf on each plate. Fill the hollow of each pear half with 2 teaspoons of the sour cream, then sprinkle each pear half with 1 teaspoon of cheese and a sprinkling of pecans. Serve immediately.

Nutritional Facts (per serving)

CALORIES: 84 CARBOHYDRATES: 15 G CHOLESTEROL: 0 MG FAT: 1.8 G FIBER: 1.7 G
PROTEIN: 2.5 G SODIUM: 47 MG CALCIUM: 57 MG GI RATING: LOW

Fabulous Fruit Salad

YIELD: 6 SERVINGS

3 large navel oranges
1 cup seedless red grapes
1 medium Red Delicious or Gala apple, unpeeled and diced
1 large banana, peeled and sliced
3 tablespoons sweetened flaked coconut

1. Peel the oranges, cutting down to the flesh. Cut the orange segments away from the membranes. Place the orange segments and the juices that have accumulated in a large bowl. Squeeze any juice from the pieces of orange rind and add it to the bowl.
2. Add the grapes and apples to the oranges and toss to mix well. Cover the mixture and refrigerate for at least 1 hour or until well chilled. Add the bananas and refrigerate for an additional hour before serving. To serve, divide the mixture among six 8-ounce bowls or goblets, and top each serving with a sprinkling of the coconut.

Nutritional Facts (per ⅞-cup serving)
CALORIES: 113 CARBOHYDRATES: 26 G CHOLESTEROL: 0 MG FAT: 1.8 G FIBER: 3.4 G
PROTEIN: 1.4 G SODIUM: 10 MG CALCIUM: 43 MG GI RATING: LOW

Two-Layer Fruit Salad

YIELD: 9 SERVINGS

Fruit Layer
1-pound can peaches in juice
8-ounce can crushed pineapple in juice
1 package (4-serving size) sugar-free orange or lime gelatin mix

Cheese Layer
1 package (4-serving size) sugar-free orange or lime gelatin mix
½ cup boiling water
1 cup orange juice
1 block (8 ounces) nonfat or reduced-fat cream cheese

1. To make the fruit layer, drain the peaches and pineapple, reserving the juice. Coarsely chop the peaches, and set aside with the drained pineapple. Place the juices in a 2-cup measure, and add enough water to bring the volume to 2 cups. Set aside.
2. Pour the gelatin in a medium-sized bowl and set aside. Pour 1 cup of the juice mixture in a small pot and bring to a boil. Pour the boiling juice over the gelatin and stir to dissolve it. Add the remaining juice to the gelatin mixture and stir to mix well.
3. Chill the gelatin mixture for about 1¼ hours or until it is the consistency of raw egg whites. Stir in the drained fruits and pour the mixture into a square 2-quart glass dish. Cover and refrigerate for about 1 hour, or until the gelatin is almost set.
4. To make the cheese layer, pour the gelatin mix in a blender and add the boiling water. Blend the mixture at low speed with the lid slightly ajar for 1 minute or until the gelatin is completely dissolved. Add the orange juice and blend to mix well. Add the cream cheese and blend until the mixture is smooth.
5. Pour the cheese mixture over the fruit mixture in the dish. Chill for at least 4 hours or until firm. Cut into squares to serve.

Nutritional Facts (per serving)

CALORIES: 88 CARBOHYDRATES: 16 G CHOLESTEROL: 2 MG FAT: 0.1 G FIBER: 1 G
PROTEIN: 6.3 G SODIUM: 194 MG CALCIUM: 97 MG GI RATING: LOW

Cherry-Apple Salad

YIELD: 5 SERVINGS

1 package (4-serving size) sugar-free cherry gelatin
1 cup boiling water
1 cup frozen pitted dark, sweet cherries, halved
¾ cup apple juice
1 cup finely chopped peeled apples
⅓ cup finely chopped celery
¼ cup chopped walnuts or pecans

1. Pour the gelatin in a large bowl, add the boiling water, and stir for 2 minutes, or until the gelatin is completely dissolved. Add the frozen cherries and the apple juice and stir for a minute or two or until the cherries thaw. Place the mixture in the refrigerator and chill for about 45 minutes or until the mixture is the consistency of raw egg whites.
2. Fold in the apples, celery, and nuts and pour the mixture into a 1-quart mold or bowl. Cover

and refrigerate for at least 6 hours or until the gelatin is firm. Unmold the salad* onto a lettuce-lined plate if desired, or simply serve from the bowl.

Nutritional Facts (per serving)

CALORIES: 100 CARBOHYDRATES: 14 G CHOLESTEROL: 0 MG FAT: 3.6 G FIBER: 1.9 G

PROTEIN: 3 G SODIUM: 51 MG CALCIUM: 16 MG GI RATING: VERY LOW

Parmesan-Peppercorn Dressing

YIELD: 1¼ CUPS

1 cup nonfat or light mayonnaise
¼ cup grated Parmesan cheese
2 tablespoons skim or low-fat milk
1 tablespoon white-wine vinegar
1½ teaspoons crushed garlic
½ teaspoon coarsely ground or cracked black pepper

1. Combine all the ingredients in a small bowl and stir to mix well. Add a little more milk if the mixture seems too thick.
2. Transfer the mixture to a covered container and refrigerate for several hours before serving.

Nutritional Facts (per tablespoon)

CALORIES: 15 CARBOHYDRATES: 2 G CHOLESTEROL: 1 MG FAT: 0.4 G FIBER: 0 G

PROTEIN: 0.6 G SODIUM: 108 MG CALCIUM: 20 MG GI RATING: LOW

Sesame-Ginger Dressing

For variety, substitute peanut butter for the sesame tahini.

YIELD: 1¼ CUPS

¼ cup plus 1 tablespoon seasoned rice vinegar
¼ cup orange juice

To unmold the salad, dip the mold in warm water for a few seconds to loosen the salad's edges. Then center a plate upside down over the mold and invert the salad onto the plate. Shake the mold gently until it loosens, then carefully lift the mold off. Repeat these steps if the salad doesn't release from the mold.

2 tablespoons reduced-sodium soy sauce

2 tablespoons roasted sesame tahini

1 tablespoon roasted dark sesame oil

1 tablespoon light brown sugar or honey

1 teaspoon crushed garlic

1 teaspoon ground ginger or 1 tablespoon grated fresh ginger

1. Combine all the ingredients in a blender and blend until smooth.
2. Cover and chill for at least 2 hours before serving.

Nutritional Facts (per tablespoon)

CALORIES: 30 CARBOHYDRATES: 2.7 G CHOLESTEROL: 0 MG FAT: 1.9 G FIBER: 0.2 G

PROTEIN: 0.5 G SODIUM: 158 MG CALCIUM: 10 MG GI RATING: MODERATE

Sun-Dried Tomato Dressing

YIELD: ⅞ CUP

¼ cup plus 2 tablespoons water

3 tablespoons white wine vinegar

3 tablespoons extra-virgin olive oil

1 tablespoon chopped sun-dried tomatoes

1 tablespoon sugar or honey

2 teaspoons crushed garlic

½ teaspoon dried oregano

¼ teaspoon dried thyme

½ teaspoon salt

¼ teaspoon ground black pepper

1. Combine all the ingredients in a blender and blend until smooth.
2. Cover and chill for at least 2 hours before serving.

Nutritional Facts (per tablespoon)

CALORIES: 30 CARBOHYDRATES: 1.2 G CHOLESTEROL: 0 MG FAT: 2.9 G FIBER: 0.1 G

PROTEIN: 0.1 G SODIUM: 89 MG CALCIUM: 2 MG GI RATING: LOW

Yogurt Ranch Dressing

YIELD: 1½ CUPS

1 cup nonfat or light mayonnaise
¼ cup plain nonfat or low-fat yogurt
¼ cup skim or low-fat milk
1 teaspoon crushed garlic
1½ teaspoons dried chives
1½ teaspoons dried parsley
¼ teaspoon ground black pepper
¼ teaspoon onion powder

1. Combine all the ingredients in a blender and blend to mix well.
2. Cover and chill for at least 2 hours before serving.

Nutritional Facts (per tablespoon)

CALORIES: 9   CARBOHYDRATES: 1.7 G   CHOLESTEROL: 0 MG   FAT: 0 G   FIBER: 0 G

PROTEIN: 0.3 G   SODIUM: 73 MG   CALCIUM: 9 MG   GI RATING: LOW

Fast and Flavorful Dry Rubs

Bursting with flavor, rubs can transform bland and boring meat, seafood, and poultry into delicious culinary creations. When time is in short supply, rubs are just what you need to perk up a meal. Use a commercial premixed blend, like Cajun seasoning or lemon pepper, or make your own mixture using one of the following recipes.

To apply the rub, rinse the meat and pat it dry with paper towels. Then, using your fingers, rub the outside surface of the meat with the seasoning blend, using 1 to 2 tablespoons of rub per pound of meat. For extra flavor, mix the rub with just enough olive oil to make a thick paste before applying it to the food. Let the food stand at room temperature for 15 to 30 minutes before cooking. This will allow the seasonings to permeate the food. (Refrigerate if you are going to let the food stand for more than 1 hour.) If you did not mix the rub with olive oil, spray the coated food lightly with nonstick cooking spray, then grill, broil, or roast the food and enjoy great flavor with a minimum of fat and salt.

The following recipes will remain flavorful for several months, so make a double or triple batch of your favorite rubs and store the mixtures in airtight containers to always have a supply on hand.

Zesty Herb Rub

YIELD: ABOUT 5 TABLESPOONS

1 tablespoon dried oregano
1 tablespoon dried thyme
1 tablespoon lemon pepper
2 teaspoons garlic powder
2 teaspoons onion powder
2 teaspoons light brown sugar
½ teaspoon salt

Combine all the ingredients in a small bowl and stir to mix well. Apply (use 1 to 2 tablespoons per pound of meat) according to the directions given above, and grill, broil, or roast the meat as desired.

Nutritional Facts (per 1-teaspoon serving)
CALORIES: 7   CARBOHYDRATES: 1.5 G   CHOLESTEROL: 0 MG   FAT: 0.1 G
FIBER: 0.3 G   PROTEIN: 0.2 G   SODIUM: 145 MG   CALCIUM: 6 MG
GI RATING: VERY LOW

Ragin' Cajun Rub

YIELD: ABOUT 5 TABLESPOONS

1½ tablespoons ground paprika
2 teaspoons dried thyme
2 teaspoons dried oregano
1½ teaspoons garlic powder
1½ teaspoons light brown sugar
1 teaspoon onion powder

1 teaspoon coarsely ground black pepper
¾ teaspoon salt
¼ teaspoon ground cayenne pepper

Combine all the ingredients in a small bowl, and stir to mix well. Apply (use 1 to 2 tablespoons per pound of meat) according to the directions given above, and grill, broil, or roast the meat as desired.

Nutritional Facts (per 1-teaspoon serving)
CALORIES: 6 CARBOHYDRATES: 1 G CHOLESTEROL: 0 MG FAT: 0.1 G FIBER: 0.4 G
PROTEIN: 0.2 G SODIUM: 117 MG CALCIUM: 7 MG GI RATING: VERY LOW

Jamaican Jerk Rub

YIELD: ABOUT 5 TABLESPOONS

1 tablespoon ground paprika
1 tablespoon light brown sugar
1 tablespoon lemon pepper
2 teaspoons onion powder
1 teaspoon garlic powder
2 teaspoons dried thyme
1 teaspoon ground allspice
½ teaspoon salt

Combine all the ingredients in a small bowl and stir to mix well. Apply (use 1 to 2 tablespoons per pound of meat) according to the directions given above, and grill, broil, or roast the meat as desired.

Nutritional Facts (per 1-teaspoon serving)
CALORIES: 8 CARBOHYDRATES: 2 G CHOLESTEROL: 0 MG FAT: 0.1 G FIBER: 0.3 G
PROTEIN: 0.2 G SODIUM: 132 MG CALCIUM: 5 MG GI RATING: VERY LOW

11. Savvy Sandwiches

Sandwiches—on a low-GI diet? Yes. Made properly, even sandwiches can fit into a low-GI eating plan. When making your sandwiches, just remember that all breads are not created equal. So instead of the soft, airy white stuff, go for the hearty whole-grain breads. Chapter 4 will guide you in selecting the best kinds. Add a lean protein filling and plenty of fresh vegetable toppings, finish off with a low-fat spread or dressing, and you have a satisfying meal that will fill you up but not out. Remember, too, that accompaniments can make or break a low-GI meal, so instead of high-GI pretzels, chips, or fries, have a cup of soup, a garden salad, or some fresh fruit with your sandwich.

This chapter offers a selection of hearty sandwiches that are versatile, portable, and quick and easy to make. So whether you are looking for a hot tuna melt, a creative wrap, or a hearty burger, you are sure to find a sensational sandwich that meets your needs deliciously.

Herbed Turkey Salad Sandwiches

Yield: 4 servings

1H cups cooked diced turkey or chicken breast; or 2 cans (6 ounces each) turkey or
    chicken breast, drained
¾ cup finely chopped celery
¼ cup thinly sliced scallions
⅓ cup chopped walnuts (optional)
8 slices firm whole-wheat or multigrain bread
2 tablespoons nonfat or light mayonnaise
4 leaves Boston or Bibb lettuce

Dressing
¼ cup plus 2 tablespoons nonfat or light mayonnaise
¼ cup nonfat or light sour cream
½ teaspoon fines herbes

1. Combine the turkey or chicken, celery, scallions, and, if desired, the walnuts in a medium-sized bowl and toss to mix well.
2. Combine the dressing ingredients in a small bowl and stir to mix well. Add the dressing to the turkey mixture and toss to mix well. Mix in a little more mayonnaise if the mixture seems too dry. Cover the salad and refrigerate for at least 2 hours before assembling the sandwiches.
3. To assemble the sandwiches, toast the bread if desired, and spread each piece with some of the mayonnaise. Place one-fourth of the turkey salad mixture on the bottom half of each bread slice and top with a lettuce leaf.
4. Place the top halves of the bread slices on the sandwiches, cut each sandwich in half, and serve immediately.

Nutritional Facts (per sandwich)

CALORIES: 256 CARBOHYDRATES: 33 G CHOLESTEROL: 47 MG FAT: 3 G FIBER: 4.5 G
PROTEIN: 24 G SODIUM: 566 MG CALCIUM: 78 MG GI RATING: MODERATE

Saucy Roast Beef Sandwiches

YIELD: 4 SERVINGS

8 slices firm multigrain bread
8 ounces thinly sliced lean roast beef
4 ounces thinly sliced nonfat or reduced-fat Swiss cheese
4 slices tomato
4 thin slices red or sweet onion
4 lettuce leaves

Sauce
¼ cup nonfat or light mayonnaise
¼ cup nonfat or light sour cream
2–3 teaspoons prepared horseradish

1. To make the sauce, combine the mayonnaise, sour cream, and horseradish in a small bowl and stir to mix well. Set aside.
2. Lay the bread slices out on a flat surface and spread each one with some of the sauce. Place 2 ounces of roast beef on each of 4 bread slices and top the roast beef with some of the cheese, a slice of tomato, a slice of onion, and a lettuce leaf.
3. Place the remaining bread slices on the sandwiches, cut each sandwich in half, and serve immediately.

Nutritional Facts (per sandwich)

CALORIES: 282 CARBOHYDRATES: 33 G CHOLESTEROL: 31 MG FAT: 4.6 G FIBER: 4.3 G
PROTEIN: 27 G SODIUM: 846 MG CALCIUM: 284 MG GI RATING: MODERATE

Turkey-Bacon Club Sandwiches

YIELD: 4 SERVINGS

8 slices firm whole-wheat or multigrain bread, toasted
¼ cup nonfat or light mayonnaise
6 ounces thinly sliced roasted turkey breast
8 slices cooked turkey bacon
4 slices (¾ ounce each) nonfat or reduced-fat Cheddar or Swiss cheese
8 thin slices tomato
4 leaves romaine lettuce

1. Place one slice of the toast on a cutting board, and spread with 1½ teaspoons of the mayonnaise. Layer a quarter of the turkey, 2 slices of the turkey bacon, 1 slice of the cheese, 2 slices of tomato, and 1 piece of lettuce over the toast. Finally, spread another piece of toast with 1½ teaspoons of mayonnaise, and place it on top of the sandwich. Repeat with the remaining ingredients to make 4 sandwiches. Cut the sandwiches in half, and serve immediately.

Nutritional Facts (per serving)

CALORIES: 286 CARBOHYDRATES: 30 G CHOLESTEROL: 77 MG FAT: 3.9 G FIBER: 4.3 G
PROTEIN: 31 G SODIUM: 854 MG CALCIUM: 211 MG GI RATING: MODERATE

Righteous Reubens

YIELD: 4 SERVINGS

8 slices whole-grain rye or pumpernickel bread
Butter-flavored nonstick cooking spray
⅓ cup bottled nonfat or light Thousand Island salad dressing
8 ounces thinly sliced corned beef or pastrami at least 97-percent lean
4 ounces thinly sliced reduced-fat Swiss cheese
1 cup very thinly sliced purple cabbage or sauerkraut, well drained

1. Spray 1 side of each slice of bread with the cooking spray. Spread the other side of each bread slice with 2 teaspoons of the salad dressing.
2. Place 4 slices of bread, cooking-spray side down, on a flat surface. Top each slice with 2 ounces of meat, 1 ounce of cheese, and ¼ cup of cabbage or sauerkraut. Top with the remaining bread slices, dressing side in.
3. Preheat a large nonstick skillet or griddle over medium-low heat and place the sandwiches in the skillet or griddle. Cook for about 3 minutes on each side or until the bread is toasted and the cheese is melted. Serve hot.

Nutritional Facts (per serving)

CALORIES: 314   CARBOHYDRATES: 36 G   CHOLESTEROL: 25 MG   FAT: 6.9 G   FIBER: 5 G
PROTEIN: 25 G   SODIUM: 1,158 MG   CALCIUM: 296 MG   GI RATING: MODERATE

Grilled Ham & Cheese Sandwiches

YIELD: 4 SERVINGS

8 slices firm whole-wheat or pumpernickel bread
Butter-flavored nonstick cooking spray
6 ounces thinly sliced ham (at least 97-percent lean)
6 ounces thinly sliced nonfat or reduced-fat American or Swiss cheese

1. Spray 1 side of each slice of bread lightly with the cooking spray.
2. Place 4 slices of bread, cooking-spray side down, on a flat surface. Top each bread slice with 1½ ounces of meat, and 1½ ounces of cheese. Top with the remaining bread slices.

3. Preheat a large nonstick skillet or griddle over medium-low heat and place the sandwiches in the skillet or griddle. Cook for about 3 minutes on each side or until the bread is toasted and the cheese is melted. Serve hot.

Nutritional Facts (per serving)

CALORIES: 244 CARBOHYDRATES: 29 G CHOLESTEROL: 15 MG FAT: 3.7 G FIBER: 4 G
PROTEIN: 25 G SODIUM: 1,031 MG CALCIUM: 360 MG GI RATING: MODERATE

Spinach and Cheese Melts

YIELD: 4 SERVINGS

1¼ cups sliced fresh mushrooms
10-ounce box frozen chopped spinach, thawed and drained
1–2 tablespoons roasted salted sunflower seeds
3 tablespoons nonfat or light mayonnaise
2 tablespoons grated Parmesan cheese
4 whole-wheat or multigrain burger buns or 8 slices pumpernickel bread
4 slices tomato
¾ cup alfalfa sprouts
4 ounces thinly sliced nonfat or reduced-fat Swiss, mozzarella, or provolone cheese
2–3 tablespoons spicy mustard

1. Coat a large nonstick skillet with cooking spray and place over medium-high heat. Add the mushrooms and cook, stirring frequently, for several minutes or until the mushrooms are nicely browned. Cover the skillet periodically during cooking as it starts to dry out (the steam released during cooking will moisten the skillet). Add a few teaspoons of water or broth to the skillet only if necessary.
2. Add the spinach to the skillet and reduce the heat to medium. Cook, stirring frequently, until the spinach is heated through and any excess liquid has evaporated. (The mixture should be fairly dry.) Add the sunflower seeds to the skillet mixture and stir to mix well. Remove the skillet from the heat and stir in first mayonnaise and then the Parmesan cheese.
3. To assemble the sandwiches, place a quarter of the spinach mixture on 4 bread slices or on the bottom half of each bun. Top the spinach on each bread slice or bun with a slice of tomato, some of the sprouts, and some of the cheese slices. Spread the remaining 4 bread slices or top half of each bun with some of the mustard, and place on the sandwiches.

4. Place each sandwich on a microwave-safe plate, and cover with a paper towel. Microwave each sandwich at high power for about 30 seconds, or until the cheese is melted. Serve hot.

Nutritional Facts (per serving)

CALORIES: 247   CARBOHYDRATES: 31 G   CHOLESTEROL: 5 MG   FAT: 5.3 G   FIBER: 7 G

PROTEIN: 19 G   SODIUM: 720 MG   CALCIUM: 387 MG   GI RATING: MODERATE

Turkey & Artichoke Melts

YIELD: 4 SERVINGS

15-ounce can artichoke hearts, well drained and finely chopped
½ cup nonfat or light mayonnaise
1 tablespoon Dijon mustard
8 slices firm multigrain or pumpernickel bread
6 ounces thinly sliced roasted turkey breast
8 thin rings red bell pepper
4 thin slices red onion
1 cup alfalfa sprouts
4 ounces thinly sliced nonfat or reduced-fat Swiss cheese

1. Place the artichokes, ¼ cup of the mayonnaise, and all the mustard in a medium-sized bowl, and stir to mix well. Set aside.
2. Place one slice of the bread on a cutting board, and spread with 1½ teaspoons of the remaining mayonnaise. Layer a quarter of the turkey, a quarter of the artichoke mixture, 2 rings of red bell pepper, an onion slice, a quarter of the sprouts, and a quarter of the cheese over the bread slice. Spread another piece of bread with 1½ teaspoons of mayonnaise, and place it on top of the sandwich.
3. Repeat with the remaining ingredients to make 4 sandwiches. Place each sandwich on a microwave-safe plate, and cover with a paper towel. Microwave each sandwich at high power for about 30 seconds, or just until the sandwich is heated through and the cheese is melted. Serve hot.

Nutritional Facts (per serving)

CALORIES: 302   CARBOHYDRATES: 41 G   CHOLESTEROL: 38 MG   FAT: 2.9 G   FIBER: 8.4 G

PROTEIN: 29 G   SODIUM: 804 MG   CALCIUM: 347 MG   GI RATING: MODERATE

Tangy Tuna Melts

YIELD: 4 SERVINGS

12-ounce can water-packed chunk light or albacore tuna, drained
½ cup finely chopped celery
½ cup finely chopped onion
¼ cup plus 2 tablespoons nonfat or light mayonnaise
1 tablespoon plus 1 teaspoon Dijon mustard
¼ teaspoon dried fines herbes or thyme
⅛ teaspoon ground black pepper
4 whole-wheat or oat bran English muffins, split and toasted
4 ounces thinly sliced reduced-fat Swiss cheese; or 1 cup shredded

1. Combine the drained tuna, celery, onion, mayonnaise, mustard, *fines herbes* or thyme, and black pepper in a medium-sized bowl, and stir to mix well. Set aside.
2. Arrange the English muffins on a baking sheet, split side up. Spread about ¼ cup of the tuna mixture over each piece and place under a preheated broiler for 2 to 3 minutes or until the mixture is hot. Top each muffin half with some of the cheese and broil for another minute or two or until the cheese is melted. Serve hot.

Nutritional Facts (per serving)

CALORIES: 329   CARBOHYDRATES: 33 G   CHOLESTEROL: 35 MG   FAT: 6 G   FIBER: 5 G
PROTEIN: 35 G   SODIUM: 870 MG   CALCIUM: 253 MG   GI RATING: MODERATE

Riviera Burgers

YIELD: 6 SERVINGS

Sauce
½ cup plus 1 tablespoon nonfat or light mayonnaise
1 tablespoon plus 1½ teaspoons Dijon mustard
1½ teaspoons honey

Burger Mixture
1 pound 95-percent lean ground beef
1 cup finely chopped fresh mushrooms

¾ cup finely chopped onion

¾ cup frozen meatless recipe crumbles, thawed

1 tablespoon Dijon mustard

1 tablespoon Worcestershire sauce

1½ teaspoons fines herbes; or ¾ teaspoon each dried thyme and marjoram

1½ teaspoons crushed garlic

½ teaspoon coarsely ground black pepper

Toppings

6 slices (¾ ounce each) nonfat or reduced-fat Swiss cheese

6 multigrain or sourdough burger buns

6 slices tomato

6 thin slices red onion

6 leaves Boston or Bibb lettuce

1. Combine the sauce ingredients in a small bowl and stir to mix well. Set aside.
2. Combine all the burger mixture ingredients in a large bowl and mix thoroughly. Shape the mixture into 6 four-inch patties.
3. Coat a large nonstick skillet with cooking spray and preheat over medium heat. Place the patties in the skillet, and cook for 4 to 5 minutes on each side or until the meat is no longer pink inside. (Alternatively, cook the burgers over medium coals or under a broiler for about 7 minutes on each side or until the meat is no longer pink inside.)
4. Lay a slice of cheese over each burger, cover the skillet, and cook for another minute or just until the cheese is melted. If you are broiling the burgers, add the cheese and broil for another 30 seconds, or until the cheese is melted.
5. Split the buns open, and spread some of the sauce over each piece. Place each burger on the bottom half of a bun, and top each burger with a slice of tomato, a slice of onion, and a lettuce leaf, and the top half of the bun. Serve hot.

Nutritional Facts (per serving)

CALORIES: 309   CARBOHYDRATES: 35 G   CHOLESTEROL: 42 MG   FAT: 5.9 G   FIBER: 6.1 G

PROTEIN: 31 G   SODIUM: 792 MG   CALCIUM: 220 MG   GI RATING: MODERATE

Zesty Crab Burgers

Nonstick cooking spray

⅓ cup finely chopped celery (include the leaves)

⅓ cup finely chopped scallions

⅓ cup finely chopped red bell pepper

1½ cups cooked crabmeat; or 2 cans (6 ounces each) crabmeat, well drained

1 tablespoon finely chopped fresh parsley or 1 teaspoon dried parsley

½ teaspoon ground paprika

⅛ teaspoon cayenne pepper

1 cup multigrain or sourdough bread crumbs*

¼ cup fat-free egg substitute; or 2 egg whites, lightly beaten

3 ounces thinly sliced or shredded reduced-fat Swiss cheese (optional)

4 whole-wheat or multigrain burger buns

4 slices tomato

1 cup shredded romaine lettuce

Sauce

¼ cup plus 1 tablespoon nonfat or light mayonnaise

1 tablespoon chili sauce

1. To make the sauce, combine the mayonnaise and chili sauce in a small dish and stir to mix well. Set aside.
2. Coat a large nonstick skillet with cooking spray, and add the celery, scallions, red bell peppers, and 1 tablespoon of water. Place the skillet over medium heat, cover, and cook, stirring occasionally, for about 3 minutes or until the vegetables are soft. (Add a little more water if the skillet begins to dry out, but only enough to prevent scorching.) Remove the skillet from the heat, add the crab, parsley, paprika, and cayenne pepper, and stir to mix well. Stir in first the bread crumbs and then the egg substitute or egg whites.
3. Coat a large baking sheet with nonstick cooking spray. Shape the crab mixture into four 3½-inch patties, and place the patties on the baking sheet. Spray the tops of the patties lightly with

*To make the bread crumbs, tear about 1½ slices of firm multigrain or sourdough bread into chunks. Put in a food processor or blender and process into crumbs.

the cooking spray. Bake at 450° F for 8 minutes, turn the patties over, and bake for an additional 8 minutes, or until golden brown. If desired, top each patty with some of the Swiss cheese during the last 2 minutes of baking to allow the cheese to melt.

4. Split the buns open, and spread some of the sauce over each piece. Place a patty on the bottom half of each bun, top with a slice of tomato, some of the lettuce, and the top half of the bun. Serve hot.

Nutritional Facts (per serving)

CALORIES: 222 CARBOHYDRATES: 34 G CHOLESTEROL: 33 MG FAT: 3 G FIBER: 5.8 G
PROTEIN: 19 G SODIUM: 695 MG CALCIUM: 97 MG GI RATING: MODERATE

Garden Veggie Bagelwiches

YIELD: 4 SERVINGS

4 small whole-wheat or oat-bran bagels; or 8 slices firm multigrain bread
6 ounces thinly sliced nonfat or reduced-fat Swiss or provolone cheese
4 thin slices red onion
4 thin slices tomato
4 rings green bell pepper
4 canned (drained) artichoke hearts, quartered
¾ cup alfalfa or spicy sprouts or 4 lettuce leaves

Dressing
¼ cup plus 2 tablespoons nonfat or light mayonnaise
1 tablespoon plus 1 teaspoon Dijon mustard
1 teaspoon honey

1. To make the dressing, combine the mayonnaise, mustard, and honey in a small bowl and stir to mix well. Set aside.
2. Toast the bagels or bread if desired. Spread both halves of each bagel or bread slice with some of the dressing. Place one-fourth of the cheese on the bottom half of each bagel or bread slice, top the cheese with a slice of onion, a slice of tomato, a bell pepper ring, some of the artichokes, and some of the sprouts or a lettuce leaf.
3. Place the top bagel halves or bread slices on the sandwiches, cut each sandwich in half, and serve immediately.

Nutritional Facts (per sandwich)

      CALORIES: 259 CARBOHYDRATES: 40 G CHOLESTEROL: 4 MG FAT: 2.3 G FIBER: 7.6 G

      PROTEIN: 20 G SODIUM: 829 MG CALCIUM: 357 MG GI rating: MODERATE

Bistro Bagelwiches

YIELD: 4 SERVINGS

½ cup plus 2 tablespoons nonfat or reduced-fat cream cheese, softened to room temperature
1 teaspoon crushed garlic
½ teaspoon fines herbes, or ¼ teaspoon each dried thyme and marjoram
4 small whole-wheat or oat-bran bagels; or 8 slices firm multigrain bread
8 ounces roasted turkey breast
4 thin slices red onion
4 slices tomato
4 Boston or Bibb lettuce leaves

1. Combine the cream cheese, garlic, and *fines herbes* in a small bowl, and stir to mix well. Set aside.
2. Toast the bagels or bread slices if desired. Spread both halves of each bagel or bread slice with some of the cream cheese spread. Place 2 ounces of turkey on the bottom half of each bagel or bread slice, top the turkey with a slice of onion, a slice of tomato, and a lettuce leaf.
3. Place the top bagel halves or bread slices on the sandwiches, cut each sandwich in half, and serve immediately.

Nutritional Facts (per sandwich)

      CALORIES: 279 CARBOHYDRATES: 35 G CHOLESTEROL: 50 MG FAT: 2.3 G FIBER: 6.4 G

      PROTEIN: 30 G SODIUM: 503 MG CALCIUM: 159 MG GI rating: MODERATE

Savory Roast Beef Subs

YIELD: 4 SERVINGS

1 medium onion, thinly sliced
2 cups sliced fresh mushrooms
¼ teaspoon dried thyme

⅛ teaspoon ground black pepper

1 tablespoon dry sherry

4 whole-wheat sub rolls (6 inches long)

8 ounces thinly sliced lean roast beef

4 ounces thinly sliced nonfat or reduced-fat Swiss or provolone cheese

Dressing

⅓ cup nonfat or light mayonnaise

1 tablespoon Dijon mustard

1. To make the dressing, combine the mayonnaise and mustard in a small bowl and stir to mix well. Set aside.

2. Coat a large nonstick skillet with cooking spray and add the onions, mushrooms, thyme, black pepper, and sherry. Place the skillet over medium-high heat. Cover and cook, stirring frequently, for about 4 minutes or until the onions and mushrooms are tender and nicely browned. Add a little more sherry during cooking if the skillet becomes too dry, but only enough to prevent scorching. Remove the skillet from the heat and set aside.

3. Place the bottom half of each roll on a flat surface and spread each with some of the dressing. Top each roll with 2 ounces of the roast beef, a quarter of the onion-mushroom mixture, and 1 ounce of the cheese. Spread the top half of each piece of roll with some of the dressing and place on the sandwiches.

4. Place each sandwich on a microwave-safe plate, and cover with a paper towel. Microwave each sandwich at high power for about 30 seconds or just until the sandwiches are heated through and the cheese is melted. Serve immediately.

Nutritional Facts (per serving)

CALORIES: 417 CARBOHYDRATES: 53 G CHOLESTEROL: 50 MG FAT: 5.8 G FIBER: 3.2 G
PROTEIN: 36 G SODIUM: 973 MG GI RATING: MODERATE

Chutney Chicken Pita Pockets

YIELD: 4 SERVINGS

4 whole-wheat or oat-bran pita pockets (6-inch rounds), cut in half

8 ounces thinly sliced chicken or turkey breast

8 leaves Boston or Bibb lettuce

4 thin slices red onion

1 medium-small cucumber, peeled and thinly sliced

Dressing
½ cup minus 1 tablespoon nonfat or light mayonnaise
2 tablespoons mango chutney

1. To make the dressing, combine the mayonnaise and chutney in a small bowl, and stir to mix well. Set aside.
2. To heat the pita pockets, place them on a microwave-safe plate. Cover with a damp paper towel, and microwave on high power for about 45 seconds, or until warm. (If heating only 1 pita at a time, microwave only 15 seconds.)
3. To assemble the sandwiches, place 1 ounce of turkey in each of the 8 pita halves. Add 1 leaf of lettuce, a few rings of onion, 3 to 4 cucumber slices, and some of the dressing. Serve immediately.

Nutritional Facts (per serving)

CALORIES: 274 CARBOHYDRATES: 38 G CHOLESTEROL: 48 MG FAT: 2.6 G FIBER: 5.4 G
PROTEIN: 25 G SODIUM: 547 MG CALCIUM: 70 MG GI RATING: MODERATE

Tuscan Tuna Pitas

YIELD: 4 SERVINGS

4 cups torn romaine lettuce
¾ cup chopped canned artichoke hearts, drained
4 slices red onion, separated into rings
¼ cup sliced black olives
2 cans (6 ounces each) albacore tuna in water, drained
¼ cup bottled nonfat or light Italian salad dressing
2 tablespoons grated Parmesan cheese
4 whole-wheat or oat-bran pita pockets (6-inch rounds), cut in half

1. Combine the lettuce, artichoke hearts, onion rings, olives, and drained tuna in a large bowl and toss to mix well. Add the Italian dressing and the Parmesan cheese, and toss again. Set aside.
2. To heat the pita pockets, place them on a microwave-safe plate. Cover with a damp paper towel, and microwave on high power for about 45 seconds, or until warm. If heating only 1 pita at a time, microwave only 15 seconds.
3. To assemble the sandwiches, place about 1 cup of the tuna mixture in each of the pita halves and serve immediately.

Crab Salad Pitas

YIELD: 4 SERVINGS

2½ cups cooked flaked crabmeat; or 3 cans (6 ounces each) crabmeat, drained
¾ cup diced, peeled, and seeded cucumber or avocado
¼ cup finely chopped celery
¼ cup sliced scallions
¼ cup diced red bell pepper
4 whole-wheat or oat-bran pita pockets (6-inch rounds), cut in half
8 leaves Boston or Bibb lettuce

Dressing
¼ cup plus 2 tablespoons nonfat or light mayonnaise
¼ cup nonfat or light sour cream
1½ teaspoons finely chopped fresh dill or ½ teaspoon dried dill

1. Combine the crabmeat, cucumber or avocado, celery, scallions, and bell pepper in a large bowl and toss to mix well. Set aside.
2. To make the dressing, combine the mayonnaise, sour cream, and dill in a small bowl, and stir to mix well. Add the dressing to the crab mixture and toss to mix well. Stir in a little more mayonnaise if the mixture seems too dry. Set aside.
3. Heat the pita pockets by placing them on a microwave-safe plate, covering with a damp paper towel, and microwaving at high power for about 45 seconds, or until soft and warm. If heating only 1 pita at a time, microwave only 15 seconds.
4. Line each pocket with a lettuce leaf, and stuff scant ½ cup of the crab salad into each pocket. Serve immediately.

Nutritional Facts (per serving)
  CALORIES: 255 CARBOHYDRATES: 35 G CHOLESTEROL: 56 MG FAT: 2 G FIBER: 4.7 G
  PROTEIN: 24 G SODIUM: 755 MG CALCIUM: 114 MG GI RATING: MODERATE

Portabella Pitas

YIELD: 4 SERVINGS

24 ½-inch-thick slices Portabella mushrooms (about 12 ounces)
4 ½-inch-thick slices red onion
¼ cup nonfat or light balsamic vinaigrette salad dressing
4 whole-wheat or oat-bran pita pockets (6-inch rounds), cut in half
7-ounce jar roasted red bell peppers, drained and cut into 8 equal pieces
4 ounces thinly sliced or shredded reduced-fat Swiss cheese

Sauce
¼ cup plus 2 tablespoons nonfat or light mayonnaise
2 tablespoons Dijon mustard

1. To make the sauce, combine the mayonnaise and mustard in a small bowl and stir to mix well. Set aside.
2. Coat a large baking sheet with nonstick cooking spray and arrange the mushroom and onion slices in a single layer on the sheet. Brush both sides of the mushroom and onion slices with some of the balsamic vinaigrette dressing. Place the sheet under a preheated broiler and broil for 4 minutes or until the mushrooms and onions are nicely browned. Turn the slices and broil for an additional 3 minutes or until the slices are tender and browned on both sides. Separate the onion slices into rings and set aside.
3. Spread some of the mayonnaise mixture inside each of the pita pockets. Fill each pocket with 3 mushroom slices, some of the onion rings, some of the roasted red peppers, and some of the cheese.
4. Arrange each sandwich on a microwave-safe plate, cover with a paper towel, and microwave each sandwich at high power for about 30 seconds, or just until the cheese is melted. Serve hot.

Nutritional Facts (per serving)

CALORIES: 287   CARBOHYDRATES: 46 G   CHOLESTEROL: 3 MG   FAT: 5.4 G   FIBER: 8.1 G
PROTEIN: 19 G   SODIUM: 851 MG   CALCIUM: 358 MG   GI RATING: MODERATE

Roasted Vegetable Wraps

YIELD: 4 SERVINGS

1¼ cups 1-inch pieces fresh asparagus spears or ⅜-inch-thick slices zucchini
1¼ cups ½-inch-thick slices baby Portabella or button mushrooms
1 small red bell pepper, cut into ¾-inch-thick strips
1 medium onion, cut into ¾-inch-thick wedges
1 medium plum tomato, sliced ⅜-inch thick
1 tablespoon balsamic vinegar
¾ teaspoon dried Italian seasoning
¼ teaspoon salt
⅛ teaspoon ground black pepper
Nonstick olive oil cooking spray
4 whole-wheat flour tortillas (8-inch rounds)
1 cup shredded nonfat or reduced-fat mozzarella or provolone cheese

1. Place the vegetables, vinegar, Italian seasoning, salt, and black pepper in a large bowl and toss to mix well. Coat a large baking sheet with the cooking spray and spread the mixture in a single layer over the pan. Spray the top of the vegetable mixture lightly with cooking spray.

2. Bake at 450° F for 10 minutes, turn the vegetables with a spatula, and bake for 8 minutes more, or until the vegetables are tender and nicely browned.

3. While the vegetables are cooking, warm the tortillas according to package directions. Arrange the warm tortillas on a flat surface. Spread a quarter of the vegetable mixture over the lower third of each tortilla, leaving a 1-inch margin on the right and left sides. Top the vegetables on each tortilla with a quarter of the cheese.

4. Fold the right and left margins in, then roll each tortilla up from the bottom jellyroll style. Cut each wrap in half and serve immediately.

Nutritional Facts (per serving)
CALORIES: 222 CARBOHYDRATES: 32 G CHOLESTEROL: 3 MG FAT: 3.3 G FIBER: 4.2 G
PROTEIN: 15 G SODIUM: 564 MG CALCIUM: 239 MG GI RATING: MODERATE

California Wraps

YIELD: 4 SERVINGS

4 whole-wheat flour tortillas (8-inch rounds)
8 ounces thinly sliced roasted turkey breast
4 ounces thinly sliced nonfat or reduced-fat Swiss or Monterey Jack cheese
12 (¼-inch-thick) slices avocado
¼ cup Yogurt Ranch Dressing (page 174) or bottled nonfat or light ranch salad
  dressing
1 small carrot, coarsely shredded with a potato peeler
2 thin slices red onion, separated into rings
1 cup alfalfa or spicy sprouts

1. Warm the tortillas according to package directions. Lay the tortillas on a flat surface and top each tortilla with a quarter of the turkey slices, covering the entire tortilla but leaving a 1-inch margin on the right and left sides.
2. Arrange a quarter of the cheese and 3 slices of avocado over the *bottom half only* of each tortilla, and drizzle 1 tablespoon of dressing over the avocados. Arrange a quarter of the carrots, onions, and sprouts over the cheese and avocados.
3. Fold the right and left margins in, then roll each tortilla up from the bottom jellyroll style. Cut each wrap in half and serve immediately.

Nutritional Facts (per serving)
CALORIES: 318 CARBOHYDRATES: 33 G CHOLESTEROL: 49 MG FAT: 6 G FIBER: 3.8 G
PROTEIN: 30 G SODIUM: 512 MG CALCIUM: 170 MG GI RATING: MODERATE

Tempting Turkey Wraps

YIELD: 4 SERVINGS

4 whole-wheat flour tortillas (8-inch rounds)
½ cup nonfat or reduced-fat garlic-and-herb-flavored cream cheese, softened at
  room temperature
8 ounces thinly sliced roasted turkey breast

1 cup chopped canned artichoke hearts, drained

2 tablespoons bottled nonfat or light balsamic vinaigrette salad dressing

8 thin rings red bell pepper

2 thin slices red onion, separated into rings

12 leaves fresh spinach or arugula leaves

1. Warm the tortillas according to package directions. Lay the tortillas on a flat surface and spread each with 2 tablespoons of the cream cheese, extending the cheese all the way to the edges. Top each tortilla with one-quarter of the turkey slices, covering the entire tortilla but leaving a 1-inch margin on the right and left sides.

2. Scatter a quarter of the artichoke hearts over the *bottom half only* of each tortilla, then drizzle 1½ teaspoons of the dressing over the artichoke hearts. Arrange some of the red bell peppers, onions, and spinach or arugula over the bottom half of the tortilla.

3. Fold the right and left margins in, then roll each tortilla up from the bottom jellyroll style. Cut each wrap in half, and serve immediately.

Nutritional Facts (per serving)

CALORIES: 279   CARBOHYDRATES: 34 G   CHOLESTEROL: 49 MG   FAT: 3.5 G   FIBER: 5.1 G

PROTEIN: 27 G   SODIUM: 455 MG   CALCIUM: 276 MG   GI RATING: MODERATE

12. Smart Side Dishes

Choosing the right side dishes can substantially lighten your glycemic load. Side dishes like baked or mashed potatoes, French fries, instant rice, and instant stuffing rank very high on the glycemic index. Pair any of these foods with high-GI bread, and you double your glycemic load.

So what can you serve alongside your favorite entrée? Fresh vegetables and whole grains are the best choices by far. Busy cooks will be happy to know that the less you do to vegetables in the way of cooking, the better off your side dish will be nutritionally. Simple cooking methods like steaming, roasting, and stir-frying are superior techniques for preserving nutrients. Or cook your vegetables in a covered skillet with a few tablespoons of broth or wine.

It is equally easy to base your side dishes on wholesome whole grains like brown rice, bulgur wheat, barley, and whole-wheat couscous. When combined with plenty of vegetables, a bit of garlic, and some flavorful herbs, you can create savory side dishes that are special enough for any occasion.

Be sure to consider your personal nutrition goals when choosing side dishes. For instance, if you are having a starchy entrée like Creamy Risotto (page 259), pair it with a fresh garden salad and a generous portion of low-carbohydrate vegetables, such as steamed broccoli or roasted asparagus. Add another starchy food like a hearty whole-grain bread if you need the extra carbohydrates and calories.

Fresh Roasted Asparagus

YIELD: 4 SERVINGS

1¼ pounds fresh asparagus spears
Nonstick olive oil or butter-flavored cooking spray
¼ teaspoon salt
⅛ teaspoon ground black pepper

1. Rinse the asparagus spears with cool water and snap off and discard the tough stem ends. Pat the asparagus spears dry with paper towels. Coat a large baking sheet with the cooking spray, and arrange the spears in a single layer on the sheet.
2. Spray the spears lightly with the cooking spray and sprinkle with the salt and black pepper. Bake at 450° F for 10 to 12 minutes or just until the spears are tender. Serve hot.

Nutritional Facts (per serving)

CALORIES: 30 CARBOHYDRATES: 5 G CHOLESTEROL: 0 MG FAT: 0.5 G FIBER: 2.4 G
PROTEIN: 2.4 G SODIUM: 145 MG CALCIUM: 24 MG GI RATING: VERY LOW

Autumn Acorn Squash

YIELD: 4 SERVINGS

2 medium acorn squash (about 1 pound each)
2 tablespoons frozen apple juice concentrate
2 tablespoons light margarine or butter
½ teaspoon dried rosemary (optional)

1. Wash the squash with cool water and trim off the ends. Slice each squash crosswise into 4 rings. Remove the seeds, then cut each ring in half to make two semicircles.
2. Coat a 9-by-13-inch pan with nonstick cooking spray and arrange the squash in a single layer in the pan.
3. Combine the juice concentrate and the margarine or butter in a small microwave-safe bowl and microwave at high power for about 30 seconds or until the margarine or butter is melted. Drizzle the juice mixture over the squash and sprinkle with the rosemary if desired.
4. Cover the pan with aluminum foil and bake at 400° F for 25 minutes, or until the squash is tender. Remove the foil, and bake for an additional 5 minutes, or until most of the liquid has evaporated. Serve hot.

Nutritional Facts (per serving)

CALORIES: 94 CARBOHYDRATES: 18 G CHOLESTEROL: 0 MG FAT: 2.6 G FIBER: 4.5 G
PROTEIN: 1.2 G SODIUM: 43 MG CALCIUM: 46 MG GI RATING: MODERATE

Green Beans with Toasted Almonds

🌿 For variety, substitute chopped walnuts for the almonds.

YIELD: 5 SERVINGS

5 cups 1-inch pieces fresh green beans (about 1¼ pounds)
¾ teaspoon dried thyme
1 tablespoon plus 1 teaspoon light margarine or butter
3–4 tablespoons sliced toasted almonds (page 78)
⅛ teaspoon salt

1. Fill a 4-quart pot half full with water and bring to a boil over high heat. Add the green beans and ½ teaspoon of the thyme and boil for about 4 minutes or just until the green beans are crisp-tender.
2. Drain the beans well and return them to the pot. Add the margarine or butter, the almonds, the remaining ¼ teaspoon of thyme, and the salt. Cook over low heat, tossing to mix, for a minute or two or until the margarine or butter is melted. Serve hot.

Nutritional Facts (per ¾-cup serving)
CALORIES: 67 CARBOHYDRATES: 8 G CHOLESTEROL: 0 MG FAT: 3.3 G FIBER: 4.1 G
PROTEIN: 2.7 G SODIUM: 91 MG CALCIUM: 50 MG GI RATING: VERY LOW

Mediterranean Green Beans

YIELD: 5 SERVINGS

4 cups 1-inch pieces fresh green beans (about 1 pound)
1 tablespoon extra-virgin olive oil
1½ teaspoons crushed garlic
1 cup chopped seeded plum tomato (about 4 medium)
¾ teaspoon dried oregano
¼ teaspoon salt
⅛ teaspoon ground black pepper

1. Fill a 3-quart pot half full with water and bring to a boil over high heat. Add the green beans and boil for about 4 minutes or just until the green beans are crisp-tender. Drain the beans well and set aside.

2. Add the olive oil to the pot used to cook the green beans and place the pot over medium heat. Add the garlic and cook for a few seconds, or just until the garlic begins to turn color and smells fragrant. Add the tomatoes and the oregano, salt, and pepper, cover, and cook for about 45 seconds or just until the tomatoes are heated through. Add the green beans to the tomato mixture and toss to mix well. Serve hot.

Nutritional Facts (per ¾-cup serving)
CALORIES: 58 CARBOHYDRATES: 8 G CHOLESTEROL: 0 MG FAT: 2.9 G FIBER: 3.4 G
PROTEIN: 1.9 G SODIUM: 124 MG CALCIUM: 34 MG GI RATING: VERY LOW

Broccoli Rabe with Garlic and Olive Oil

Broccoli rabe looks and tastes like a cross between broccoli and greens. Like all cruciferous vegetables, it is packed with nutrients.

YIELD: 5 SERVINGS

1 pound broccoli rabe
3–4 teaspoons extra-virgin olive oil
2–3 teaspoons crushed garlic
¼ teaspoon salt
⅛ teaspoon ground black pepper
Grated Parmesan cheese (optional)

1. Rinse the broccoli rabe with cool water and shake off the excess water, but do not dry. Cut off about 1½ inches from the bottoms to remove the tough stem ends. Cut the broccoli rabe into 1-inch pieces and set aside. (There should be about 8 cups.)

2. Place 2 tablespoons of water in a large, deep nonstick skillet and add the broccoli rabe. Place the skillet over medium-high heat and cook, tossing frequently, for several minutes or until the leaves are wilted and the stems are crisp-tender. Periodically place a lid over the skillet if it becomes too dry. Add a little more water to the skillet during cooking if necessary, but only enough to prevent scorching. (Note that if you prefer a milder flavor, you can cook the broccoli

rabe in a large pot of boiling water for about 2 minutes, or until crisp-tender. Then drain the broccoli rabe and toss it with the sautéed garlic and olive oil in step 3.)

3. Push the broccoli rabe to one side of the skillet and add the oil and garlic. Sauté the garlic in the oil for a few seconds or just until it smells fragrant and begins to turn color. Remove the skillet from the heat and sprinkle the salt and black pepper over the top. Toss the broccoli rabe to coat it with the oil and garlic. Serve hot, topping each serving with a sprinkling of Parmesan cheese if desired.

Nutritional Facts (per ⅔-cup serving)

CALORIES: 49 CARBOHYDRATES: 4 G CHOLESTEROL: 0 MG FAT: 3.3 G FIBER: 2.8 G
PROTEIN: 2.6 G SODIUM: 165 MG CALCIUM: 27 MG GI RATING: VERY LOW

Braised Cabbage & Onions

YIELD: 4 SERVINGS

½ medium-large head cabbage
2 teaspoons extra-virgin olive oil
1 medium yellow onion, thinly sliced
¼ teaspoon dried thyme
¼ cup water
¼ teaspoon salt

1. Cut the piece of cabbage in half and trim away the core. Cut the cabbage into ½-inch slices and set aside.

2. Coat a large nonstick skillet with the olive oil and place over medium heat. Add the onions and thyme, cover, and cook, stirring occasionally, for about 3 minutes or until the onions start to soften (do not let them brown).

3. Add the cabbage, water, and salt to the skillet and reduce the heat to medium-low. Cover and cook, stirring occasionally, for about 10 minutes or until the cabbage is wilted and tender. Add a little more water during cooking if the skillet becomes too dry, keeping only enough liquid in the skillet to prevent scorching. Serve hot.

Nutritional Facts (per ¾-cup serving)

CALORIES: 63 CARBOHYDRATES: 9 G CHOLESTEROL: 0 MG FAT: 2.6 G FIBER: 3.4 G
PROTEIN: 2.1 G SODIUM: 167 MG CALCIUM: 63 MG GI RATING: VERY LOW

Sweet and Sour Cabbage

2 teaspoons canola or walnut oil
1 medium yellow onion, chopped
1 medium Granny Smith apple, peeled and chopped
4 cups coarsely shredded red cabbage (about ½ medium head)
¼ cup vegetable or chicken broth
3 tablespoons frozen apple juice concentrate
2 tablespoons apple cider vinegar
¼ teaspoon salt
⅛ teaspoon ground black pepper

1. Coat a large nonstick skillet with the oil and place over medium heat. Add the onions, cover, and cook, stirring occasionally, for about 3 minutes or until the onions start to soften. Add a few teaspoons of water if the skillet begins to dry out.

2. Add the remaining ingredients to the skillet and stir to mix well. Reduce the heat to medium-low, cover, and cook, stirring occasionally, for about 12 minutes or until the cabbage is tender. Add a little more broth during cooking if the skillet becomes too dry, but only enough to prevent scorching. If there is excess liquid in the skillet at the end of cooking, remove the lid and cook, stirring frequently, for a minute or two or until most of the liquid evaporates. Serve hot.

Nutritional Facts (per ⅔-cup serving)

CALORIES: 75 CARBOHYDRATES: 14 G CHOLESTEROL: 0 MG FAT: 2.4 G FIBER: 2.4 G
PROTEIN: 1.3 G SODIUM: 162 MG CALCIUM: 36 MG GI RATING: VERY LOW

Asian-Style Collard Greens

For variety, substitute fresh spinach leaves for the collard greens.

1 pound fresh collard greens
3 tablespoons orange juice

2 teaspoons toasted (dark) sesame oil
1½ teaspoons crushed garlic
1 tablespoon reduced-sodium soy sauce

1. Rinse the greens with cool water and shake off the excess water. Trim the leaves away from the tough stalks that run through the center. Stack the leaves and cut them into ¾-inch strips. Set them aside. There should be about 6 cups (packed) of greens.
2. Pour the orange juice in a large, deep nonstick skillet and add the greens. Place the skillet over medium-high heat and cook, tossing frequently, for a couple of minutes or just until the leaves turn bright green and are wilted but still crisp-tender. Add a little more juice to the skillet during cooking if necessary.
3. Push the greens to one side of the skillet and add the oil and garlic. Sauté the garlic in the oil for a few seconds, or just until it smells fragrant and begins to turn color. Remove the skillet from the heat and sprinkle the soy sauce over the top. Toss the greens to coat them with the soy sauce, oil, and garlic, and serve immediately.

Nutritional Facts (per ¾-cup serving)

CALORIES: 61 CARBOHYDRATES: 8 G CHOLESTEROL: 0 MG FAT: 2.7 G FIBER: 4.1 G
PROTEIN: 3.1 G SODIUM: 174 MG CALCIUM: 165 MG GI RATING: VERY LOW

Variation: Mediterranean-Style Collard Greens
Substitute extra-virgin olive oil for the sesame oil and substitute ¼ teaspoon salt and ⅛ teaspoon ground black pepper for the soy sauce.

Nutritional Facts (per ¾-cup serving)

CALORIES: 59 CARBOHYDRATES: 7 G CHOLESTEROL: 0 MG FAT: 2.7 G FIBER: 4.1 G
PROTEIN: 2.9 G SODIUM: 168 MG CALCIUM: 165 MG GI RATING: VERY LOW

Sautéed Snow Peas

YIELD: 4 SERVINGS

1 tablespoon plus 1 teaspoon reduced-fat margarine or light butter
4 cups fresh snow peas
¼ teaspoon dried dill
⅛ teaspoon salt

1. Put the margarine or butter in a large nonstick skillet and preheat over medium-high heat.
2. Add all the remaining ingredients, cover, and cook, stirring frequently, for several minutes or until the snow peas are crisp-tender. Serve hot.

Nutritional Facts (per ¾-cup serving)

CALORIES: 41 CARBOHYDRATES: 5 G CHOLESTEROL: 0 MG FAT: 1.8 G FIBER: 1.6 G
PROTEIN: 1.8 G SODIUM: 108 MG CALCIUM: 27 MG GI RATING: VERY LOW

Summer Garden Sauté

YIELD: 5 SERVINGS

2 tablespoons reduced-fat margarine or light butter
2 large zucchini squash (about 1 pound), halved lengthwise and sliced ¼ inch thick
½ medium onion, cut into ½-inch wedges
1 cup fresh or frozen whole-kernel corn, thawed
½ cup matchstick-sized pieces red bell pepper
1 teaspoon crushed garlic
½ teaspoon dried thyme or oregano
¼ teaspoon salt

1. Put the margarine or butter in a large nonstick skillet and preheat over medium-high heat.
2. Add the remaining ingredients and cook, stirring frequently, for about 4 minutes or until the vegetables are crisp-tender. Place a lid over the skillet periodically if it becomes too dry. (The steam released from the cooking vegetables will moisten the skillet.) Serve hot.

Nutritional Facts (per ¾-cup serving)

CALORIES: 66 CARBOHYDRATES: 11 G CHOLESTEROL: 0 MG FAT: 2.4 G FIBER: 2.5 G
PROTEIN: 2.1 G SODIUM: 160 MG CALCIUM: 16 MG GI RATING: LOW

Zucchini & Mushroom Sauté

YIELD: 4 SERVINGS

2–3 teaspoons extra-virgin olive oil
3 cups sliced zucchini squash (about 3 medium)

2 cups sliced fresh mushrooms

1½ teaspoons crushed garlic

¼ teaspoon salt

⅛ teaspoon coarsely ground black pepper

1. Coat a large nonstick skillet with the olive oil and preheat over medium-high heat.
2. Add all the remaining ingredients and cook, stirring frequently, for about 4 minutes, or until the vegetables are crisp-tender. Place a lid over the skillet periodically if it becomes too dry. (The steam released from the cooking vegetables will moisten the skillet.)

Nutritional Facts (per ¾-cup serving)

CALORIES: 42 CARBOHYDRATES: 4.5 G CHOLESTEROL: 0 MG FAT: 2.5 G FIBER: 1.6 G
PROTEIN: 2 G SODIUM: 149 MG CALCIUM: 16 MG GI RATING: VERY LOW

Broccoli-Macaroni Bake

YIELD: 8 SERVINGS

5 ounces elbow macaroni (about 1¼ cups)

2 cups skim or low-fat milk

2 tablespoons plus 1 ½ teaspoons unbleached flour

2 tablespoons instant nonfat dry milk powder

¾ teaspoon dry mustard

8 ounces diced reduced-fat process Cheddar cheese (like Velveeta Light) or finely shredded reduced-fat Cheddar cheese (about 2 cups)

10-ounce package frozen chopped broccoli, thawed and squeezed dry

2 tablespoons dried bread crumbs

Butter-flavored nonstick cooking spray

1. Cook the macaroni al dente according to package directions. Drain well and return to the pot. Set aside.
2. While the macaroni is cooking, combine ½ cup of the milk and all the flour, milk powder, and dry mustard in a jar with a tight-fitting lid. Shake until smooth and set aside.
3. Pour the remaining 1½ cups of milk into a 2-quart pot and bring to a boil over medium heat, stirring constantly. Add the flour mixture and cook, still stirring, for about 1 minute or until bubbly. Reduce the heat to medium-low, add the cheese, and stir just until the cheese melts. Remove the pot from the heat.

4. Pour the cheese sauce over the macaroni and toss to mix well. Add the broccoli and toss to mix well. Coat a 2-quart casserole dish with nonstick cooking spray and spread the macaroni mixture evenly in the dish. Sprinkle the bread crumbs over the top and spray lightly with the cooking spray. Bake at 350° F for about 30 minutes or until the top is lightly browned and the dish is hot and bubbly around the edges. Remove the dish from the oven and let sit for 15 minutes before serving.

Nutritional Facts (per ¾-cup serving)

CALORIES: 174   CARBOHYDRATES: 24 G   CHOLESTEROL: 11 MG   FAT: 3.5 G   FIBER: 1.6 G
PROTEIN: 12 G   SODIUM: 485 MG   CALCIUM: 263 MG   GI RATING: LOW

Roasted Portabella Mushrooms

YIELD: 4 SERVINGS

Nonstick olive oil cooking spray
20 ½-inch-thick slices Portabella mushrooms (about 12 ounces)
¼ teaspoon salt
⅛ teaspoon ground black pepper
¾ teaspoon fines herbes or dried thyme

1. Coat a large baking sheet with the cooking spray and arrange the mushroom slices in a single layer on the sheet. Spray the mushrooms lightly with the cooking spray and sprinkle with the salt, black pepper, and herbs.
2. Bake at 450° F for 10 minutes, turn the slices over, and bake for an additional 5 minutes or until the mushrooms are tender and nicely browned. Serve hot.

Nutritional Facts (per serving)

CALORIES: 21   CARBOHYDRATES: 4 G   CHOLESTEROL: 0 MG   FAT: 0.4 G   FIBER: 1 G
PROTEIN: 1.8 G   SODIUM: 148 MG   CALCIUM: 4 MG   GI RATING: VERY LOW

Roasted Peppers, Onions, and Mushrooms

YIELD: 6 SERVINGS

1 medium-large onion, cut into 1-inch wedges
8 ounces sliced baby Portabella mushrooms or ½-inch-thick slices button
    mushrooms (about 3 cups)
1 green bell pepper, cut into ¾-inch-thick strips
1 red bell pepper, cut into ¾-inch-thick strips
1 tablespoon balsamic vinegar
1 tablespoon extra-virgin olive oil
1½ teaspoons crushed garlic
1 teaspoon dried Italian seasoning
¼ teaspoon salt
¼ teaspoon coarsely ground black pepper

1. Place all ingredients in a large bowl and toss to mix well. Coat a large shallow roasting pan (at least 11 by 13 inches) with nonstick cooking spray and spread the mixture evenly in the pan.
2. Bake at 450° F for about 30 minutes, stirring every 10 minutes, or until the vegetables are tender and nicely browned. Serve hot.

Nutritional Facts (per ¾-cup serving)
CALORIES: 55 CARBOHYDRATES: 7 G CHOLESTEROL: 0 MG FAT: 2.6 G FIBER: 1.8 G
PROTEIN: 1.5 G SODIUM: 100 MG CALCIUM: 12 MG GI RATING: VERY LOW

Sautéed Mushrooms with Sherry

YIELD: 4 SERVINGS

2–3 teaspoons extra-virgin olive oil
1 teaspoon crushed garlic
1 pound sliced fresh mushrooms
¼ teaspoon salt
¼ teaspoon ground black pepper
2–3 tablespoons dry sherry, red wine, or white wine

1. Coat a large nonstick skillet with the olive oil and preheat over medium-high heat. Add the garlic, mushrooms, salt, and black pepper, and cook, stirring frequently, for several minutes or until the mushrooms are tender and nicely browned. Place a lid over the skillet periodically if it begins to dry out. (The steam released from the cooking mushrooms will moisten the skillet.)
2. Add the sherry or wine to the skillet, and cook for another minute or two, or until most of the sherry or wine has evaporated. Serve hot.

Nutritional Facts (per ¾-cup serving)

CALORIES: 58 CARBOHYDRATES: 5 G CHOLESTEROL: 0 MG FAT: 2.7 G FIBER: 1 G

PROTEIN: 2.4 G SODIUM: 151 MG CALCIUM: 7 MG GI RATING: VERY LOW

Savory Black-Eyed Peas

YIELD: 6 SERVINGS

1½ cups dried black-eyed peas
2½ teaspoons instant vegetable, ham, or chicken bouillon granules; or 1½ teaspoons
    bouillon granules plus ¾ cup diced smoked turkey or lean ham (about 4
    ounces)
½ cup chopped onion
1 teaspoon dried sage
⅛ teaspoon ground black pepper
⅛ teaspoon ground cayenne pepper
4 cups water

1. Combine all the ingredients in a 3-quart pot and bring to a boil over high heat.
2. Reduce the heat to low, cover, and simmer for about 1 hour or until the beans are soft and the liquid is thick. Serve hot.

Nutritional Facts (per ¾-cup serving)

CALORIES: 147 CARBOHYDRATES: 26 G CHOLESTEROL: 0 MG FAT: 0.6 G FIBER: 4.7 G

PROTEIN: 10 G SODIUM: 273 MG CALCIUM: 48 MG GI RATING: LOW

Rosemary Roasted Sweet Potatoes

YIELD: 6 SERVINGS

5 cups ¼-inch-thick peeled sweet potato slices (about 1¾ pounds)
1 teaspoon dried rosemary
1½ teaspoons crushed garlic
¼ teaspoon salt
1 tablespoon extra-virgin olive oil

1. Place the potatoes in a large bowl. Sprinkle with the rosemary, garlic, and salt and drizzle with the olive oil. Toss well to coat.
2. Coat a 9-by-13-inch pan with nonstick cooking spray and spread the potatoes evenly in the pan. Cover the pan with aluminum foil and bake at 400° F for 15 minutes. Remove the foil and bake for 10 additional minutes. Turn the potatoes and bake for 10 minutes more or until tender. Serve hot.

Nutritional Facts (per ⅔-cup serving)
CALORIES: 104 CARBOHYDRATES: 19 G CHOLESTEROL: 0 MG FAT: 2.3 G FIBER: 2.4 G
PROTEIN: 1.4 G SODIUM: 105 MG CALCIUM: 23 MG GI RATING: LOW

Parsley New Potatoes

YIELD: 6 SERVINGS

4½ cups 1-inch chunks small new potatoes (about 1¼ pounds)
¼ to ⅓ cup finely chopped fresh parsley
1 tablespoon plus 1 teaspoon extra-virgin olive oil
¼ teaspoon salt

1. Place the potatoes in a 4-quart pot and cover with water. Bring to a boil over high heat. Reduce the heat to medium and cook for about 12 minutes or until the potatoes are tender. Drain the potatoes and return them to the pot.
2. Add the parsley, olive oil, and salt to the potatoes, and toss to mix well. Serve hot.

Nutritional Facts (per ¾-cup serving)

CALORIES: 110 CARBOHYDRATES: 19 G CHOLESTEROL: 0 MG FAT: 3.1 G FIBER: 2 G
PROTEIN: 1.8 G SODIUM: 104 MG CALCIUM: 11 MG GI RATING: MODERATE

Unfried Green Tomatoes

YIELD: 5 SERVINGS

1½ cups Special K cereal
¼ cup plus 2 tablespoons grated Parmesan cheese
1 teaspoon dried basil
¼ teaspoon ground black pepper
¼ cup plus 2 tablespoons fat-free egg substitute
1 pound green tomatoes (about 3 medium-large), sliced ¼-inch thick
Nonstick olive oil or garlic-flavored cooking spray

1. Place the cereal in a food processor and process into coarse crumbs. (Alternatively, place the crumbs in a plastic zip-type bag and crush with a rolling pin or the bottom of a glass.) There should be ¾ cup of crumbs.
2. Combine the cereal crumbs, Parmesan cheese, basil, and black pepper in a shallow bowl and stir to mix well. Pour the egg substitute into another shallow bowl.
3. Dip the tomato slices first in the egg substitute and then in the crumb mixture, turning to coat both sides well. Coat a large baking sheet with nonstick cooking spray and arrange the slices in a single layer on the sheet. Spray the tops lightly with the cooking spray.
4. Bake at 450° F for 8 minutes. Turn the slices with a spatula and bake for an additional 8 to 10 minutes or until golden brown and tender. Serve hot.

Nutritional Facts (per serving)

CALORIES: 93 CARBOHYDRATES: 10 G CHOLESTEROL: 6 MG FAT: 2.5 G FIBER: 1.2 G
PROTEIN: 7.5 G SODIUM: 248 MG CALCIUM: 115 MG GI RATING: LOW

Mushroom & Herb Pilaf

YIELD: 5 SERVINGS

1½ cups sliced fresh mushrooms
¼ cup finely chopped onion

¼ cup finely chopped celery

½ teaspoon dried thyme

2 tablespoons light margarine or butter

3 cups cooked brown rice, wild rice, barley, or bulgur wheat

⅛ teaspoon salt

1. Coat a large nonstick skillet with nonstick cooking spray and add the mushrooms, onion, celery, and thyme. Place the skillet over medium-high heat, cover, and cook, stirring frequently, for several minutes or until the vegetables are tender. Add a little water or broth if the skillet becomes too dry.

2. Reduce the heat to medium, add the margarine or butter, and stir until it melts. Add the grain and salt to the skillet mixture and cook and stir for a minute or two or until the mixture is heated through. Serve hot.

Nutritional Facts (per ¾-cup serving)

CALORIES: 155 CARBOHYDRATES: 28 G CHOLESTEROL: 0 MG FAT: 3.1 G FIBER: 2.5 G

PROTEIN: 3.5 G SODIUM: 107 MG CALCIUM: 15 MG GI RATING: LOW

Sesame Fried Rice

YIELD: 6 SERVINGS

1 tablespoon sesame oil

1 teaspoon crushed garlic

¾ teaspoon freshly grated ginger root; or ¼ teaspoon dried ginger

2 cups finely chopped fresh broccoli

1 cup coarsely chopped fresh mushrooms

½ cup finely chopped carrots

2 tablespoons vegetable or chicken broth

3 cups cooked brown rice

2 tablespoons reduced-sodium soy sauce

1. Pour the oil in a large nonstick skillet, and preheat over medium-high heat. Add the garlic and ginger and stir-fry for a few seconds or just until the garlic begins to turn color and smells fragrant. Add the broccoli, mushrooms, carrots, and broth to the skillet. Cover and cook, stirring frequently, for about 3 minutes or until the vegetables are crisp-tender. Add a little more broth if the skillet becomes too dry.

2. Reduce the heat to medium and add the rice, and soy sauce. Cook and stir for a minute or two or until the mixture is heated through. Serve hot.

Nutritional Facts (per ⅞-cup serving)

CALORIES: 147 CARBOHYDRATES: 25 G CHOLESTEROL: 0 MG FAT: 3.3 G FIBER: 3.1 G
PROTEIN: 4 G SODIUM: 218 MG CALCIUM: 27 MG GI RATING: LOW

Garden Pilaf

YIELD: 4 SERVINGS

2 tablespoons reduced-fat margarine or light butter
⅓ cup chopped onion
⅓ cup chopped red bell pepper
1 cup frozen chopped broccoli, thawed
⅔ cup frozen whole-kernel corn, thawed
1 tablespoon finely chopped fresh parsley; or 1 teaspoon dried parsley
¼ teaspoon salt
2 cups prepared bulgur wheat

1. Place the margarine or butter in a large nonstick skillet and preheat over medium-high heat. Add the onions and bell peppers, cover, and cook, stirring frequently, for a couple of minutes or until the vegetables are crisp-tender.
2. Add the broccoli, corn, parsley, and salt to the skillet mixture and reduce the heat to medium. Cook, stirring frequently, for a couple of minutes or until the vegetables are heated through. Add the bulgur wheat and cook covered for another minute or two or until heated through. Serve hot.

Nutritional Facts (per ⅞-cup serving)

CALORIES: 140 CARBOHYDRATES: 26 G CHOLESTEROL: 0 MG FAT: 3 G FIBER: 6.4 G
PROTEIN: 5 G SODIUM: 198 MG CALCIUM: 37 MG GI RATING: LOW

Curried Couscous

⅓ cup finely chopped onion
⅓ cup finely chopped celery
1½ cups reduced-sodium chicken or vegetable broth
1½ teaspoons curry paste
1 cup whole-wheat couscous
¼ cup chopped dried apricots or golden raisins
¼ cup sliced toasted almonds (page 78) or chopped roasted peanuts

1. Coat a large nonstick skillet with cooking spray and preheat over medium heat. Add the onion and celery to the skillet, cover, and cook, stirring frequently, for about 3 minutes or until the vegetables are crisp-tender. Add a few teaspoons of water if the skillet becomes too dry.
2. Add the broth and curry paste and stir to mix well. Add the couscous, apricots or raisins, and the almonds or peanuts, and stir to mix well. Bring the mixture to a boil, then reduce the heat to low, cover, and cook for 2 minutes without stirring. Remove the skillet from the heat and let sit for 5 minutes. Fluff with a fork and serve hot.

Nutritional Facts (per ¾-cup serving)
CALORIES: 196 CARBOHYDRATES: 35 G CHOLESTEROL: 0 MG FAT: 4.2 FIBER: 6.1 G
PROTEIN: 6.8 G SODIUM: 151 MG CALCIUM: 34 MG GI RATING: MODERATE

Confetti Couscous

For variety, add 1 to 1½ teaspoons of mild curry paste along with the water.

2 tablespoons reduced-fat margarine or light butter
½ cup finely chopped celery
½ cup finely chopped onion
½ cup finely chopped carrot
¾ teaspoon crushed garlic

1½ cups water
¼ teaspoon salt
1 cup whole-wheat couscous
¾ cup frozen green peas

1. Coat a large nonstick skillet with the margarine or butter and preheat over medium heat. Add the celery, onion, carrot, and garlic to the skillet, cover, and cook, stirring frequently, for several minutes or until the vegetables are crisp-tender.
2. Add the water, salt, couscous, and peas to the skillet and stir to mix well. Bring the mixture to a boil, then reduce the heat to low, cover, and cook for 2 minutes without stirring. Remove the skillet from the heat and let sit for 5 minutes. Fluff with a fork, and serve hot.

Nutritional Facts (per ¾-cup serving)

CALORIES: 180   CARBOHYDRATES: 35 G   CHOLESTEROL: 0 MG   FAT: 2.5 G   FIBER: 6.2 G
PROTEIN: 6.6 G   SODIUM: 163 MG   CALCIUM: 27 MG   GI RATING: MODERATE

Broccoli Couscous

YIELD: 6 SERVINGS

1½ cups water
2 tablespoons reduced-fat margarine or light butter
¼ teaspoon salt
10-ounce package frozen chopped broccoli, thawed and drained
1 cup whole-wheat couscous

1. Put the water, margarine or butter, and salt in a 2½-quart pot and bring to a boil over high heat. Stir in the broccoli and couscous and let the mixture come to a boil.
2. Reduce the heat to low, cover, and cook for 2 minutes without stirring. Remove the pot from the heat and let sit for 5 minutes. Fluff with a fork, and serve hot.

Nutritional Facts (per ⅞-cup serving)

CALORIES: 166   CARBOHYDRATES: 32 G   CHOLESTEROL: 0 MG   FAT: 2.4 G   FIBER: 5.9 G
PROTEIN: 6.6 G   SODIUM: 140 MG   CALCIUM: 35 MG   GI RATING: MODERATE

13. Pasta Perfection

Pasta is proof that all carbohydrates are not alike. With a glycemic index in the 35 to 50 range, pasta has a mild effect on blood sugar and insulin levels; perhaps this is why pasta is such a prominent player in some of the world's most healthful cuisines.

The dishes in this chapter have been developed with both taste and nutrition in mind. Pasta is combined with lean meats, seafood, plenty of garden vegetables, and light sauces to provide dishes that allow for generous portions without blowing your fat, calorie, or carbohydrate budgets. Many of these dishes can also be whipped up in a matter of minutes, making them perfect for busy cooks.

While the pasta entrées in this chapter rank low on the glycemic index, realize that, like all starchy foods, pasta is a fairly concentrated source of carbohydrate. So when planning pasta meals, be sure to keep your calorie and carbohydrate goals in mind. For instance, if you are watching your weight, balance your pasta entrée with lower-carbohydrate side dishes like nonstarchy vegetables and a fresh garden salad. Add some crusty whole-grain bread to your meal if you need the extra carbohydrates and calories.

Italian Beef with Bow Ties

YIELD: 4 SERVINGS

8 ounces bow tie pasta (about 4 cups) or penne pasta (about 3 cups)
12 ounces 95-percent lean ground beef
1 cup chopped onion
1 teaspoon crushed garlic
½ teaspoon dried oregano
14½-ounce can Italian-style stewed tomatoes, undrained
¾ cup beef broth

¼ cup tomato paste with roasted garlic
1 medium-large zucchini, halved lengthwise and sliced ¼-inch thick
¼ cup grated Parmesan cheese (optional)

1. Cook the pasta al dente according to package directions. Drain well, return to the pot, and cover to keep warm.
2. Coat a large, deep nonstick skillet with cooking spray and add the ground beef. Place the skillet over medium heat and cook, stirring to crumble, until the meat is no longer pink. Drain off and discard any excess fat. Add the onions, garlic, and oregano. Cover and cook for about 4 minutes more or until the onions start to soften. Add a little water if the skillet becomes too dry. Add the undrained tomatoes, broth, tomato paste, and zucchini, cover, and cook for about 5 minutes more, stirring occasionally, until the zucchini are tender.
3. Add the pasta to the skillet mixture and toss over low heat to mix well. Add a little more broth if the mixture seems too dry. Serve hot, topping each serving with some of the Parmesan cheese if desired.

Nutritional Facts (per 2-cup serving)
CALORIES: 392   CARBOHYDRATES: 57 G   CHOLESTEROL: 57 MG   FAT: 5.3 G   FIBER: 3.9 G
PROTEIN: 26 G   SODIUM: 457 MG   CALCIUM: 58 MG   GI RATING: LOW

Saucy Spaghetti & Meatballs

YIELD: 5 SERVINGS

Meatballs
1 pound 95-percent lean ground beef
1 cup whole-wheat or multigrain bread crumbs*
1 cup finely chopped fresh mushrooms
¼ cup plus 2 tablespoons finely chopped onion
2 tablespoons fat-free egg substitute; or 1 egg white, lightly beaten
2 tablespoons finely chopped fresh parsley; or 2 teaspoons dried parsley
1 teaspoon crushed garlic

To make whole-wheat bread crumbs, tear about 1½ slices of firm stone-ground, whole-wheat, or multigrain bread into chunks, place in a blender or food processor, and process into crumbs.

¼ teaspoon salt
¼ teaspoon ground black pepper

10 ounces thin spaghetti
1 tablespoon extra-virgin olive oil (optional)
*1 jar (26 ounces) marinara sauce (choose a brand that contains little or no added
    sugar and fat)*

¼ cup plus 2 tablespoons grated Parmesan cheese (optional)

1. To make the meatballs, combine all the meatball ingredients in a large bowl and mix together. Lightly shape the mixture into 20 1¼-inch meatballs. Coat a large baking sheet with nonstick cooking spray and lay the meatballs on the sheet, spacing them evenly apart. Spray the tops of the meatballs lightly with the cooking spray. Bake at 350° F for 30 minutes or until the meatballs are no longer pink inside. Set aside.
2. While the meatballs are baking, cook the spaghetti al dente according to package directions. Drain the pasta, return it to the pot, toss in the olive oil if desired, and cover to keep warm. Set aside.
3. Pour the sauce into a large nonstick skillet. Add the meatballs to the sauce and, using a spatula, scrape up any browned bits from the baking sheet and add them to the sauce. Place the skillet over medium-high heat and bring the mixture to a boil. Reduce the heat to low, cover, and simmer for about 10 minutes or until the flavors are well blended.
4. Serve hot, topping each serving with some of the Parmesan cheese if desired.

Nutritional Facts (per serving)

CALORIES: 404 CARBOHYDRATES: 56 G CHOLESTEROL: 48 MG FAT: 5.4 G FIBER: 4 G
PROTEIN: 29 G SODIUM: 708 MG CALCIUM: 78 MG GI RATING: LOW

Penne with Ham and Asparagus

YIELD: 4 SERVINGS

1¼ cups evaporated skim or low-fat milk
¼ cup fat-free egg substitute
¼ teaspoon coarsely ground black pepper
8 ounces penne pasta (about 3 cups)
1½ cups 1-inch pieces fresh asparagus (about ½ pound)
½ cup frozen (unthawed) green peas

1 teaspoon crushed garlic
4 ounces thinly sliced ham (at least 97-percent lean) cut into thin strips
¼ cup plus 2 tablespoons grated Parmesan cheese, divided

1. Pour the evaporated milk, egg substitute, and black pepper in a small bowl and stir to mix well. Set aside.
2. Cook the pasta al dente according to package directions. One minute before the pasta is done, add the asparagus and peas and cook for 1 minute more or until the asparagus is crisp-tender and the pasta is al dente. Drain well, return to the pot, and cover to keep warm.
3. Coat a large nonstick skillet with cooking spray and preheat over medium-high heat. Add the garlic and ham and cook, stirring frequently, for a couple of minutes or until the ham starts to brown.
4. Reduce the heat under the skillet to medium-low and add the pasta to the skillet. Slowly pour the evaporated milk mixture over the pasta and toss gently for a minute or two or until the sauce thickens slightly. Add a little more evaporated milk if the sauce seems too dry.
5. Remove the skillet from the heat and toss in half of the Parmesan cheese. Serve hot, topping each serving with some of the remaining Parmesan cheese.

Nutritional Facts (per 1¾-cup serving)
CALORIES: 378 CARBOHYDRATES: 58 G CHOLESTEROL: 18 MG FAT: 4.8 G FIBER: 3.3 G
PROTEIN: 26 G SODIUM: 584 MG CALCIUM: 396 MG GI RATING: LOW

Bow Ties with Chicken and Broccoli

YIELD: 4 SERVINGS

Sauce
1¼ cups evaporated skim or low-fat milk
3 tablespoons fat-free egg substitute
2 tablespoons dry sherry
¼ teaspoon lemon pepper or coarsely ground black pepper

8 ounces bow tie pasta (about 4 cups) or penne pasta (about 3 cups)
2 cups small broccoli florets
1½ cups diced or shredded cooked chicken breast
1 cup sliced fresh mushrooms
1 teaspoon crushed garlic
½ cup grated Parmesan cheese

1. Combine all the sauce ingredients in a small bowl and stir to mix well. Set aside.
2. Cook the pasta al dente according to package directions. One minute before the pasta is done, add the broccoli florets and cook for 1 minute more or until the broccoli is crisp-tender and the pasta is al dente. Drain well, return the pasta mixture to the pot, and toss in the chicken.
3. Coat a large nonstick skillet with cooking spray, and place the pot over medium heat. Add the mushrooms and garlic, cover and cook for about 2 minutes, or until the mushrooms start to soften and release their juices. (Do not brown.) Add the pasta mixture to the skillet and pour the sauce over the pasta mixture. Toss gently for a minute or two or until the sauce is heated through and thickens slightly. Add a little more milk if the mixture seems too dry.
4. Remove the skillet from the heat and toss in the Parmesan cheese. Serve hot.

Nutritional Facts (per 2-cup serving)

CALORIES: 442 CARBOHYDRATES: 54 G CHOLESTEROL: 57 MG FAT: 6.5 G FIBER: 2.9 G
PROTEIN: 37 G SODIUM: 398 MG CALCIUM: 449 MG GI RATING: LOW

Greek Chicken Pasta

YIELD: 4 SERVINGS

8 ounces tricolor rotini pasta (about 3 cups)
1 tablespoon extra-virgin olive oil
4 boneless, skinless chicken breast halves (4 ounces each)
¼ teaspoon coarsely ground black pepper
½ cup chicken broth (plus more if needed)
1 teaspoon dried oregano
1 teaspoon crushed garlic
14½-ounce can stewed tomatoes, crushed, undrained
½ cup nonfat or reduced-fat feta cheese
¼ cup sliced black olives
¼ cup sliced scallions

1. Cook the pasta al dente according to package directions. Drain and return it to the pot. Toss in the olive oil. Set aside.
2. While the pasta is cooking, rinse the chicken with cool water, and pat it dry with paper towels. Sprinkle both sides of the chicken pieces with the black pepper. Coat a large nonstick skillet with cooking spray, and preheat over medium-high heat. Add the chicken and cook for about 2 minutes on each side or until nicely browned.

3. Reduce the heat under the skillet to medium-low. Combine ¼ cup of the broth and all the oregano and garlic in a small bowl and stir to mix well. Pour the broth mixture around the chicken. Cover the skillet and cook for about 10 minutes or until the chicken is tender and no longer pink inside. Add a little more broth if the skillet becomes too dry, but only enough to keep the skillet barely moist. Remove the chicken to a cutting board and cover to keep warm.

4. Add the undrained tomatoes and the remaining broth to the skillet. Raise the heat under the skillet to bring the mixture to a boil, then reduce the heat to low.

5. Add the rotini to the skillet and toss over low heat for a minute or two, or until the mixture is heated through. Add a little more broth if the mixture seems too dry.

6. To serve, place one-fourth (about 1⅛ cups) of the rotini mixture on each of 4 serving plates. Slice the chicken at an angle and arrange one sliced chicken breast half over the pasta on each plate. Sprinkle some of the feta cheese, olives, and scallions over each serving. Serve hot.

Nutritional Facts (per serving)

CALORIES: 430 CARBOHYDRATES: 52 G CHOLESTEROL: 66 MG FAT: 6.5 G FIBER: 2.6 G
PROTEIN: 38 G SODIUM: 680 MG CALCIUM: 125 MG GI RATING: LOW

Chicken Pasta Puttanesca

YIELD: 4 SERVINGS

8 ounces thin spaghetti
¾ pound boneless, skinless chicken breast, cut into bite-size pieces
¼ teaspoon salt
1 tablespoon extra-virgin olive oil
2 teaspoons crushed garlic
1 cup chicken broth
½ cup dry white wine
1 teaspoon anchovy paste
¾ teaspoon dried oregano
½ teaspoon crushed red pepper
1 tablespoon small capers
¼ cup sliced black olives
1 cup chopped fresh tomato (about 1 large)
¼ cup grated Parmesan cheese

1. Cook the pasta al dente according to package directions. Drain well, return to the pot, and cover to keep warm.
2. Sprinkle the chicken with the salt and set aside.
3. Pour the olive oil in a large nonstick skillet and preheat over medium-high heat. Add the garlic and chicken and stir-fry for about 4 minutes or until the chicken is nicely browned and no longer pink inside. Remove the chicken to a bowl, cover to keep warm, and set aside.
4. Add the broth, wine, anchovy paste, oregano, and crushed red pepper to the skillet and place the skillet over medium-high heat. Cook, stirring frequently, for several minutes or until the mixture is reduced by half. Add the capers, olives, and tomato to the skillet, cover, and cook for about 1 minute or just until the tomatoes are heated through and are starting to soften.
5. Add the pasta and chicken to the skillet mixture and toss over low heat to mix well. Serve hot, topping each serving with some of the Parmesan cheese.

Nutritional Facts (per 1¾-cup serving)

CALORIES: 402 CARBOHYDRATES: 45 G CHOLESTEROL: 57 MG FAT: 8.3 G FIBER: 2.3 G
PROTEIN: 32 G SODIUM: 696 MG CALCIUM: 61 MG GI RATING: LOW

Spicy Pork Lo Mein

For variety, substitute boneless, skinless chicken breast or shrimp for the pork.

YIELD: 4 SERVINGS

¾ pound pork tenderloin, cut into ¾-inch cubes; or ¾ pound boneless lean pork
    loin chops, cut into thin strips
8 ounces fettuccine pasta or udon noodles
2 cups small broccoli florets
1 cup sliced fresh mushrooms
¾ cup matchstick-sized pieces of red bell pepper
½ cup sliced scallions

Sauce
¾ cup plus 2 tablespoons chicken broth
3 tablespoons reduced-sodium soy sauce
3 tablespoons dry sherry
1 tablespoon plus 1½ teaspoons dark brown sugar

2 teaspoons toasted (dark) sesame oil
3 to 4 teaspoons Szechuan seasoning*
1 teaspoon cornstarch

1. To make the sauce, combine all the sauce ingredients except the cornstarch in a small bowl and stir to mix well.
2. Pour ¼ cup of the sauce mixture over the pork, toss to mix well, and set aside for 20 minutes.
3. Dissolve the cornstarch into 1 tablespoon of the remaining sauce, then add the cornstarch mixture to the sauce and set aside.
4. While the meat is marinating, cook the pasta according to package directions, drain well, and set aside.
5. Coat a large, deep nonstick skillet or wok with cooking spray and preheat over medium-high heat. Add the pork, along with the sauce it is marinating in, and stir-fry for about 4 minutes or until all the liquid evaporates and the meat is thoroughly cooked and nicely browned. Remove the meat from the skillet and set aside to keep warm.
6. Respray the skillet and add the broccoli, mushrooms, bell pepper pieces, and scallions. Stir-fry for about 3 minutes or until the vegetables are crisp-tender. Cover the skillet periodically during cooking as it starts to dry out (the steam released during cooking will moisten the skillet). Add a little water or broth during cooking if needed.
7. Place the pork back in the skillet and toss to mix well. Add the pasta and toss to mix well. Stir the sauce and pour it over the pasta mixture. Cook and stir for a minute or two or until the sauce comes to a boil and thickens slightly. Serve hot.

Nutritional Facts (per 2-cup serving)
CALORIES: 390 CARBOHYDRATES: 54 G CHOLESTEROL: 50 MG FAT: 6.5 G FIBER: 3.9 G
PROTEIN: 28 G SODIUM: 574 MG CALCIUM: 50 MG GI RATING: LOW

Shells and Crab Carbonara

YIELD: 4 SERVINGS

1¼ cups evaporated skim or low-fat milk
¼ cup fat-free egg substitute

*A mixture of ginger, garlic, pepper, and Asian seasonings, Szechuan seasoning can be found in the spice section of most grocery stores. Or combine 1 teaspoon ground ginger, ¾ teaspoon dry mustard, ¾ teaspoon lemon pepper, ½ teaspoon garlic powder, and ½ teaspoon crushed red pepper.

⅛ teaspoon ground white pepper

Pinch ground nutmeg

8 ounces medium seashell pasta (about 3 cups)

1 cup frozen (unthawed) green peas

1 teaspoon crushed garlic

1 tablespoon dry white wine or chicken broth

1 cup sliced fresh mushrooms

1½ cups cooked crabmeat (about 8 ounces); or 2 cans (6 ounces each) crabmeat, drained

½ cup grated Parmesan cheese, divided

1. Combine the evaporated milk, egg substitute, white pepper, and nutmeg in a small bowl and stir to mix well. Set aside.

2. Cook the pasta al dente according to package directions. One minute before the pasta is done, add the peas and cook for 1 minute more or until the peas are heated through and the pasta is al dente. Drain well, return to the pot, and cover to keep warm.

3. Coat a large nonstick skillet with cooking spray and preheat over medium-high heat. Add the garlic, wine or broth, and mushrooms and cook, stirring frequently, for a couple of minutes or until the mushrooms are tender. (Do not brown.)

4. Reduce the heat under the skillet to medium-low and add the pasta mixture and the crabmeat to the skillet. Slowly pour the evaporated milk mixture over the pasta, and toss gently for a minute or two or until the sauce thickens slightly. Add a little more evaporated milk if the sauce seems too dry.

5. Remove the skillet from the heat and toss in half of the Parmesan cheese. Serve hot, topping each serving with a tablespoon of the remaining Parmesan cheese.

Nutritional Facts (per 1½-cup serving)

CALORIES: 420 CARBOHYDRATES: 58 G CHOLESTEROL: 46 MG FAT: 5.6 G FIBER: 3.3 G

PROTEIN: 32 G SODIUM: 568 MG CALCIUM: 454 MG GI RATING: LOW

Mediterranean Tuna Pasta

YIELD: 4 SERVINGS

8 ounces thin spaghetti

1 tablespoon extra-virgin olive oil

2 teaspoons crushed garlic

1 cup chicken broth

½ cup thinly sliced sun-dried tomatoes (not packed in oil)

½ teaspoon dried oregano

½ teaspoon dried basil

¼ teaspoon coarsely ground black pepper

1 cup coarsely chopped frozen (thawed) or canned (drained) artichoke hearts

9-ounce can albacore tuna, drained

¼ cup sliced black olives

½ cup nonfat or reduced-fat crumbled feta cheese

1. Cook the pasta al dente according to package directions. Drain well, and return the pasta to the pot. Add the olive oil, and toss to mix. Cover the pot and set aside to keep warm.

2. Coat a large nonstick skillet with cooking spray and preheat over medium-high heat. Add the garlic and stir-fry for a few seconds or just until the garlic begins to turn color and smells fragrant. Add the broth, tomatoes, oregano, basil, and black pepper to the skillet, and bring the mixture to a boil. Reduce the heat to low, cover, and simmer for about 3 minutes or until the tomatoes are soft.

3. Add the artichoke hearts, drained tuna, and olives to the skillet mixture. Cover and cook for a minute or two or just until heated through. Add the pasta and toss gently to mix. Add a little more broth if the mixture seems too dry. Serve hot, topping each serving with some of the feta cheese.

Nutritional Facts (per 1¾-cup serving)

CALORIES: 386   CARBOHYDRATES: 52 G   CHOLESTEROL: 28 MG   FAT: 7.3 G   FIBER: 4.9 G
PROTEIN: 28 G   SODIUM: 806 MG   CALCIUM: 108 MG   GI RATING: LOW

Sesame-Ginger Scallops and Noodles

YIELD: 4 SERVINGS

1 pound medium-large scallops or peeled and deveined shrimp

8 ounces fettuccine pasta or udon noodles

1½ cups sliced fresh mushrooms

1 cup matchstick-sized carrots

⅓ cup sliced scallions

3 cups (packed) coarsely chopped fresh spinach

Sauce

½ cup orange juice

3 tablespoons reduced-sodium soy sauce

2 teaspoons crushed garlic

1 teaspoon ground ginger

1 tablespoon plus 1 teaspoon light brown sugar

⅛ teaspoon ground white pepper

2 to 3 teaspoons toasted (dark) sesame oil

1 teaspoon cornstarch

½ cup chicken broth

1. To make the sauce, place the orange juice, soy sauce, garlic, ginger, brown sugar, pepper, and sesame oil in a small bowl and stir to mix well. Pour 2 tablespoons of the mixture over the scallops or shrimp, toss to mix well, and set aside for 20 minutes. Dissolve the cornstarch into a tablespoon of the broth, then add the cornstarch mixture and the remaining broth to the sauce. Set aside.

2. While the scallops are marinating, cook the pasta al dente according to package directions, drain well, and set aside.

3. Coat a large, deep nonstick skillet or wok with cooking spray and preheat over medium-high heat. Add the scallops along with the sauce they are marinating in and stir-fry for about 4 minutes or until all the liquid evaporates and the scallops turn opaque. Remove the scallops from the skillet and set aside to keep warm.

4. Respray the skillet and add the mushrooms, carrots, and scallions. Stir-fry for about 3 minutes or until the vegetables are crisp-tender. Cover the skillet periodically during cooking as it starts to dry out (the steam released during cooking will moisten the skillet). Add a little water or broth during cooking if needed. Add the spinach and cook, stirring frequently, for another minute or two or just until the spinach is wilted.

5. Return the scallops to the skillet and toss to mix well. Add the pasta and toss to mix well. Stir the sauce and pour it over the pasta mixture. Cook and stir for a minute or two or until the sauce comes to a boil and thickens slightly. Add a little more broth if the mixture seems too dry. Serve hot.

Nutritional Facts (per 2-cup serving)

CALORIES: 394 CARBOHYDRATES: 59 G CHOLESTEROL: 37 MG FAT: 4.4 G FIBER: 3.5 G
PROTEIN: 29 G SODIUM: 657 MG CALCIUM: 83 MG GI RATING: LOW

Linguine with Spicy Clam Sauce

YIELD: 4 SERVINGS

8 ounces linguine pasta

2 cans (6 ounces each) chopped clams

1–2 tablespoons extra-virgin olive oil

2 teaspoons crushed garlic

14½-ounce can Italian-style stewed tomatoes, undrained

2 cups sliced fresh mushrooms

¼ cup tomato paste with roasted garlic or Italian seasonings

⅛–¼ teaspoon crushed dried red pepper flakes

¼ cup sliced scallions or finely chopped fresh parsley

¼ cup grated Parmesan cheese

1. Cook the pasta al dente according to package directions. Drain well, return to the pot, and cover to keep warm.
2. Drain the clams, reserving the juice, and set aside.
3. Pour the olive oil in a large, deep nonstick skillet and preheat over medium-high heat. Add the garlic and cook for a few seconds or just until the garlic begins to turn color and smell fragrant. Add the clam juice, undrained tomatoes, mushrooms, tomato paste, and crushed red pepper and bring to a boil. Reduce the heat to medium-low, cover, and cook for about 5 minutes or until the mushrooms are tender. Add the clams to the sauce and cook for an additional minute.
4. Add the pasta to the sauce, and toss over low heat to mix well. Serve hot, topping each serving with a sprinkling of scallions or parsley and some of the Parmesan cheese.

Nutritional Facts (per 1½-cup serving)

CALORIES: 400 CARBOHYDRATES: 57 G CHOLESTEROL: 35 MG FAT: 7.6 G FIBER: 3.3 G
PROTEIN: 24 G SODIUM: 642 MG CALCIUM: 183 MG GI RATING: LOW

Ratatouille Pasta

YIELD: 4 SERVINGS

Vegetable Mixture

1 pound plum tomatoes, quartered lengthwise (about 8 medium-small)

2 cups ¾-inch cubes peeled eggplant (about 1 small)

1 medium zucchini, halved lengthwise and sliced ½ inch thick
1 medium green bell pepper, cut into ½-inch strips
1 medium yellow onion, cut into ½-inch-thick wedges
1 cup sliced fresh mushrooms
2–3 teaspoons crushed garlic
1 teaspoon dried thyme
½ teaspoon salt
½ teaspoon coarsely ground black pepper
1 tablespoon balsamic vinegar
1–2 tablespoons extra-virgin olive oil

8 ounces fusilli twists (about 3¼ cups) or rotini pasta (about 3 cups)
½ cup hot vegetable or chicken broth
¼ cup grated Parmesan cheese
1 cup shredded nonfat or reduced-fat mozzarella cheese
¼ cup finely chopped fresh parsley

1. Combine all the vegetable mixture ingredients in a large bowl and toss to mix well. Coat an 11-by-13-inch nonstick roasting pan with nonstick olive oil cooking spray, and spread the mixture evenly in the pan. Cover the pan with aluminum foil.
2. Bake at 450° F for 15 minutes. Then remove the foil and bake for 15 additional minutes. Turn the vegetables and bake for 15 minutes more or until the tomatoes are soft and the vegetables are nicely browned.
3. While the vegetables are roasting, cook the pasta according to package directions. Drain and return it to the pot.
4. When the vegetables are done, add the mixture to the pasta.
5. Pour the broth in the roasting pan and rinse it around to mix the residue from the vegetables with the broth. Add this liquid to the pasta mixture and toss to mix well. Add the Parmesan cheese, and toss to mix well.
5. Divide the pasta mixture among 4 serving dishes. Top each serving with ¼ cup of the mozzarella cheese and a tablespoon of the parsley. Serve hot.

Nutritional Facts (per 2-cup serving)

CALORIES: 375   CARBOHYDRATES: 60 G   CHOLESTEROL: 7 MG   FAT: 6.8 G   FIBER: 5.8 G
PROTEIN: 20 G   SODIUM: 650 MG   CALCIUM: 320 MG   GI RATING: LOW

Gemelli with Spinach, Mushrooms, and Mozzarella

YIELD: 4 SERVINGS

8 ounces gemelli pasta (about 2⅔ cups)

Olive oil nonstick cooking spray; or 1 tablespoon extra-virgin olive oil

2 teaspoons crushed garlic

2 cups sliced fresh mushrooms

½ teaspoon dried thyme

½ teaspoon dried oregano

¼ teaspoon coarsely ground black pepper

1 cup vegetable or chicken broth (plus more if needed)

4 cups (packed) coarsely chopped fresh spinach

¼ cup toasted pine nuts

¼ cup sliced black olives

¼ cup grated Parmesan cheese

1 cup shredded nonfat or reduced-fat mozzarella cheese

¼ cup sliced scallions

1. Cook the pasta al dente according to package directions. Drain well, return to the pot, and cover to keep warm.

2. While the pasta is cooking, coat a large nonstick skillet with the cooking spray or olive oil and add the garlic, mushrooms, thyme, oregano, and black pepper. Place the skillet over medium-high heat and cook, stirring frequently, for several minutes, or until the mushrooms have released their juices and are nicely browned. Cover the skillet periodically if it begins to dry out. (The steam released from the mushrooms will moisten the skillet.) Add a few teaspoons of broth if needed.

3. Add the broth to the skillet and cook, stirring occasionally, for several minutes or until the broth is reduced by half. Add the spinach, pine nuts, and olives, and cook, stirring frequently, for a minute or two or until the spinach is wilted. Add the pasta, and toss to mix well. Add a little more broth if the mixture seems too dry.

4. Remove the skillet from the heat and toss in the Parmesan cheese. Divide the mixture among 4 serving dishes and top each serving with ¼ cup of the mozzarella cheese and a tablespoon of the scallions. Serve hot.

CALORIES: 361   CARBOHYDRATES: 53 G   CHOLESTEROL: 7 MG   FAT: 6.4 G   FIBER: 3.4 G

PROTEIN: 23 G   SODIUM: 525 MG   GI RATING: LOW

Rigatoni with Arugula and Sun-Dried Tomatoes

For variety, substitute broccoli rabe or spinach for the arugula.

YIELD: 4 SERVINGS

8 ounces rigatoni pasta (about 3¼ cups)

1 tablespoon extra-virgin olive oil

2 teaspoons crushed garlic

2 cups sliced fresh mushrooms

1 teaspoon dried Italian seasoning

¼ teaspoon coarsely ground black pepper

1¼ cups vegetable or chicken broth (plus more if needed)

½ cup chopped sun-dried tomatoes (not packed in oil)

3 cups (moderately packed) coarsely chopped arugula

⅓ cup sliced black olives

¼ cup chopped walnuts (optional)

¼ cup grated Parmesan cheese

1 cup shredded nonfat or reduced-fat mozzarella or provolone cheese

¼ cup finely chopped fresh parsley

1. Cook the pasta al dente according to package directions. Drain well, return to the pot, and cover to keep warm.
2. While the pasta is cooking, coat a large nonstick skillet with the olive oil and add the garlic, mushrooms, Italian seasoning, and black pepper. Place the skillet over medium-high heat and cook, stirring frequently, for several minutes, or until the mushrooms have released their juices and are nicely browned. Cover the skillet periodically if it begins to dry out. (The steam released from the mushrooms will moisten the skillet.) Add a few teaspoons of broth if needed.
3. Add the broth and tomatoes to the skillet and reduce the heat to medium. Cover and cook for 2 to 3 minutes or until the tomatoes are plumped. Add the arugula and cook uncovered, stirring

frequently, for a minute or two, or until the arugula is wilted. Add the pasta, olives, and if desired, the walnuts, and toss to mix well. Add a little more broth if the mixture seems too dry.

4. Remove the skillet from the heat, and toss in the Parmesan cheese. Divide the mixture among 4 serving dishes and top each serving with ¼ cup of the mozzarella or provolone cheese and a tablespoon of the parsley. Serve hot.

Nutritional Facts (per 2-cup serving)

CALORIES: 346 CARBOHYDRATES: 50 G CHOLESTEROL: 7 MG FAT: 7.8 G FIBER: 3.3 G
PROTEIN: 18 G SODIUM: 600 MG CALCIUM: 333 MG GI RATING: LOW

Orecchiette with Broccoli and Italian Sausage

YIELD: 4 SERVINGS

8 ounces orecchiette pasta (about 2 cups)
8 ounces turkey Italian sausage, casings removed
10-ounce package frozen chopped broccoli, thawed and undrained
½ cup grated Parmesan cheese

1. Cook the pasta al dente according to package directions. Drain well, return to the pot, and cover to keep warm.
2. While the pasta is cooking, coat a large nonstick skillet with cooking spray and add the sausage to the skillet. Cook over medium heat, stirring to crumble, until the meat is no longer pink. Drain off and discard any excess fat.
3. Add the undrained broccoli to the skillet, cover, and cook for a couple of minutes or just until the broccoli is heated through. Add the pasta to the skillet mixture and toss gently over low heat to mix well.
4. Remove the skillet from the heat and toss in half of the Parmesan cheese. Serve hot, topping each serving with some of the remaining Parmesan cheese.

Nutritional Facts (per 1½-cup serving)

CALORIES: 361 CARBOHYDRATES: 46 G CHOLESTEROL: 46 MG FAT: 6.9 G FIBER: 3.5 G
PROTEIN: 28 G SODIUM: 421 MG CALCIUM: 222 MG GI RATING: LOW

Summertime Rotini

8 ounces rotini pasta (about 3 cups)

1 tablespoon extra-virgin olive oil

2 cups diced fresh zucchini (about 2 medium)

2 teaspoons crushed garlic

¼ teaspoon coarsely ground black pepper

¼ teaspoon salt

2 cups chopped fresh tomatoes (about 2½ medium)

¼ cup chopped fresh basil

¼ cup coarsely chopped black olives

½ cup grated Parmesan cheese

¾ cup diced nonfat or reduced-fat mozzarella cheese

1. Cook the pasta al dente according to package directions. Drain well, return to the pot, and cover to keep warm.
2. While the pasta is cooking, coat a large nonstick skillet with the olive oil and preheat over medium-high heat. Add the zucchini, garlic, black pepper, and salt. Cover and cook, stirring occasionally, for about 3 minutes or until the zucchini is crisp-tender.
3. Add the tomatoes, basil, and olives to the skillet mixture and reduce the heat to medium. Cover and cook for a couple of minutes or just until the tomatoes are heated through and begin to soften. Add the pasta and toss to mix well.
4. Remove the skillet from the heat and toss in half of the Parmesan cheese and then all of the mozzarella. Serve hot, topping each serving with some of the remaining Parmesan cheese.

Nutritional Facts (per 1⅞-cup serving)

CALORIES: 361 CARBOHYDRATES: 50 G CHOLESTEROL: 11 MG FAT: 9 G FIBER: 3.5 G

PROTEIN: 19 G SODIUM: 641 MG CALCIUM: 350 MG GI RATING: LOW

Fettuccine with Fresh Tomatoes

YIELD: 4 SERVINGS

3 cups diced fresh tomatoes (about 3 medium)
½ cup finely chopped fresh basil
1–2 tablespoons extra-virgin olive oil
2 teaspoons crushed garlic
½ teaspoon coarsely ground black pepper
½ teaspoon salt
8 ounces fettuccine or linguine pasta
¼ cup grated Parmesan cheese

1. Combine the tomatoes, basil, olive oil, garlic, black pepper, and salt in a medium-sized bowl. Toss to mix well and let sit at room temperature for 30 minutes.
2. Cook the pasta al dente according to package directions. Drain the pasta and return it to the pot. Add the tomato mixture to the pasta and toss to mix well. Serve immediately, topping each serving with a tablespoon of the Parmesan cheese.

Nutritional Facts (per 1¾-cup serving)
CALORIES: 298   CARBOHYDRATES: 49 G   CHOLESTEROL: 5 MG   FAT: 6.6 G   FIBER: 3.2 G
PROTEIN: 11.1 G   SODIUM: 423 MG   CALCIUM: 111 MG   GI RATING: LOW

Slim Spaghetti Pie

YIELD: 6 SERVINGS

Crust
6 ounces thin spaghetti
⅓ cup grated Parmesan cheese
¼ cup plus 2 tablespoons fat-free egg substitute
Butter-flavored nonstick cooking spray

Sauce
12 ounces 95-percent lean ground beef
1½ cups sliced fresh mushrooms

1 cup chopped onion
½ teaspoon dried Italian seasoning or oregano
1 can (14½ ounces) Italian-style stewed tomatoes, undrained
½ cup tomato paste with roasted garlic or Italian seasonings

Filling
1 cup nonfat or low-fat ricotta cheese
1 cup shredded nonfat or reduced-fat mozzarella cheese

1. To make the crust, cook the spaghetti al dente according to package directions. Drain well and return to the pot. Add the Parmesan cheese and toss to mix well. Add the egg substitute and toss again. Coat a 10-inch pie pan with nonstick cooking spray and spread the mixture evenly over the bottom and up the sides of the pan. Set aside.
2. To make the sauce, coat a large nonstick skillet with cooking spray and preheat over medium heat. Add the ground beef and cook, stirring to crumble, until the meat is no longer pink. Drain off any excess fat. Add the mushrooms, onions, and Italian seasoning or oregano, cover, and cook for about 4 minutes more or until the onion starts to soften. Add the undrained tomatoes and the tomato paste, cover, and cook over medium-low heat for 5 minutes more, stirring occasionally, until the flavors are blended. Remove the skillet from the heat and set aside.
3. To assemble the pie, spread the ricotta cheese over the bottom of the crust, then cover the ricotta layer with the sauce. Spray the exposed edges of the crust lightly with the cooking spray, and bake uncovered at 350° F for 25 minutes or until heated through. Spread the mozzarella over the sauce, and bake for 5 minutes more or until the cheese is melted. Remove the pie from the oven and let sit for 10 minutes before cutting into wedges and serving.

Nutritional Facts (per serving)

CALORIES: 341 CARBOHYDRATES: 37 G CHOLESTEROL: 37 MG FAT: 5.4 G FIBER: 2.6 G
PROTEIN: 33 G SODIUM: 737 MG CALCIUM: 388 MG GI RATING: LOW

Pastitsio (Greek Macaroni Casserole)

YIELD: 6 SERVINGS

6 ounces elbow macaroni (about 1½ cups)
¼ cup plus 2 tablespoons grated Parmesan cheese
Butter-flavored nonstick cooking spray

Meat Mixture

12 ounces 95-percent lean ground beef

½ cup chopped onion

¾ teaspoon dried oregano

⅛ teaspoon ground cinnamon or allspice

14½-ounce can stewed tomatoes, crushed, undrained

¼ cup tomato paste with roasted garlic

Sauce

3 tablespoons unbleached flour

2 cups skim or low-fat milk

¼ cup plus 2 tablespoons fat-free egg substitute

Pinch ground nutmeg

⅛ teaspoon salt

1. Cook the macaroni al dente according to package directions. Drain well and return to the pot. Set aside.
2. To make the meat mixture, put the ground beef in a large nonstick skillet and place the skillet over medium heat. Cook, stirring to crumble, until the meat is no longer pink. Drain off any excess fat. Add the onions, oregano, cinnamon or allspice, undrained tomatoes, and tomato paste and bring the mixture to a boil over medium-high heat. Reduce the heat to low, cover, and simmer for about 10 minutes or until the onions are soft and the flavors are well blended. Set aside to keep warm.
3. To make the sauce, put the flour in a 2-quart microwave-safe bowl, add ¼ cup of the milk, and whisk until smooth. Slowly whisk in the remaining milk and then the egg substitute, nutmeg, and salt. Microwave at high power for 2 minutes, then whisk until smooth. (Note that the mixture may appear curdled at first but will become smooth as you keep whisking.) Microwave for about 3 minutes more, whisking after each minute, until the mixture is thickened and bubbly.
4. To assemble the casserole, add the meat mixture to the macaroni and toss to mix well. Toss in ¼ cup of the Parmesan cheese. Spread the macaroni mixture evenly in an 8-by-8-inch (2-quart) casserole dish. Pour the sauce evenly over the macaroni mixture, sprinkle the remaining Parmesan over the sauce, and spray the top lightly with the cooking spray.
5. Bake at 350° F for about 35 minutes or until bubbly around the edges. Remove the dish from the oven and let sit for 20 minutes before serving. To serve, cut into squares and, using a spatula, carefully lift each square onto a serving plate. Serve hot.

Nutritional Facts (per serving)

CALORIES: 296 CARBOHYDRATES: 37 G CHOLESTEROL: 37 MG FAT: 5.2 G FIBER: 1.9 G
PROTEIN: 23 G SODIUM: 530 MG CALCIUM: 221 MG GI RATING: LOW

Baked Spaghetti Florentine

For variety, substitute broccoli for the spinach.

YIELD: 8 SERVINGS

12 ounces thin spaghetti

15-ounce container nonfat or reduced-fat ricotta cheese

2 cups skim or low-fat milk

¾ cup grated Parmesan cheese

¼ cup fat-free egg substitute

1½ teaspoons crushed garlic

½ teaspoon coarsely ground black pepper

Pinch ground nutmeg

10 ounces frozen chopped spinach, thawed and squeezed dry

2 cups shredded nonfat or reduced-fat mozzarella cheese

8 slices extra-lean turkey bacon, cooked, drained, and crumbled (optional)

Nonstick butter-flavored cooking spray

1. Cook the spaghetti al dente according to package directions, drain well, and return to the pot.
2. Combine the ricotta, milk, ½ cup of the Parmesan cheese, the egg substitute, garlic, pepper, and nutmeg in a large bowl and stir with a wire whisk to mix well. Add the ricotta mixture to the spaghetti and toss to mix well. Add the spinach, mozzarella cheese, and, if desired, bacon, and toss again.
3. Coat a 9-by-13-inch pan with nonstick cooking spray and spread the spaghetti mixture evenly in the pan. Sprinkle the remaining ¼ cup of Parmesan cheese over the top, then spray the top lightly with the cooking spray.
4. Bake uncovered at 350° F for about 30 minutes or until the edges are bubbly and the top is lightly browned. Remove the dish from the oven and let sit for 10 minutes. Cut into squares and serve hot.

Nutritional Facts (per serving)

CALORIES: 331 CARBOHYDRATES: 42 G CHOLESTEROL: 12 MG FAT: 3.7 G FIBER: 2.1 G
PROTEIN: 29 G SODIUM: 530 MG CALCIUM: 714 MG GI RATING: LOW

Sicilian Baked Fusilli

YIELD: 6 SERVINGS

8 ounces fusilli or pasta twists (about 3 cups)
¾ cup nonfat or low-fat ricotta cheese
¾ cup evaporated skim or low-fat milk
8 ounces Italian turkey sausage, casings removed
½ cup chopped onion
½ teaspoon dried thyme
¾ cup chopped seeded plum tomatoes (about 3 medium)
¾ cup chopped commercial roasted red bell pepper (about 5 ounces)
¼ cup grated Parmesan cheese
Olive oil nonstick cooking spray

1. Cook the pasta al dente according to package directions, drain well, and return to the pot.
2. Combine the ricotta and evaporated milk in a medium-sized bowl and stir with a wire whisk to mix well. Set aside.
3. Coat a large nonstick skillet with cooking spray and add the sausage. Cook over medium heat, stirring to crumble, until the meat is no longer pink. Drain off and discard any excess fat. Add the onion and thyme to the skillet, cover, and cook, stirring occasionally, for an additional 3 minutes or until the onions start to soften. Add the tomatoes, cover, and cook for another minute or two or until the tomatoes start to soften. Stir the bell peppers into the skillet mixture.
4. Add the sausage mixture to the pasta and toss to mix well. Add the ricotta mixture, and toss again.
5. Coat a 9-by-13-inch baking dish with nonstick cooking spray and spread the pasta mixture evenly in the dish. Sprinkle the Parmesan cheese over the top, and spray the top lightly with the cooking spray. Bake at 425° F for about 15 to 20 minutes or until hot and bubbly. Serve immediately.

Nutritional Facts (per serving)
CALORIES: 292 CARBOHYDRATES: 37 G CHOLESTEROL: 37 MG FAT: 5.5 G FIBER: 1.6 G
PROTEIN: 21 G SODIUM: 468 MG CALCIUM: 320 MG GI RATING: LOW

14. Hearty Home-Style Entrées

*M*any people believe that adopting a healthy low-GI diet means spending hours in the kitchen learning complicated cooking techniques or perusing specialty stores for exotic and expensive ingredients. This chapter will prove that nothing could be further from the truth. The following pages present a wide range of hearty home-style entrées guaranteed to provide a tempting answer to that age-old question, "What's for dinner?" Whether you're looking for a simple baked chicken dish, a hearty pot roast, or a crispy oven-fried fish recipe, you will be sure to find a dish that meets your need deliciously.

As you glance through the pages of this chapter, remember that these are just some of the savory low-GI entrées that are within your reach. Delicious pasta entrées are presented in chapter 13, a wide variety of main dish salads can be found in chapter 10, and hearty soups are featured in chapter 9.

When planning low-GI meals, remember to balance your entrée with the appropriate side dishes. For instance, if you are having a starch-based entrée like Shrimp & Sausage Jambalaya, pair it with low-carbohydrate vegetables such as steamed cabbage, broccoli, or green beans (see pages 20–21 for a list of low-carb vegetables) and a fresh garden salad. Add some crusty whole-grain bread or another starchy side dish only if you need the extra carbohydrates and calories.

Baked Chicken Dijon

For variety, substitute pork tenderloin for the chicken.

YIELD: 4 SERVINGS

4 boneless skinless chicken breast halves (4 ounces each)

Marinade
¼ cup Dijon mustard
1 tablespoon extra-virgin olive oil

1 tablespoon frozen apple juice concentrate, thawed

2 teaspoons crushed garlic

1 teaspoon dried rosemary

1. Place all the marinade ingredients in a small bowl and stir to mix well. Place the chicken in a nonmetal container and spoon the marinade over the chicken. Turn the chicken to coat all sides with the marinade. Cover and refrigerate for 6 to 24 hours.

2. Coat a 9-by-13-inch pan with nonstick cooking spray, and place the chicken in the pan. Spoon the marinade remaining in the container over the chicken.

3. Bake uncovered at 375° F for about 25 minutes or until the chicken is tender and no longer pink inside. Serve hot.

Nutritional Facts (per serving)

CALORIES: 183   CARBOHYDRATES: 4 G   CHOLESTEROL: 65 MG   FAT: 6.2 G   FIBER: 0.3 G
PROTEIN: 27 G   SODIUM: 453 MG   CALCIUM: 40 MG   GI RATING: VERY LOW

Chicken Breasts with Savory Apple Stuffing

YIELD: 4 SERVINGS

4 skinless chicken breast halves with bone (about 6 ounces each)

¼ teaspoon salt

¼ teaspoon ground black pepper

Butter-flavored nonstick cooking spray

Stuffing

4 slices firm whole-wheat, multigrain, or sourdough bread

¼ cup finely chopped onion

¼ cup finely chopped celery (include the leaves)

1 cup chopped, peeled Granny Smith apple (about 1 medium-large)

½ teaspoon fines herbes; or ¼ teaspoon each dried thyme and sage

¼ cup plus 2 tablespoons chicken broth

1. Rinse the chicken with cool water, and pat it dry with paper towels. Lightly sprinkle both sides with the salt and black pepper and set aside.

2. Tear the bread into pieces, put in a blender or food processor, and process into coarse crumbs. Set aside.

3. Coat a large nonstick skillet with cooking spray. Add the onion, celery, apple, herbs, and 2 tablespoons of the broth and place the skillet over medium heat. Cover the skillet and cook, stirring occasionally, for about 2 minutes or until the vegetables and apples start to soften. Remove the skillet from the heat, and toss in the bread crumbs.

4. Tossing gently, slowly add enough of the remaining broth to make a moist but not wet stuffing that holds together. Set the stuffing aside.

5. Coat a 9-by-13-inch pan with nonstick cooking spray, and lay the chicken in the pan with the bone side up. Mound a quarter of the stuffing into the depression of the breastbone of each piece of chicken. Spray the tops of the stuffing lightly with the cooking spray.

6. Cover the pan with aluminum foil, and bake at 350° F for 40 minutes. Remove the foil and bake for 20 additional minutes or until the chicken is tender, the juices run clear, and the stuffing is lightly browned. Serve hot.

Nutritional Facts (per serving)

CALORIES: 248   CARBOHYDRATES: 18 G   CHOLESTEROL: 82 MG   FAT: 3.1 G   FIBER: 2.9 G
PROTEIN: 36 G   SODIUM: 435 MG   CALCIUM: 48 MG   GI RATING: LOW

Citrus-Sauced Chicken

YIELD: 4 SERVINGS

Sauce
½ teaspoon cornstarch
½ cup orange juice
½ cup chicken broth
¼ cup dry white wine

Chicken and Seasonings
1 pound boneless, skinless chicken breast
1 teaspoon lemon pepper
½ teaspoon garlic powder
1 teaspoon dried rosemary
¼ teaspoon salt
3–4 teaspoons extra-virgin olive oil

Garnish
2 tablespoons sliced scallions
2 tablespoons finely chopped fresh parsley

1. To make the sauce, put the cornstarch in a 2-cup measure, add a tablespoon of the juice, and stir to dissolve the cornstarch. Add the remaining juice, the broth, and the wine and stir to mix well. Set aside.
2. Rinse the chicken and pat it dry with paper towels. Cut the chicken crosswise into 8 equal pieces. With the cut side up, use the palm of your hand to flatten each piece to slightly less than ½-inch thickness. Sprinkle both sides of the chicken pieces with some of the lemon pepper, garlic powder, rosemary, and salt and set aside.
3. Coat a large nonstick skillet with the olive oil and preheat over medium-high heat. Add the chicken and cook for about 2 to 3 minutes on each side or until nicely browned and no longer pink inside. Remove the chicken from the skillet. Set aside and keep warm.
4. Pour the sauce into the skillet and cook, stirring constantly, for several minutes or until the sauce thickens slightly and is reduced to about ½ cup.
5. To serve, place some of the chicken on each of 4 serving plates, drizzle with some of the sauce, and top with a sprinkling of the scallions and parsley. Serve hot.

Nutritional Facts (per serving)

CALORIES: 182 CARBOHYDRATES: 4 G CHOLESTEROL: 65 MG FAT: 4.8 G FIBER: 0.3 G
PROTEIN: 26 G SODIUM: 416 MG CALCIUM: 24 MG GI RATING: LOW

Sonoma Chicken

YIELD: 4 SERVINGS

1 pound boneless, skinless chicken breast
1 teaspoon dried rosemary
½ teaspoon garlic powder
¼ teaspoon salt
¼ teaspoon ground black pepper
3–4 teaspoons extra-virgin olive oil
1 medium onion, cut into ¼-inch-thick slices, and separated into rings
1½ cups sliced fresh mushrooms
1 cup chicken broth
¼ cup dry white wine
3 tablespoons chopped sun-dried tomatoes (not packed in oil)
¼ cup finely chopped fresh parsley

1. Rinse the chicken and pat it dry with paper towels. Cut it crosswise into 8 equal pieces. With the cut side up, use the palm of your hand to flatten each piece to slightly less than ½-inch thickness. Sprinkle both sides of the chicken pieces with some of the rosemary, garlic powder, salt, and black pepper, and set aside.

2. Coat a large nonstick skillet with the olive oil and preheat over medium-high heat. Add the chicken and cook for about 2 to 3 minutes on each side or until nicely browned and no longer pink inside. Remove the chicken from the skillet and set aside to keep warm.

3. Add the onion rings, mushrooms, and 1 tablespoon of the broth to the skillet. Cover and cook, stirring frequently, for a couple of minutes or until the onions and mushrooms start to brown and begin to soften. Add a little more broth if the skillet becomes too dry, but only enough to prevent scorching.

4. Add the remaining broth, wine, and tomatoes to the skillet mixture and bring to a boil. Reduce the heat to medium-low, cover, and cook for about 3 minutes or until the tomatoes have softened. Raise the heat to medium-high and cook uncovered, stirring frequently, for several minutes or until about ¼ to ⅓ cup of liquid remains in the skillet.

5. To serve, place some of the chicken on each of 4 serving plates. Top each serving with some of the vegetable mixture, pan juices, and a sprinkling of parsley. Serve hot.

Nutritional Facts (per serving)

CALORIES: 189 CARBOHYDRATES: 5 G CHOLESTEROL: 65 MG FAT: 4.8 G FIBER: 1.2 G
PROTEIN: 27 G SODIUM: 436 MG CALCIUM: 32 MG GI RATING: VERY LOW

Pecan Chicken

YIELD: 4 SERVINGS

1 pound boneless, skinless chicken breast
1 cup nonfat or low-fat buttermilk or yogurt
2 cups Special K cereal
¼ to ⅓ cup finely chopped pecans
1 teaspoon lemon pepper
¾ teaspoon poultry seasoning
¼ teaspoon salt
Butter-flavored nonstick cooking spray

1. Rinse the chicken and pat it dry with paper towels. Cut the chicken crosswise into 8 equal pieces, then, with the cut side up, use the palm of your hand to flatten each piece to ½-inch thickness.

2. Place the chicken in a shallow nonmetal container and cover with the buttermilk or yogurt. Turn the chicken to coat. Cover and refrigerate for 6 to 24 hours, turning occasionally.

3. Put the cereal in a food processor and process into coarse crumbs. (Alternatively, put the cereal in a plastic zip-type bag and crush with a rolling pin or the bottom of a glass.) There should be 1 cup of crumbs. Put the crumbs in a shallow dish and add the pecans, lemon pepper, poultry seasoning, and salt. Stir to mix well.

4. Remove the chicken from the buttermilk or yogurt and shake off the excess. Dip the chicken pieces in the crumb mixture, turning to coat both sides well.

5. Coat a large baking sheet with nonstick cooking spray, and arrange the chicken pieces in a single layer on the sheet. Spray the tops lightly with the cooking spray and bake at 400° F for about 25 minutes or until the chicken is crisp and golden on the outside and is cooked through. Serve hot.

Nutritional Facts (per serving)

CALORIES: 221 CARBOHYDRATES: 10 G CHOLESTEROL: 65 MG FAT: 6.8 G FIBER: 0.9 G
PROTEIN: 29 G SODIUM: 415 MG CALCIUM: 17 MG GI RATING: LOW

Savory Roast Turkey

Don't wait for Thanksgiving to roast a turkey. Making a turkey is really quite easy, and this is a great year-round recipe that provides plenty of leftovers for salads and sandwiches.

YIELD: ABOUT 12 SERVINGS

12-pound turkey, fresh or defrosted
½ cup water
½ cup dry sherry

Basting Sauce
2 tablespoons dry sherry
1½ teaspoons ground paprika
1 teaspoon crushed garlic
1 teaspoon brown sugar
¾ teaspoon poultry seasoning
½ teaspoon lemon pepper

1. Remove the packet containing the giblets and neck from the cavity of the turkey. (You may have to release the legs from a wire or plastic lock in order to do this.) Rinse the turkey inside and out, and dry it with paper towels. Trim away any excess fat.
2. Transfer the turkey to a rack in a large roasting pan. Return the legs to the wire or plastic lock or loosely tie them together with sturdy string. Fold the wings back and underneath the bird.
3. Pour the water and sherry into the bottom of the roasting pan. Combine the basting sauce ingredients in a small bowl and stir to mix well. Brush the sauce over the skin of the bird. Completely enclose the bird in aluminum foil, crimping the foil around the edges of the pan to seal it tightly.
4. Bake at 325° F for 2½ hours. Remove the foil and cook for an additional 30 minutes, basting occasionally with the pan juices, until the turkey is nicely browned, the drumsticks move easily in the sockets, and a thermometer inserted in the thigh reads 180 to 185° F. Remove from the oven and let sit loosely covered with foil for 20 minutes before carving. Retain the drippings left in the pan to make Savory Roast Turkey Gravy (below).

Nutritional Facts (per 3-ounce serving, skinless white meat)
CALORIES: 114 CARBOHYDRATES: 0 G CHOLESTEROL: 70 MG FAT: 0.6 G FIBER: 0 G
PROTEIN: 26 G SODIUM: 44 MG CALCIUM: 10 MG GI RATING: VERY LOW

Nutritional Facts (per 3-ounce serving, skinless dark meat)
CALORIES: 163 CARBOHYDRATES: 0 G CHOLESTEROL: 68 MG FAT: 6.6 G FIBER: 0 G
PROTEIN: 24 G SODIUM: 64 MG CALCIUM: 25 MG GI RATING: VERY LOW

Savory Roast Turkey Gravy

YIELD: 2½ CUPS

2 cups turkey drippings
Pinch ground white pepper
¼ teaspoon poultry seasoning
1½ teaspoons instant chicken bouillon granules
¼ cup plus 1 tablespoon whole-wheat pastry flour or unbleached flour
½ cup skim or low-fat milk (for a richer gravy use evaporated skim or low-fat milk)

1. Defat the Savory Roast Turkey drippings by placing them in a fat separator cup. Measure out 2 cups of the defatted drippings, place them in a 1-quart pot, and add the white pepper, poultry

seasoning, and bouillon granules. Bring the mixture to a boil over high heat, then reduce the heat to low, and simmer covered for 5 minutes.

2. Combine the flour and milk in a jar with a tight-fitting lid and shake until smooth. Slowly add the milk mixture to the simmering broth, stirring constantly with a wire whisk. Continue to cook and stir until the gravy is thick and bubbly. Serve hot.

Nutritional Facts (per ¼-cup serving)

CALORIES: 25 CARBOHYDRATES: 3.7 G CHOLESTEROL: 0 MG FAT: 0.1 G FIBER: 0.5 G
PROTEIN: 2.1 G SODIUM: 136 MG CALCIUM: 19 MG GI RATING: MODERATE

Shrimp & Sausage Jambalaya

YIELD: 4 SERVINGS

2 to 3 teaspoons extra-virgin olive oil
1 cup diced smoked sausage or kielbasa (about 5 ounces)
½ cup chopped onion
½ cup sliced celery
1 teaspoon crushed garlic
14½-ounce can stewed tomatoes, crushed, undrained
8 ounces peeled and deveined raw shrimp
1½–2 teaspoons Cajun seasoning
1½ teaspoons ground paprika
3 cups cooked brown rice

1. Coat a large nonstick skillet with the olive oil and preheat over medium heat. Add the sausage, onion, celery, and garlic. Cover and cook, stirring frequently, for about 4 minutes or until the vegetables start to soften.

2. Add the undrained tomatoes, shrimp, Cajun seasoning, and paprika to the skillet mixture and cook covered, stirring occasionally, for an additional 5 minutes or until the shrimp turn pink and are thoroughly cooked. Stir the rice into the skillet mixture and cook and stir for another minute or two, or until the rice is heated through. Serve hot.

Nutritional Facts (per 1½-cup serving)

CALORIES: 318 CARBOHYDRATES: 47 G CHOLESTEROL: 93 MG FAT: 4.9 G FIBER: 4.4 G
PROTEIN: 18 G SODIUM: 650 MG CALCIUM: 89 MG GI RATING: LOW

Variation: Red Bean & Sausage Jambalaya
Omit the shrimp, and add 1¼ cups of canned drained red kidney beans along with the rice.

Nutritional Facts (per 1½-cup serving)
CALORIES: 347   CARBOHYDRATES: 60 G   CHOLESTEROL: 12 MG   FAT: 4.8 G
FIBER: 8 G   PROTEIN: 14 G   SODIUM: 714 MG   CALCIUM: 88 MG   GI RATING: LOW

Curried Shrimp with Brown Rice

YIELD: 4 SERVINGS

1 pound peeled and deveined raw shrimp
¼ cup finely chopped onion
1 teaspoon crushed garlic
1 cup frozen green peas
¼ cup vegetable or chicken broth
2–3 teaspoons mild curry paste
3 cups cooked brown rice
1–2 teaspoons roasted (dark) sesame oil

1. Coat a large, deep nonstick skillet with cooking spray and preheat over medium-high heat. Add the shrimp, onion, and garlic and cook, stirring frequently, for about 4 minutes or until the shrimp turn pink and are thoroughly cooked. Periodically place a lid over the skillet if it becomes too dry (the steam released during cooking will moisten the skillet) or add a few teaspoons of water or broth as needed.

2. Add the peas and broth to the skillet and reduce the heat to medium. Cover and cook for a minute or two or just until the peas are thawed and heated through.

3. Add the rice and the sesame oil. Toss the mixture gently over medium heat for a minute or two or until heated through. Add a little more broth if the mixture seems too dry. Serve hot.

Nutritional Facts (per 1¼-cup serving)
CALORIES: 338   CARBOHYDRATES: 40 G   CHOLESTEROL: 172 MG   FAT: 5.9 G   FIBER: 4.7 G
PROTEIN: 28 G   SODIUM: 328 MG   CALCIUM: 83 MG   GI RATING: LOW

Saucy Stuffed Cabbage

YIELD: 5 SERVINGS

1 pound 95-percent lean ground beef

⅔ cup uncooked bulgur wheat or orzo pasta

¾ cup finely chopped onion

1½ teaspoons crushed garlic

¾ teaspoon dried thyme

¼ teaspoon ground black pepper

¾ cup beef broth

10 large cabbage leaves

1-pound can tomato sauce

1. Combine the ground beef, uncooked bulgur wheat or orzo, onion, garlic, thyme, black pepper, and broth in a large bowl and mix well. Set aside.

2. Place the cabbage leaves, two or three at a time, in a microwave steamer or conventional stovetop steamer and cook at high power or over high heat for about 3 minutes or until the leaves are pliable enough to roll up. (Alternatively, plunge the leaves, two or three at a time, into a large pot of boiling water for a couple of minutes. Remove the leaves, drain off any excess water, and set aside.)

3. Lay one cabbage leaf out on a flat surface. Trim away about 1 inch of the thickest part of the center vein so the leaf will roll up more easily.

4. Spread ⅓ cup of the meat mixture along the bottom of each leaf, leaving a 1½-inch margin on each side. Fold the sides in and roll the leaf up to enclose the filling. Coat a 9-by-13-inch pan with nonstick cooking spray, and lay the cabbage rolls seam side down in the pan. Pour the tomato sauce over the cabbage rolls.

5. Cover the pan with aluminum foil, and bake at 350° F for 1 hour or until the meat is thoroughly cooked and the rice is tender. (An instant-read thermometer should read at least 160° F when inserted through the center of a roll.) Serve hot.

Nutritional Facts (per serving)

CALORIES: 227   CARBOHYDRATES: 25 G   CHOLESTEROL: 48 MG   FAT: 4.6 G   FIBER: 6.4 G
PROTEIN: 22 G   SODIUM: 575 MG   CALCIUM: 50 MG   GI RATING: LOW

Spinach and Beef Burritos

YIELD: 6 SERVINGS

1 pound 95-percent lean ground beef

¾ teaspoon crushed garlic

½ cup chopped onion

1½ cups canned enchilada sauce, or bottled mild chunky-style salsa

3 cups (packed) coarsely chopped fresh spinach

6 flour tortillas (8-inch rounds), warmed to room temperature

1 cup plus 2 tablespoons shredded nonfat or reduced-fat Monterey Jack or Cheddar cheese

Toppings

¾ cup nonfat or light sour cream

¼ cup plus 2 tablespoons sliced scallions

¼ cup plus 2 tablespoons sliced black olives

1. Coat a large nonstick skillet with cooking spray and add the ground beef and garlic. Place the skillet over medium heat and cook, stirring to crumble, until the meat is no longer pink. Add the onions and ½ cup of the enchilada sauce or salsa, cover and cook, stirring occasionally, for about 3 minutes or until the onions start to soften.

2. Add the spinach to the skillet. Cook, stirring frequently, for a minute or two or until the spinach is wilted and any excess liquid evaporates.

3. Lay the tortillas on a flat surface and spoon one-sixth of the meat mixture along the right side of each tortilla, stopping 1½ inches from the bottom. Top the filling on each burrito with 1 tablespoon of the cheese. Fold the bottom edge of each tortilla up about 1 inch. (This fold will prevent the filling from falling out.) Then, beginning at the right edge, roll each tortilla up jellyroll style. (See diagram on page 94.)

4. Coat a 9-by-13-inch pan with nonstick cooking spray, and lay the filled tortillas seam side down in a single layer in the pan. Spread the remaining 1 cup of enchilada sauce or salsa down the center of the burritos, and sprinkle with the remaining ¾ cup of cheese.

5. Cover the pan with aluminum foil. Bake at 350° F for 20 minutes or until the burritos are heated through and the cheese is melted. Top each burrito with 2 tablespoons of the sour cream, 1 tablespoon of scallions, and 1 tablespoon of olives. Serve hot.

Nutritional Facts (per serving)

CALORIES: 341 CARBOHYDRATES: 35 G CHOLESTEROL: 42 MG FAT: 7.5 G FIBER: 3.1 G
PROTEIN: 26 G SODIUM: 676 MG CALCIUM: 207 MG GI RATING: LOW

Mexican Lasagna

YIELD: 8 SERVINGS

1 cup nonfat or reduced-fat ricotta cheese
¼ cup plus 2 tablespoons fat-free egg substitute
1 pound 95-percent lean ground beef
14½-ounce can Mexican-style stewed tomatoes, crushed, undrained
2 tablespoons tomato paste
15-ounce can black or pinto beans, drained
4-ounce can chopped green chilies, drained
1 tablespoon chili powder
10 corn tortillas (6-inch rounds)
2½ cups shredded nonfat or reduced-fat Monterey Jack or Cheddar cheese

1. Combine the ricotta and egg substitute in a small bowl and stir to mix well. Set aside.
2. Put the ground beef in a large nonstick skillet over medium heat. Cook, stirring to crumble, until the meat is no longer pink. Add the tomatoes, tomato paste, beans, chilies, and chili powder and stir to mix well. Cook uncovered, stirring frequently, for about 10 minutes or until the mixture is thick. Remove the skillet from the heat and set aside.
3. Coat a 9-by-13-inch pan with nonstick cooking spray, and line the bottom of the pan with 5 of the tortillas, slightly overlapping them. (You will need to cut one of the tortillas in half). Spread half of the meat mixture over the tortillas, dot with half of the ricotta mixture, and top with half of the cheese. Repeat the layers using the remaining ingredients.
4. Cover the dish with aluminum foil and bake at 350° F for 25 minutes. Remove the foil and bake for 5 minutes more or until the dish is heated through and the cheese is melted. Remove the dish from the oven, and let sit for 10 minutes before cutting into squares and serving.

Nutritional Facts (per serving)

CALORIES: 275 CARBOHYDRATES: 32 G CHOLESTEROL: 34 MG FAT: 3.4 G FIBER: 5 G
PROTEIN: 29 G SODIUM: 660 MG CALCIUM: 482 MG GI RATING: LOW

Classic Meatloaf

YIELD: 8 SERVINGS

1½ pounds 95-percent lean ground beef
1 cup finely chopped fresh mushrooms
½ cup finely chopped onion
⅓ cup finely chopped celery (include the leaves)
2 teaspoons crushed garlic
¾ cup old-fashioned rolled oats
¼ cup fat-free egg substitute or 2 egg whites
½ teaspoon ground black pepper
1 tablespoon Dijon mustard
1 tablespoon Worcestershire sauce
½ cup vegetable juice cocktail (like V•8)
½ cup ketchup or chili sauce

1. Combine all the ingredients except the ketchup or chili sauce in a large bowl and mix well. Coat a 9-by-5-inch meatloaf pan with nonstick cooking spray and press the mixture into the pan to form a loaf.
2. Bake at 350° F for 30 minutes. Spread the ketchup or chili sauce over the top of the loaf, and bake for an additional 35 minutes or until the meat is no longer pink inside and an instant-read thermometer inserted in the center of the loaf reads 160° F.
3. Remove the loaf from the oven and let sit for 10 minutes before slicing and serving.

Nutritional Facts (per serving)
CALORIES: 166 CARBOHYDRATES: 12 G CHOLESTEROL: 45 MG FAT: 4.5 G FIBER: 1.5 G
PROTEIN: 19 G SODIUM: 397 MG CALCIUM: 20 MG GI RATING: LOW

Beef and Barley Skillet

YIELD: 5 SERVINGS

1 pound 95-percent lean ground beef
1¼ cups sliced fresh mushrooms
½ cup chopped onion

1½ teaspoons dried thyme
¼ teaspoon ground black pepper
1 cup hulled or pearled barley
2½ cups water
2½ teaspoons instant beef bouillon granules
1 cup frozen green peas, thawed

1. Put the ground beef in a large, deep nonstick skillet, and cook over medium heat, stirring to crumble, until the meat is no longer pink. Drain off and discard any fat.
2. Add the remaining ingredients except for the peas and bring to a full boil over high heat. Remove the skillet from the heat, cover with aluminum foil, and bake at 350° F for 55 minutes.
3. Carefully remove the foil (steam will escape), and stir in the peas. (Add a little water if the mixture seems too dry.) Place the foil back over the skillet, and return to the oven for 5 additional minutes, or until the barley is tender and the peas are heated through. Serve hot.

Nutritional Facts (per 1⅓-cup serving)

CALORIES: 288 CARBOHYDRATES: 37 G CHOLESTEROL: 49 MG FAT: 4.7 G FIBER: 8 G
PROTEIN: 24 G SODIUM: 417 MG CALCIUM: 22 MG GI RATING: VERY LOW

Braised Beef with Sun-Dried Tomatoes

YIELD: 4 SERVINGS

1 pound extra-lean stew beef
½ cup water
⅓ cup dry red wine
2 teaspoons dark brown sugar
1 teaspoon dried rosemary
2 teaspoons instant beef bouillon granules
¼ teaspoon coarsely ground black pepper
2 cups halved fresh mushrooms
1 cup chopped onion
½ cup chopped sun-dried tomatoes (not oil-packed)
3 tablespoons chopped fresh parsley

1. Rinse the meat with cool water and pat it dry with paper towels. Set aside. Place the water, wine, brown sugar, rosemary, bouillon granules, and black pepper in a small bowl, stir to mix well, and set aside.

2. Coat a large nonstick skillet with cooking spray and preheat over medium-high heat. Add the meat and cook, stirring frequently, for several minutes or until the meat is nicely browned. Remove the skillet from the heat, add the mushrooms, onions, and sun-dried tomatoes, and stir to mix well. Add the wine mixture and stir to mix well.

3. Cover the skillet with aluminum foil and bake at 325° F for 1½ hours or until the meat is very tender.

4. Serve hot over brown rice, noodles, or whole-wheat couscous, if desired. Sprinkle some of the parsley over each serving.

Nutritional Facts (per serving)

CALORIES: 213 CARBOHYDRATES: 12 G CHOLESTEROL: 64 MG FAT: 4.2 G FIBER: 2 G
PROTEIN: 28 G SODIUM: 391 MG CALCIUM: 32 MG GI RATING: LOW

Beef Paprikash

YIELD: 4 SERVINGS

1 pound extra-lean stew beef
¾ cup water
1 tablespoon paprika
2 teaspoons instant beef bouillon granules
¼ teaspoon ground black pepper
2 cups sliced fresh mushrooms
1 cup chopped onion
½ cup finely chopped green bell pepper
¾ cup nonfat or light sour cream
1 tablespoon whole-wheat pastry flour or unbleached flour

1. Rinse the meat with cool water and pat it dry with paper towels. Set aside. Combine the water, paprika, bouillon granules, and black pepper in a small bowl, stir to mix well, and set aside.

2. Coat a large nonstick skillet with cooking spray, and preheat over medium-high heat. Add the meat and cook, stirring frequently, for several minutes, or until the meat is nicely browned. Remove the skillet from the heat. Add the mushrooms, onions, and bell pepper, and stir to mix well. Add the water mixture and stir to mix well.

3. Cover the skillet with aluminum foil and bake at 325° F for 1½ hours or until the meat is very tender. Remove the skillet from the oven and carefully remove the foil (steam will escape).

4. Put the sour cream in a small bowl, add the flour, and stir to mix well. Add ¼ cup of the pan juices from the skillet and stir to mix well. Set aside.

5. Place the skillet over medium heat, and bring the mixture to a boil. Add the sour cream mixture to the skillet and cook, stirring constantly, until the mixture comes to a boil and thickens slightly.
6. Serve hot over noodles, brown rice, or whole-wheat couscous, if desired.

Nutritional Facts (per serving)

CALORIES: 231 CARBOHYDRATES: 16 G CHOLESTEROL: 64 MG FAT: 4.2 G FIBER: 2 G
PROTEIN: 30 G SODIUM: 415 MG CALCIUM: 64 MG GI RATING: VERY LOW

Pot Roast with Sour Cream Gravy

YIELD: 8 SERVINGS

2½ pounds eye round roast
½ teaspoon coarsely ground black pepper
10½-ounce can condensed French onion soup or condensed beef broth, undiluted
¾ cup water
½ cup dry sherry
½ teaspoon dried thyme
½ teaspoon dried marjoram

Gravy
½ cup nonfat or light sour cream
3 tablespoons whole-wheat pastry flour or unbleached flour
2 cups sliced fresh mushrooms

1. Trim the meat of visible fat, rinse with cool water, and pat it dry with paper towels. Sprinkle all sides of the roast with some of the black pepper.
2. Coat a large nonstick Dutch oven or 4-quart pot with nonstick cooking spray and preheat over medium-high heat. Place the meat in the Dutch oven or pot and cook for several minutes or until all sides are nicely browned.
3. Add the undiluted soup, water, sherry, thyme, and marjoram to the pot, and let the mixture come to a boil. Reduce the heat to low, cover, and simmer for about 2½ hours, turning the roast occasionally, until it is tender. Remove the roast to a cutting board, cover loosely with foil, and set aside.
4. To make the gravy, combine the sour cream and ½ cup of the pan juices in a blender and blend until smooth. Add flour and blend until smooth. Set aside.

5. Pour the remaining pan juices into a measuring cup. Add water, if necessary, to bring the volume up to 1 cup. (If there is more than 1 cup of liquid, return it to the pot, and cook uncovered over medium-high heat for a few minutes to reduce the volume to 1 cup.) Return the pan juices to the pot and add the mushrooms. Bring the mixture to a boil, then reduce the heat to medium-low, cover, and cook for about 5 minutes or until the mushrooms are tender. Slowly add the flour mixture while stirring constantly with a wire whisk. Cook and stir for a minute or two, or until the gravy is thickened and bubbly.
6. Slice the roast thinly across the grain, and serve accompanied by the gravy.

Nutritional Facts (per serving)

CALORIES: 229 CARBOHYDRATES: 9 G CHOLESTEROL: 70 MG FAT: 5.9 G FIBER: 0.9 G
PROTEIN: 30 G SODIUM: 369 MG CALCIUM: 31 MG GI RATING: VERY LOW

Pork Medallions with Sherry-Mushroom Sauce

YIELD: 4 SERVINGS

1 pork tenderloin (1 pound)
1 teaspoon lemon pepper
¾ teaspoon dried rosemary
¼ teaspoon garlic powder
⅛ teaspoon salt
Olive oil nonstick cooking spray
½ cup dry sherry
2 cups sliced fresh mushrooms

Sauce
¼ cup chicken broth
1 teaspoon cornstarch
½ cup nonfat or light sour cream

1. Rinse the meat and pat it dry with paper towels. Cut the tenderloin crosswise into 8 slices. Using your palm, flatten each piece to about ½-inch thickness. Combine the lemon pepper, rosemary, garlic powder, and salt in a small bowl and stir to mix well. Rub some of this mixture over both sides of the pork medallions.

2. To make the sauce, pour 1 tablespoon of the broth and all of the cornstarch in a small bowl and stir with a wire whisk to dissolve the cornstarch. Add the remaining broth and the sour cream and whisk until smooth. Set aside.

3. Coat a large nonstick skillet with olive oil cooking spray and preheat over medium-high heat. Add the pork medallions to the skillet and cook for about 3 minutes or until nicely browned. Spray the tops of the medallions lightly with the cooking spray, turn, and cook for 2 to 3 minutes more, or until nicely browned on both sides and cooked through. Remove the medallions to a plate, and cover to keep warm.

4. Add half of the sherry to the skillet used to cook the pork, and cook over medium-high heat, stirring frequently, until most of the sherry has evaporated. Add the mushrooms and cook, stirring frequently, for about 3 minutes or until the mushrooms begin to brown and release their juices. Add the remaining sherry and cook, stirring frequently, until the sherry is reduced by half.

5. Reduce the heat to medium and pour any juices that have accumulated on the plate containing the cooked tenderloins into the skillet. Add the sour cream mixture to the skillet and stir to mix well. Cook, stirring constantly, until the mixture comes to a boil and thickens slightly. To serve, place 2 of the pork medallions on each of 4 serving plates and cover with some of the sauce. Serve hot.

Nutritional Facts (per serving)

CALORIES: 200 CARBOHYDRATES: 8 G CHOLESTEROL: 73 MG FAT: 4 G FIBER: 0.5 G
PROTEIN: 26 G SODIUM: 310 MG CALCIUM: 46 MG GI RATING: VERY LOW

Cantonese Roast Pork

YIELD: 8 SERVINGS

2 pork tenderloins (1 pound each)

Marinade
½ cup orange juice
3 tablespoons reduced-sodium soy sauce
3 tablespoons hoisin sauce*
2 teaspoons crushed garlic
2¼ teaspoons freshly grated gingerroot; or ¾ teaspoon ground ginger

1. Combine all the marinade ingredients in a small bowl and stir to mix well. Remove 3 tablespoons of the marinade to a small bowl, and refrigerate until ready to cook the tenderloins.

*Hoisin sauce is available in the Asian foods section of most grocery stores.

2. Rinse the tenderloins and pat them dry with paper towels. Trim away any excess fat. Place the tenderloins in a shallow nonmetal container and pour the remaining marinade over the meat. Lift the meat to allow the marinade to flow underneath. Cover and refrigerate for 6 to 24 hours, turning occasionally.

3. Coat the rack of a broiler pan with nonstick cooking spray and fill the bottom of the pan with a half-inch of water. Lay the tenderloins on the pan, spacing them at least 3 inches apart (discard the marinade used to soak the meat). Bake at 450° F for about 25 to 30 minutes or until a thermometer inserted in the thickest part of the meat reads 155 to 160° F. Baste with the reserved marinade several times during the last 15 minutes of cooking.

4. Remove the tenderloins from the oven, cover loosely with foil, and let sit for 5 minutes before slicing thinly at an angle and serving.

Nutritional Facts (per serving)

CALORIES: 149   CARBOHYDRATES: 2 G   CHOLESTEROL: 73 MG   FAT: 3.9 G   FIBER: 0 G
PROTEIN: 24 G   SODIUM: 280 MG   CALCIUM: 7 MG   GI RATING: VERY LOW

Slow-Simmered Pork Roast

YIELD: 6 SERVINGS

2 pounds boneless extra-lean pork sirloin roast
1 cup water
1 tablespoon instant chicken bouillon granules
1 teaspoon dried rosemary
1 teaspoon dried sage
½ teaspoon coarsely ground black pepper
¾ pound small new potatoes, halved
3 medium carrots, peeled and cut into 2-inch pieces, or 1½ cups baby carrots
18 whole fresh mushrooms

Gravy
½ cup evaporated skim milk
¼ cup whole-wheat pastry flour or unbleached flour

1. Trim the visible fat from the roast, rinse the roast with cool water, and pat it dry with paper towels. Coat a nonstick 4-quart pot with cooking spray and preheat over medium-high heat. Add the roast to the pot and cook for a couple of minutes on each side or until nicely browned.

2. Combine the water, bouillon granules, rosemary, sage, and black pepper, and pour over the roast. Reduce the heat to low, cover, and simmer for 1 hour and 15 minutes.

3. Place the potatoes, carrots, and mushrooms around the roast and raise the heat to return the mixture to a boil. Reduce the heat to low, cover, and simmer for an additional 30 minutes or until the meat and vegetables are tender.

4. Remove the meat to a serving platter and, using a slotted spoon, transfer the vegetables to the platter. Pour the pan juices into a fat separator cup, then pour the defatted broth into a 2-cup measure. If necessary, add water to bring the volume up to 1½ cups.

5. To make the gravy, pour the defatted broth into a 1-quart pot, and bring to a boil over medium heat. Combine the evaporated milk and flour in a jar with a tight-fitting lid and shake until smooth. Slowly pour the milk mixture into the boiling broth, while whisking constantly. Cook and stir for a minute or two or until the mixture is thickened and bubbly. Pour the gravy into a warmed gravy boat, and serve hot with the meat and vegetables.

Nutritional Facts (per serving)

CALORIES: 288 CARBOHYDRATES: 24 G CHOLESTEROL: 95 MG FAT: 5.6 G FIBER: 3.3 G
PROTEIN: 37 G SODIUM: 509 MG CALCIUM: 77 MG GI RATING: MODERATE

Unfried Fish

YIELD: 4 SERVINGS

2 cups Special K cereal
2 teaspoons Cajun or Old Bay seasoning
¼ cup plus 2 tablespoons fat-free egg substitute
1 pound orange roughy, cod, flounder, or other whitefish fillets, cut into 8 equal
    pieces
Butter-flavored nonstick cooking spray

Sauce
¼ cup nonfat or light mayonnaise
1 tablespoon finely chopped onion
1½ teaspoons finely chopped capers
¼ teaspoon Dijon mustard

1. To make the sauce, combine all the sauce ingredients in a small bowl, and stir to mix well. Set aside.

2. Put the cereal in a food processor and process into coarse crumbs. (Alternatively, place the cereal in a plastic zip-type bag and crush with a rolling pin or the bottom of a glass.) There should be 1 cup of crumbs. Pour the crumbs into a shallow dish, add the Cajun or Old Bay seasoning, and stir to mix well. Pour the egg substitute in another shallow dish.

3. Dip the fish pieces first in the egg substitute and then in the crumb mixture, turning to coat both sides well.

4. Coat a large baking sheet with nonstick cooking spray, and arrange the fish fillets on the sheet in a single layer. Spray the tops lightly with the cooking spray and bake at 450° F for 12 to 15 minutes or until the outside is crisp and golden and the fish flakes easily with a fork. Serve hot, accompanied by the sauce.

Nutritional Facts (per serving)

CALORIES: 146 CARBOHYDRATES: 12 G CHOLESTEROL: 22 MG FAT: 1.3 G FIBER: 0.6 G
PROTEIN: 21 G SODIUM: 519 MG CALCIUM: 43 MG GI RATING: MODERATE

Almond-Dill Fish

YIELD: 4 SERVINGS

1½ cups Special K cereal
1 teaspoon lemon pepper
½ teaspoon dried dill
¼ cup sliced almonds
¼ cup plus 2 tablespoons fat-free egg substitute
1 pound orange roughy, cod, flounder, or other whitefish fillets, cut into 8 equal
    pieces
Butter-flavored nonstick cooking spray
Lemon wedges (garnish)

1. Put the cereal in a food processor and process into coarse crumbs. (Alternatively, place the cereal in a plastic zip-type bag and crush with a rolling pin or the bottom of a glass.) There should be ¾ cup of crumbs. Pour the crumbs in a shallow dish, add the lemon pepper and dill, and stir to mix well. Crush the almonds into small bits and add to the crumb mixture. Pour the egg substitute in another shallow dish.

2. Dip the fish pieces first in the egg substitute and then in the crumb mixture, turning to coat both sides well.

3. Coat a large baking sheet with nonstick cooking spray, and arrange the fish fillets on the sheet

in a single layer. Spray the tops lightly with the cooking spray and bake at 450° F for 12 to 15 minutes or until the outside is crisp and golden and the fish flakes easily with a fork. Serve hot, accompanied by the lemon wedges.

Nutritional Facts (per serving)

CALORIES: 164 CARBOHYDRATES: 9 G CHOLESTEROL: 22 MG FAT: 4.6 G FIBER: 0.8 G

PROTEIN: 21 G SODIUM: 299 MG CALCIUM: 57 MG GI RATING: MODERATE

Grouper El Greco

YIELD: 4 SERVINGS

4 grouper, snapper, or orange roughy fillets (6 ounces each)
1 teaspoon lemon pepper
2–3 teaspoons extra-virgin olive oil
1½ cups sliced fresh mushrooms
½ cup chopped green bell pepper
½ cup chopped onion
1 teaspoon crushed garlic
½ teaspoon dried oregano
¼ teaspoon salt
¼ cup dry white wine
1 cup chopped seeded plum tomatoes (about 4 medium)
¼ cup crumbled nonfat or reduced-fat feta cheese (optional)

1. Rinse the fish and pat it dry with paper towels. Coat a medium-sized baking sheet with non-stick cooking spray, and place the fillets on the sheet. Sprinkle each fillet with some of the lemon pepper. Bake uncovered at 450° F for about 10 minutes or until the fish flakes easily with a fork.

2. While the fish is cooking, coat a large nonstick skillet with the olive oil. Add the mushrooms, bell peppers, onion, garlic, oregano, and salt and place the skillet over medium-high heat. Cook, stirring frequently, for about 4 minutes or until the vegetables are crisp-tender. Periodically place a lid over the skillet if it begins to dry out. (The steam released during cooking will moisten the skillet.) Add the wine to the skillet and cook uncovered for a couple of minutes or until the wine is reduced by half.

3. Add the tomatoes to the skillet, and reduce the heat to medium. Cover and cook for a minute or two, or just until the tomatoes are heated through and begin to soften.

4. Place a fish fillet on each of 4 serving plates and top each fillet with a quarter of the vegetable mixture. Top each serving with some of the feta cheese if desired. Serve immediately.

Nutritional Facts (per serving)

CALORIES: 203 CARBOHYDRATES: 6 G CHOLESTEROL: 63 MG FAT: 4.3 G FIBER: 1.4 G
PROTEIN: 34 G SODIUM: 356 MG CALCIUM: 54 MG GI RATING: VERY LOW

Salmon Cakes with Cucumber-Dill Sauce

YIELD: 4 SERVINGS

¼ cup plus 2 tablespoons finely chopped celery (include the leaves)
¼ cup plus 2 tablespoons finely chopped scallions
1½ cups flaked cooked salmon or 2 cans (6 ounces each) boneless, skinless salmon, drained
¾ teaspoon lemon pepper
¾ teaspoon finely chopped fresh dill; or ¼ teaspoon dried dill
1 cup whole-wheat bread or multigrain crumbs*
2 tablespoons fat-free egg substitute; or 1 egg white, lightly beaten
2 tablespoons nonfat or light mayonnaise
Olive oil nonstick cooking spray

Sauce
¼ cup nonfat or light mayonnaise
¼ cup nonfat or light sour cream or plain yogurt
1 tablespoon finely chopped fresh dill; or 1 teaspoon dried dill
½ cup finely chopped seeded cucumber

1. To make the sauce, combine all the sauce ingredients in a small bowl and stir to mix well. Set aside.
2. Put the celery and scallions in a large nonstick skillet and add a tablespoon of water. Place the skillet over medium heat, cover, and cook, stirring occasionally, for about 3 minutes or until the vegetables are soft. Add a little more water if the skillet becomes too dry.
3. Remove the skillet from the heat and stir in first the drained salmon, lemon pepper, and dill, then the bread crumbs, and finally the egg substitute and mayonnaise. Shape the salmon mixture into four 3½-inch patties.

*To make whole-wheat bread crumbs, tear about 1¼ slices of firm stone-ground whole-wheat or multigrain bread into chunks. Place in a food processor or blender and process into crumbs.

4. Coat a large nonstick skillet with cooking spray and preheat over medium heat. Cook the patties for about 3 minutes or until the bottoms are nicely browned. Spray the tops of the patties lightly with the cooking spray, turn, and cook for an additional 3 minutes or until the patties are nicely browned on the second side. Serve hot, accompanied by the sauce.

Nutritional Facts (per serving)

CALORIES: 167 CARBOHYDRATES: 11 G CHOLESTEROL: 32 MG FAT: 4.5 G FIBER: 1.2 G
PROTEIN: 18 G SODIUM: 355 MG CALCIUM: 69 MG GI rating: low

Grilled Ginger Fish

YIELD: 4 SERVINGS

4 firm-fleshed fish steaks or fillets, such as tuna, salmon, mahi mahi, grouper, or
  amberjack (5 ounces each)

Marinade
3 tablespoons dry sherry
3 tablespoons reduced-sodium soy sauce
2 tablespoons frozen (thawed) orange juice concentrate
1 tablespoon freshly grated ginger; or 1 teaspoon dried ground ginger
1 tablespoon toasted (dark) sesame oil
1 teaspoon crushed garlic

1. Combine all the marinade ingredients in a shallow nonmetal dish and stir to mix well. Remove 2 tablespoons of the marinade, transfer to a covered container, and refrigerate until ready to cook the fish.
2. Place the fish in the dish, and turn to coat all sides with the marinade. Cover and marinate in the refrigerator, turning occasionally, for 1–2 hours.
3. Grill the fish, covered, over medium coals, or broil 6 inches under a preheated broiler for about 5 minutes on each side or until the meat is easily flaked with a fork. Baste with the reserved marinade during the last few minutes of cooking. Serve hot.

Nutritional Facts (per serving)

CALORIES: 170 CARBOHYDRATES: 1 G CHOLESTEROL: 63 MG FAT: 2.5 G FIBER: 0 G
PROTEIN: 33 G SODIUM: 278 MG CALCIUM: 25 MG GI rating: VERY LOW

Citrus Grilled Fish

4 firm-fleshed fish steaks or fillets (5 ounces each), such as tuna, salmon, mahi
   mahi, grouper, or amberjack

Marinade
⅓ cup orange juice
1 tablespoon plus 1½ teaspoons extra-virgin olive oil
1 tablespoon lemon juice
1 teaspoon dried dill, thyme, or oregano
1 teaspoon crushed garlic
½ teaspoon coarsely ground black pepper
¼ teaspoon salt

1. Combine all the marinade ingredients in a shallow nonmetal dish and stir to mix well. Remove 2 tablespoons of the marinade, transfer to a covered container, and refrigerate until ready to cook the fish.
2. Place the fish in the dish, and turn to coat all sides with the marinade. Cover, and marinate in the refrigerator, turning occasionally, for 1–2 hours.
3. Grill the fish, covered, over medium coals, or broil 6 inches under a preheated broiler for about 5 minutes on each side or until the meat is easily flaked with a fork. Baste with the reserved marinade during the last few minutes of cooking. Serve hot.

Nutritional Facts (per serving)
   CALORIES: 170 CARBOHYDRATES: 1 G CHOLESTEROL: 63 MG FAT: 2.5 G FIBER: 0 G
   PROTEIN: 33 G SODIUM: 278 MG CALCIUM: 25 MG GI RATING: VERY LOW

Creamy Risotto

2 tablespoons reduced-fat margarine or light butter
1½ cups sliced fresh mushrooms
¼ cup finely chopped onion
1 teaspoon crushed garlic

1½ cups long-grain or basmati white rice

2½ cups reduced-sodium chicken broth

1½ cups skim or low-fat milk

1 tablespoon dried parsley

⅛ teaspoon ground white pepper

¼ cup grated Parmesan cheese

Toppings
3 tablespoons finely chopped scallions

Additional Parmesan cheese (optional)

1. Put the margarine or butter in a 3-quart nonstick pot and melt over medium-high heat. Add the mushrooms, onions, and garlic and cook, stirring frequently, for a couple of minutes or until the mushrooms and onions start to soften (do not brown).

2. Add the rice, broth, milk, parsley, and white pepper to the pot, and bring to a boil. Stir to mix well, and reduce the heat to low. Cover and simmer, stirring occasionally, for about 20 minutes or until most of the liquid has been absorbed and the rice is tender but still a little firm to the bite.

3. Add the Parmesan cheese to the pot and stir to mix well. Add a little more milk if necessary to bring the mixture to a moist and creamy consistency. Serve hot, topping each serving with a sprinkling of scallions and some additional Parmesan cheese if desired.

Nutritional Facts (per 1-cup serving)

CALORIES: 300 CARBOHYDRATES: 53 G CHOLESTEROL: 5 MG FAT: 4.2 G FIBER: 1.2 G PROTEIN: 10.2 G SODIUM: 245 MG CALCIUM: 195 MG GI RATING: LOW

For variety, try any of the following:

• Stir ¾ cup of frozen green peas, fresh cut asparagus, or chopped frozen (thawed) artichoke hearts into the rice mixture 3 to 5 minutes before it is done.

• Stir 1 cup (packed) chopped fresh spinach into the rice mixture along with the Parmesan cheese. Cook and stir for a minute or two or just until the spinach wilts.

• Place 3 to 4 tablespoons of chopped sun-dried tomatoes in a small bowl and cover with boiling water. Let sit for 10 minutes or until the tomatoes plump. Drain off the excess liquid and add the tomatoes to the finished risotto.

• Add 1 cup of diced roasted chicken along with the Parmesan cheese.

• Add ½ pound of steamed or sautéed scallops or shrimp along with the Parmesan cheese.

Pepperoni Pizza

Oat Bran Pizza Crust (page 262)
¾ cup bottled marinara sauce
15–20 turkey pepperoni slices
1 cup shredded reduced-fat mozzarella cheese (or use half mozzarella plus half
    white Cheddar)
½ cup sliced mushrooms
½ small yellow onion cut into thin wedges

1. Spread the sauce over the crust to within one-half inch of the edges, and top with the pepper-oni. Sprinkle the cheese over the top, then top with the mushrooms and onions.
2. Bake at 425° F for about 12 minutes, or until the cheese is melted and the crust is lightly browned. Slice and serve immediately.

Nutritional Facts (per slice)
   CALORIES: 136   CARBOHYDRATES: 21 G   CHOLESTEROL: 12 MG   FAT: 3 G   FIBER: 2 G
   PROTEIN: 10 G   SODIUM: 295 MG   CALCIUM: 77 MG   GI RATING: MODERATE

Portabella Pizza

YIELD: 8 SLICES

Oat Bran Pizza Crust (page 262)
2 medium-large Portabella mushrooms, sliced ½ inch thick
Nonstick olive oil cooking spray
⅛ teaspoon salt
⅛ teaspoon ground black pepper
¼ teaspoon dried oregano
¾ cup bottled marinara sauce
2 tablespoons grated Parmesan cheese
1 cup shredded reduced-fat mozzarella cheese (or use half mozzarella plus half
    provolone)

Oat-Bran Pizza Crust

✎ Pizza is perhaps one of the most requested meals in many families. And contrary to popular belief, pizza doesn't have to be junk food. Start out with a wholesome crust, like Oat-Bran Pizza Crust, in which oat bran replaces part of the flour to lower the GI and boost nutrition. When you add plenty of vegetable toppings and top it off with reduced-fat cheese, you actually have a respectable main dish. Keep the GI of your meal low by adding a fresh green salad with vinaigrette dressing. If you have a bread machine, you will find that making pizza is so easy, you will want to make your own crust on a regular basis.

When time is in short supply, you can also use rounds of whole-wheat or oat-bran pita bread for pizza crusts. Simply divide the toppings in the pizza recipes among four 6-inch pita rounds and bake at 400° F for about 10 minutes.

YIELD: ONE 14-INCH CRUST

1¼ cups wheat blend or regular bread flour
½ cup oat bran
3 tablespoons instant buttermilk powder or nonfat dry milk powder
1½ teaspoons rapid rising yeast
1 teaspoon sugar
¼ teaspoon salt
¾ cup water

1. Place all the dough ingredients in the pan of a bread machine. Set the machine to "rise," "dough," "manual," or equivalent setting so that the machine will mix and knead the dough and let it rise once. Check the mixture 5 minutes after the machine has started. It should form a soft, satiny dough. If the dough seems too sticky, add a little more flour, a tablespoonful at a time. Be careful not to add too much flour or the crust will be hard to roll out.

2. When the dough is ready, remove it from the machine and place it on a lightly floured surface. Roll the crust into a 14-inch circle, then transfer it to a 14-inch pizza pan. Set the crust aside for 10 minutes (to allow it to rise slightly) before adding the toppings.

1. Combine ¾ cup of the flour and all the oat bran, milk powder, yeast, sugar, and salt in a large bowl and stir to mix well. Pour the water in a small saucepan and heat until very warm (125 to 130° F). Add the water to the flour mixture and stir for 1 minute. Stir in enough of the remaining flour, 2 tablespoonsful at a time, to form a soft dough.
2. Sprinkle 2 tablespoons of the remaining flour over a flat surface and turn the dough onto the surface. Knead the dough for 5 minutes, gradually adding enough flour to form a smooth, satiny dough. (Be careful not to make the dough too stiff, or it will be hard to roll out.)
3. Coat a large bowl with nonstick cooking spray, and place the ball of dough in the bowl. Cover the bowl with a clean kitchen towel, and let rise in a warm place for about 35 minutes or until doubled in size.
4. When the dough has risen, punch it down, shape it into a ball, turn it onto a lightly floured surface, and roll into a 14-inch circle.

Nutritional Facts (per ⅛ crust)

CALORIES: 84 CARBOHYDRATES: 19 G CHOLESTEROL: 0 MG FAT: 0.5 G

FIBER: 1.6 G PROTEIN: 4 G SODIUM: 81 MG CALCIUM: 23 MG

GI RATING: MODERATE

1. Coat a medium-sized baking sheet with the cooking spray and lay the mushroom slices on the sheet. Spray the tops of the mushroom slices lightly with the cooking spray and sprinkle with the salt, black pepper, and oregano. Bake at 450° F for 10 minutes, turn the slices, and bake for 5 additional minutes, or until the slices are tender and nicely browned. Remove the mushroom slices from the oven and set aside.
2. Spread the sauce over the crust to within one-half inch of the edges. Sprinkle the Parmesan cheese over the sauce and top the pizza with the mushroom slices, arranging them like the spokes of a wheel. Sprinkle the mozzarella cheese over the top.
3. Bake at 425° F for about 12 minutes or until the cheese is melted and the crust is lightly browned. Slice and serve immediately.

Nutritional Facts (per slice)

CALORIES: 135 CARBOHYDRATES: 21 G CHOLESTEROL: 9 MG FAT: 3 G FIBER: 2 G

PROTEIN: 9.7 G SODIUM: 264 MG CALCIUM: 97 MG GI RATING: MODERATE

Saucy Spinach Pizza

YIELD: 8 SLICES

Oat Bran Pizza Crust (page 262)
1 cup sliced fresh mushrooms
2 cups coarsely chopped fresh spinach
¾ cup bottled marinara sauce
¼ cup nonfat or reduced-fat feta cheese
1 cup shredded reduced-fat mozzarella cheese

1. Coat a large nonstick skillet with nonstick olive oil cooking spray and add the mushrooms. Place the skillet over medium-high heat and cook, stirring frequently, for about 3 minutes or until the mushrooms are nicely browned and have released their juices. Place a lid over the skillet periodically if it begins to dry out. (The steam released during cooking will moisten the skillet.) Or add a few teaspoons of water if needed. Add the spinach to the skillet and cook, stirring frequently, for another minute or two or until the spinach is wilted. Remove the skillet from the heat and set aside.

2. Spread the sauce over the crust to within one-half inch of the edges. Spread the spinach mixture over the sauce, then sprinkle first with the feta cheese and then with the mozzarella cheese.

3. Bake at 425° F for about 12 minutes or until the cheese is melted and the crust is lightly browned. Slice and serve immediately.

Nutritional Facts (per slice)

CALORIES: 132 CARBOHYDRATES: 21 G CHOLESTEROL: 8 MG FAT: 2.3 G FIBER: 2 G
PROTEIN: 10 G SODIUM: 310 MG CALCIUM: 103 MG GI RATING: MODERATE

15. Delectable Desserts

Y ou may be happy to learn that living a low-GI lifestyle does not have to mean waving good-bye to dessert. Some desserts, however, are definitely better choices than others. For instance, dairy products and most fruits naturally rank low on the glycemic index, so desserts that feature these ingredients—like baked fruits, fruit crisps, puddings, custard, and ice cream—are better choices than flour-based desserts like cakes and cookies. As a bonus, fruit and dairy desserts can also offer a respectable amount of nutrition.

Of course, sugar is an essential ingredient in most desserts. And while sugar has a moderate glycemic index, remember that it is still pure refined carbohydrate and so should be eaten in reasonable amounts. The recipes in this chapter were written with this in mind, and I strove to keep fat and calories to a minimum.

Many of the recipes in this chapter take advantage of the natural sweetness of fruit, so only a small amount of added sugar is needed. Others combine sugar-free products with a small amount of sugar to produce sweet and satisfying treats with a delightfully low calorie and carbohydrate density. Some of the recipes in this chapter give you a choice of using sugar-free or sugar-sweetened products like pudding or yogurt. This will help you prepare dishes that best suit your taste and your personal nutritional needs.

So get ready to enjoy sweet satisfaction without an excess of fat, calories, or sugar. Whether you are looking for a simple baked custard, a flavorful fruit crisp, or a show-stopping trifle, here you will find a delightful array of deceptively decadent desserts that are right for any occasion.

Peach-Almond Crisp

YIELD: 8 SERVINGS

3–4 tablespoons sugar
1 tablespoon cornstarch
5 cups peeled sliced peaches (about 5 medium); or frozen peaches (thawed and undrained)

Topping
½ cup old-fashioned rolled oats
3 tablespoons whole-wheat pastry flour
¼ cup plus 2 tablespoons light brown sugar
½ teaspoon ground cinnamon
2 tablespoons chilled margarine or butter, cut into small pieces
2 teaspoons frozen (thawed) white grape or orange juice concentrate
⅓ cup chopped almonds

1. Combine the sugar and cornstarch in a small bowl and stir to mix well. Place the peaches in a large bowl, sprinkle with the sugar-cornstarch mixture, and toss to mix well. Coat a 9-inch deep-dish pie pan with nonstick cooking spray and spread the fruit mixture evenly in the dish.

2. To make the topping, combine the oats, flour, brown sugar, and cinnamon in a medium-sized bowl and stir to mix well. Using a pastry cutter or two knives, cut in the margarine or butter until the mixture is crumbly. Add the juice concentrate and stir lightly until the mixture is moist and crumbly. Add a little more juice concentrate if the mixture seems too dry. Add the almonds and toss lightly to mix.

3. Spread the oat mixture over the fruit and bake at 375° F for about 35 minutes or until the fruit is bubbly around the edges and the topping is golden brown. Cover the dish loosely with foil during the last few minutes of baking if the topping starts to brown too quickly. Remove the dish from the oven and let sit for at least 20 minutes before serving warm.

Nutritional Facts (per serving)

CALORIES: 192 CARBOHYDRATES: 33 G CHOLESTEROL: 0 MG FAT: 6.2 G FIBER: 3.6 G
PROTEIN: 3.2 G SODIUM: 48 MG CALCIUM: 33 MG GI RATING: LOW

Variations

• **Pear and Walnut Crisp:** Substitute sliced peeled pears for the peaches and walnuts or pecans for the almonds.

• **Apple Crisp:** Substitute sliced peeled Golden Delicious apples for the peaches and walnuts or pecans for the almonds. Add 3 tablespoons of apple juice to the fruit filling along with the sugar and cornstarch.

• **Apricot or Plum Crisp:** Substitute sliced fresh unpeeled apricots or plums for the peaches.

Summer Fruit Cobbler

YIELD: 8 SERVINGS

¼ to ⅓ cup sugar
1 tablespoon plus 1 teaspoon cornstarch
5 cups fresh or frozen (thawed and undrained) blueberries;
   dark, sweet pitted cherries; or mixed berries
¼ cup orange or white grape juice

Topping
½ cup unbleached flour
½ cup oat bran
3 tablespoons plus 1½ teaspoons sugar
1½ teaspoons baking powder
½ cup plus 2 tablespoons nonfat or low-fat vanilla yogurt
2 tablespoons canola oil

1. Combine the sugar and cornstarch in a small bowl and stir to mix well. Place the fruit in a large bowl, add the sugar-cornstarch mixture, and toss to mix well. Add the orange or white grape juice and toss again.

2. Coat a 2-quart casserole dish with nonstick cooking spray and spread the fruit mixture evenly in the dish. Cover the dish with aluminum foil and bake at 375° F for 30 minutes or until hot and bubbly.

3. To make the topping, combine the flour, oat bran, 3 tablespoons of the sugar, and the baking powder in a medium-sized bowl and stir to mix well. Add the yogurt and oil and stir to mix well.

4. Drop heaping tablespoonfuls of the batter onto the hot fruit filling to make 8 biscuits. Sprinkle the remaining 1½ teaspoons of sugar over the tops of the biscuits.

5. Bake uncovered at 375° F for 15 minutes or just until the biscuits are lightly browned around the edges. Remove the dish from the oven and let sit for at least 30 minutes before serving warm.

Nutritional Facts (per serving)
CALORIES: 192 CARBOHYDRATES: 39 G CHOLESTEROL: 0 MG FAT: 4.2 G FIBER: 3.5 G
PROTEIN: 3.4 G SODIUM: 87 MG CALCIUM: 107 MG GI RATING: LOW

Glorious Grapes

✍ For variety, substitute fresh blueberries for the grapes.

YIELD: 4 SERVINGS

2⅔ cups seedless red or green grapes, rinsed, patted dry, and chilled
½ cup nonfat or light sour cream
2 tablespoons plus 2 teaspoons light brown sugar

1. Rinse the grapes and thoroughly pat them dry with paper towels. Transfer to a covered container and refrigerate until well chilled.
2. Combine the grapes and sour cream in a medium-sized bowl and toss to coat the grapes with the sour cream.
3. Spoon the mixture into four 8-ounce dessert dishes and sprinkle 2 teaspoons of the brown sugar over the top of each dessert. Serve immediately.

Nutritional Facts (per serving)

CALORIES: 141 CARBOHYDRATES: 33 G CHOLESTEROL: 0 MG FAT: 0.6 G FIBER: 1.1 G
PROTEIN: 2.5 G SODIUM: 27 MG CALCIUM: 55 MG GI RATING: LOW

Glazed Summer Berries

YIELD: 4 SERVINGS

Glaze
¼ cup seedless raspberry fruit spread or jam
1 tablespoon orange, cranberry, or white grape juice

2 cups sliced fresh strawberries
1 cup fresh raspberries, rinsed, patted dry, and chilled
1 cup fresh blueberries or blackberries, rinsed, patted dry, and chilled
½ cup nonfat or light whipped topping (optional)
2 tablespoons sliced almonds (optional)

1. To make the glaze, put the fruit spread in a 1-cup glass measure or a small microwave-safe bowl and microwave at high power for about 1 minute or until hot and runny. Stir the juice into the hot fruit spread. Cover the glaze and refrigerate for at least 2 hours or until well chilled.
2. Place the berries in a large bowl, pour the glaze over the berries, and toss to mix well. Divide the berries among four 10-ounce balloon wineglasses and serve immediately, topping each serving with some of the whipped topping and almonds if desired.

Nutritional Facts (per serving)

CALORIES: 118 CARBOHYDRATES: 29 G CHOLESTEROL: 0 MG FAT: 0.7 G FIBER: 5.2 G
PROTEIN: 1.2 G SODIUM: 5 MG CALCIUM: 25 MG GI RATING: LOW

Chocolate-Covered Strawberries

YIELD: 24 PIECES

24 fresh large strawberries (about 1½ pounds)
8 ounces semisweet chocolate

1. Rinse the berries with cool water (leave the stems on), and pat dry thoroughly with paper towels. Set aside.
2. Fill a 2-quart pot one-third full with water and bring to a boil over high heat. Reduce the heat to low to maintain the water at a low simmer. Break the chocolate into pieces and put in a 2-cup glass measure. Place the measuring cup in the simmering water and stir frequently for several minutes or until the chocolate melts. Remove the pot from the heat.
3. Insert a toothpick into the stem end of a strawberry and dip the berry into the melted chocolate to coat the lower three-quarters of the berry. Place the other end of the toothpick into a piece of Styrofoam or place the chocolate-coated berry on a small baking sheet lined with waxed paper. Refrigerate the berries for at least 30 minutes and up to 12 hours before serving.

Nutritional Facts (per piece)

CALORIES: 53 CARBOHYDRATES: 6 G CHOLESTEROL: 0 MG FAT: 3.8 G FIBER: 1 G
PROTEIN: 0.9 G SODIUM: 0 MG CALCIUM: 9 MG GI RATING: LOW

All-Fruit Applesauce

YIELD: 8 SERVINGS

8 cups (about 10 medium) coarsely chopped, peeled cooking apples, such as Golden
   Delicious, Winesap, Crispin, Jonathan, Braeburn, Cortland, Gravenstein, or Ida
   Red (for best results, use a mixture of two or more varieties)
1 cup apple juice
½ teaspoon ground cinnamon (optional)
½ teaspoon ground nutmeg (optional)

1. Combine the apples, apple juice, and, if desired, the spices in a 4-quart pot. Cover and cook over medium-high heat for 5 minutes, stirring occasionally, until the mixture comes to a boil and the apples begin to soften and release some of their juices. Reduce the heat to low, and simmer, stirring occasionally, for about 25 minutes more or until the apples are very soft and break down.
2. Use a potato masher to mash the apples to the desired consistency, adding a little more apple juice if the mixture seems too thick. Transfer the applesauce to a covered container and refrigerate for several hours or until well chilled before serving.

Nutritional Facts (per ½-cup serving)
CALORIES: 73 CARBOHYDRATES: 18 G CHOLESTEROL: 0 MG FAT: 0.3 G FIBER: 2.1 G
PROTEIN: 0.2 G SODIUM: 2 MG GI RATING: VERY LOW

Harvest Baked Apples

YIELD: 4 SERVINGS

4 medium cooking apples, such as Golden Delicious or Rome
3 tablespoons chopped dried apricots or mixed dried fruit
3 tablespoons chopped walnuts or pecans
1 tablespoon light brown sugar
¼ teaspoon ground cinnamon
⅛ teaspoon ground nutmeg
4 teaspoons reduced-fat margarine or light butter
½ cup orange, apple, or cranberry juice
Low-fat vanilla ice cream (optional)

1. Starting at the stem end, use a melon baller to scoop the core out of each apple, taking care not to cut all the way through the opposite end. Peel the top third of each apple.
2. Place the apples in a nonstick 8-inch square pan. Combine the dried apricots or mixed fruit, nuts, brown sugar, cinnamon, and nutmeg in a small dish and toss to mix well. Spoon a quarter of the fruit mixture into the cavity of each apple. Dot the top of each apple with 1 teaspoon of the margarine or butter. Pour the juice into the bottom of the pan.
3. Cover the pan with aluminum foil and bake at 350° F for 30 minutes. Uncover the pan and baste the apples with the pan juices. Then bake uncovered, basting occasionally with the pan juices, for 15 additional minutes or until the apples are tender when pierced with a sharp knife.
4. Transfer the apples to serving dishes and spoon some of the pan juices over the tops. Serve warm. Top with a scoop of low-fat vanilla ice cream if desired.

Nutritional Facts (per serving)

CALORIES: 171 CARBOHYDRATES: 32 G CHOLESTEROL: 0 MG FAT: 5.2 G FIBER: 4.5 G
PROTEIN: 1.7 G SODIUM: 36 MG CALCIUM: 16 MG GI RATING: LOW

Variation

To make **Harvest Baked Pears,** cut the tops off 4 large pears so they have a roundish shape like an apple. Scoop the core out of each pear, fill, and bake as directed above, reducing the baking time to 20 minutes covered and about 10 minutes uncovered.

Nutritional Facts (per serving)

CALORIES: 179 CARBOHYDRATES: 33 G CHOLESTEROL: 0 MG FAT: 5.2 G
FIBER: 4.5 G PROTEIN: 1.9 G SODIUM: 36 MG CALCIUM: 32 MG

Sweet Cherry Mousse

YIELD: 5 SERVINGS

2 cups fresh or frozen (thawed and undrained) pitted dark, sweet cherries, halved
1 cup vanilla yogurt cheese (page 272)
2 cups nonfat or light whipped topping

1. Put the cherries in a 1-quart pot and place the pot over medium heat. Cover and cook, stirring occasionally, for about 5 minutes or until the cherries break down and release their juices. Re-

move the lid and cook uncovered, stirring frequently, for about 5 to 8 additional minutes or until the cherries reduce to about ¾ cup in volume. Transfer the cherries to a covered container and refrigerate for several hours or until well chilled.

2. When the cherries are chilled, place the yogurt cheese in a medium-sized bowl. Add the cherries and stir to mix well. Gently fold in the whipped topping.

3. Divide the mousse among five 8-ounce wineglasses or dessert dishes. Cover the desserts and refrigerate for at least 1 hour before serving.

Nutritional Facts (per ¾-cup serving)

CALORIES: 134 CARBOHYDRATES: 25 G CHOLESTEROL: 1 MG FAT: 1.1 G FIBER: 1.6 G
PROTEIN: 4.5 G SODIUM: 54 MG CALCIUM: 112 MG GI RATING: LOW

Variation

To make **Peach or Apricot Mousse,** substitute 2 cups chopped peeled peaches or apricots plus 2 tablespoons orange or white-grape juice for the cherries.

Nutritional Facts (per serving)

CALORIES: 122 CARBOHYDRATES: 24 G CHOLESTEROL: 1 MG FAT: 1.1 G FIBER: 1.7 G
PROTEIN: 4.2 G SODIUM: 50 MG CALCIUM: 95 MG GI RATING: LOW

Making Yogurt Cheese

A good substitute for cream cheese in desserts, dips, and spreads, yogurt cheese can be made at home with any brand of yogurt that does not contain gelatin, modified food starch, or vegetable gums like carrageenan and guar gum. (These ingredients will prevent the yogurt from draining.) Yogurts that contain pectin will drain nicely and can be used for making cheese.

To make yogurt cheese, start with twice as much yogurt as the amount of cheese that you will need. For instance, if your recipe calls for 1 cup of yogurt cheese, start with 2 cups of yogurt. Place the yogurt in a funnel lined with cheesecloth (or use a specially designed yogurt-cheese funnel that can be purchased in cooking shops) and let the yogurt drain in the refrigerator for 8 hours or overnight. When the yogurt is reduced by half, it is ready to use.

Very Blueberry Mousse

YIELD: 5 SERVINGS

1-pound can blueberries in juice or light syrup, undrained
1 packet (¼-ounce) unflavored gelatin
¾ cup vanilla yogurt cheese (page 272)
2 cups nonfat or light whipped topping

1. Drain the berries, reserving the juice. Pour the juice in a small pot and bring to a boil over high heat.

2. Pour the boiling juice into a blender. Sprinkle the gelatin over the top and carefully blend at low speed with the lid slightly ajar (to allow steam to escape) for 1 minute or until the gelatin is completely dissolved. Pour the mixture into a large bowl and set aside for about 30 minutes or until it reaches room temperature.

3. When the gelatin mixture has cooled to room temperature, whisk in the yogurt cheese. Chill for 25 minutes. Stir the mixture. It should be the consistency of pudding. If it is too thin, return it to the refrigerator for a few minutes.

4. When the gelatin mixture has reached the proper consistency, stir it with a wire whisk until smooth. Gently fold in first the blueberries and then the whipped topping.

5. Divide the mixture among five 8-ounce wineglasses, cover, and chill for at least 3 hours, or until set before serving.

Nutritional Facts (per ¾-cup serving)
CALORIES: 154 CARBOHYDRATES: 33 G CHOLESTEROL: 1 MG FAT: 1.3 G FIBER: 1.4 G
PROTEIN: 3.5 G SODIUM: 48 MG CALCIUM: 72 MG GI RATING: LOW

Lemon Chiffon Pudding

YIELD: 5 SERVINGS

½ cup boiling water or orange juice
1 package sugar-free lemon gelatin mix (4-serving size)
½ cup nonfat or reduced-fat cream cheese
1½ cups sugar-free or regular nonfat or low-fat lemon yogurt
2 cups nonfat or light whipped topping

1. Pour the boiling water or juice into a blender and sprinkle the gelatin over the top. Place the lid on and, leaving the lid slightly ajar (to allow steam to escape), carefully blend the mixture at low speed for 1 minute or until the gelatin is completely dissolved. Remove the lid and set the blended mixture aside for 10 minutes to cool slightly.

2. Add the cheese to the blender mixture, place the lid on, and blend at low speed until the mixture is smooth. Transfer the blended mixture to a large bowl and whisk in the yogurt. Place the mixture in the refrigerator and chill for 15 minutes. Stir the mixture. It should be the consistency of pudding. If it is too thin, return it to the refrigerator for a few minutes.

3. When the gelatin mixture has reached the proper consistency, stir it with a wire whisk until smooth. Using a wooden spoon, gently fold in the whipped topping.

4. Divide the mixture among five 8-ounce wineglasses, cover, and chill for at least 3 hours or until set before serving.

Nutritional Facts (per ⅞-cup serving)

CALORIES: 131 CARBOHYDRATES: 20 G CHOLESTEROL: 3 MG FAT: 1 G FIBER: 0 G
PROTEIN: 9 G SODIUM: 251 MG CALCIUM: 220 MG GI RATING: LOW

Mandarin Mousse

YIELD: 5 SERVINGS

11-ounce can mandarin oranges in juice or light syrup, undrained
1 package sugar-free orange gelatin mix (4-serving size)
1¼ cups sugar-free or regular nonfat or low-fat vanilla yogurt
2 cups nonfat or light whipped topping

1. Drain the oranges, reserving the juice. Crush the oranges slightly, adding any juice that accumulates to the reserved juice, and set the oranges aside. Pour the juice in a small pot and bring to a boil over high heat.

2. Pour the boiling juice into a large bowl. Sprinkle the gelatin over the top and stir with a wire whisk for 3 minutes or until the gelatin is completely dissolved. Set the mixture aside for about 15 minutes or until it reaches room temperature.

3. When the gelatin mixture has cooled to room temperature, whisk in the yogurt. Place the mixture in the refrigerator and chill for 15 minutes. Stir the mixture. It should be the consistency of pudding. If it is too thin, return it to the refrigerator for a few minutes.

4. When the gelatin mixture has reached the proper consistency, stir it with a wire whisk until smooth. Gently fold in first the oranges and then the whipped topping.

5. Divide the mixture among five 8-ounce wineglasses, cover, and chill for at least 3 hours or until set before serving.

Sourdough Bread Pudding

YIELD: 6 SERVINGS

4 cups ½-inch sourdough bread cubes (about 4 slices)
¼ cup plus 3 tablespoons sugar
¼ cup plus 2 tablespoons fat-free egg substitute; or 2 large eggs
12-ounce can evaporated skim or low-fat milk
½ cup nonfat or low-fat milk
1½ teaspoons vanilla extract
3 tablespoons finely chopped dried apricots
⅛ teaspoon ground cinnamon

Sauce (Optional)
3 tablespoons apricot fruit spread or preserves
1 tablespoon plus 1½ teaspoons brandy
1 tablespoon plus 1½ teaspoons butter

1. Put the bread cubes in a large bowl and set aside.
2. Combine ¼ cup plus 2 tablespoons of the sugar and the egg substitute or eggs in a large bowl and stir with a wire whisk until the sugar is completely dissolved. Whisk in the evaporated milk, the nonfat or low-fat milk, and the vanilla extract. Pour the milk mixture over the bread cubes and set aside for 10 minutes to allow the bread to soften and soak up some of the milk. Stir in the apricots.
3. Coat a 1½-quart casserole dish with nonstick cooking spray and pour the mixture into the dish. Combine the remaining tablespoon of sugar and cinnamon in a small bowl, stir to mix well, and sprinkle over the pudding.
4. Place the dish in a large pan filled with 1 inch of hot tap water. Bake uncovered at 350° F for about 55 minutes or until a sharp knife inserted halfway between the center of the dish and the rim comes out clean. Allow to cool at room temperature for 45 minutes before serving.

5. To make the sauce, place all the sauce ingredients in a small pot. Cook and stir over medium heat for a minute or two or until hot and runny. Serve the pudding warm or at room temperature, topping each serving with a tablespoon of the sauce if desired. Refrigerate any leftovers.

Nutritional Facts (per ¾-cup serving)

CALORIES: 171 CARBOHYDRATES: 32 G CHOLESTEROL: 2 MG FAT: 0.8 G FIBER: 0.6 G
PROTEIN: 8 G SODIUM: 230 MG CALCIUM: 215 MG GI RATING: LOW

Basmati Rice Pudding

YIELD: 5 SERVINGS

⅓ cup basmati or long-grain white rice
3 cups skim or low-fat milk
¼ cup sugar
⅛ teaspoon salt
⅓ cup chopped dried apricots or golden raisins
3 tablespoons fat-free egg substitute; or 1 large egg, beaten
¾ teaspoon vanilla extract
Ground nutmeg or cinnamon (optional)

1. Combine the rice and milk in a nonstick 2½-quart pot and bring to a boil over medium-high heat. Reduce the heat to low, cover, and simmer for 20 minutes. Add the sugar, salt, and apricots or raisins, re-cover, and simmer, stirring occasionally, for an additional 10 to 15 minutes or until the rice is tender and about ¾ of the milk has been absorbed.

2. Pour ¼ cup of the rice mixture in a bowl and stir in the egg substitute or egg. Add to the pot, while stirring constantly. Cook and stir for an additional 2 minutes or until the mixture thickens slightly.

3. Remove the pot from the heat, stir in the vanilla extract, and let sit for 20 minutes. Stir the pudding and add a little milk if it seems too thick. Serve warm, or refrigerate and serve chilled, topping each serving with a sprinkling of nutmeg or cinnamon if desired.

Nutritional Facts (per ⅔-cup serving)

CALORIES: 168 CARBOHYDRATES: 34 G CHOLESTEROL: 3 MG FAT: 0.5 G FIBER: 1 G
PROTEIN: 7 G SODIUM: 154 MG CALCIUM: 190 MG GI RATING: LOW

Baked Egg Custard

¾ cup fat-free egg substitute; or 4 large eggs
¼ cup sugar
12-ounce can evaporated skim or low-fat milk
1 cup nonfat or low-fat milk
3 tablespoons honey
2 teaspoons vanilla extract
Ground nutmeg

Topping (optional)
¾ cup Summer Berry Sauce (page 103) or canned light (reduced-sugar) cherry pie
    filling (optional)

1. Combine the egg substitute or eggs and the sugar in a large bowl and stir with a wire whisk until the sugar is dissolved. Whisk in the remaining ingredients.
2. Coat six 6-ounce custard cups with nonstick cooking spray and divide the custard mixture evenly among the cups. Sprinkle the top of each cup of custard lightly with nutmeg. Place the cups in a large roasting pan filled with 1 inch of hot tap water.
3. Bake uncovered at 350° F for about 50 minutes or until a sharp knife inserted midway between the center of the custards and the rim of the cup comes out clean. Remove the custards to a wire rack and allow to cool to room temperature. Then cover and chill for at least 1 hour before serving. Serve plain, in the cups, or run a knife around the edges of the custards, invert onto serving plates, and top each custard with 2 tablespoons of Summer Berry Sauce or light (reduced-sugar) canned cherry pie filling.

Nutritional Facts (per serving)
CALORIES: 132 CARBOHYDRATES: 24 G CHOLESTEROL: 3 MG FAT: 0.2 G FIBER: 0 G
PROTEIN: 8.7 G SODIUM: 137 MG CALCIUM: 241 MG GI RATING: LOW

Really Raspberry Parfaits

For variety, try other fresh fruits and yogurt flavors such as blueberry, peach, and strawberry in this recipe. Or substitute chocolate, white chocolate, lemon, or vanilla pudding for the yogurt.

YIELD: 4 SERVINGS

2 cups sugar-free or regular raspberry or vanilla yogurt
2 cups chilled fresh raspberries
3 tablespoons sliced toasted almonds (see page 78)

1. Place 1½ tablespoons of the yogurt in the bottoms of each of four 8-ounce wineglasses, parfait glasses, or goblets. Top the yogurt in each glass with ¼ cup of the raspberries and 3 more table-spoons yogurt.
2. Repeat the berry-and-yogurt-mixture layers, then top each parfait with some of the almonds. Serve immediately.

Nutritional Facts (per serving)

CALORIES: 130 CARBOHYDRATES: 20 G CHOLESTEROL: 3 MG FAT: 2.7 G FIBER: 4.7 G
PROTEIN: 7.2 G SODIUM: 92 MG CALCIUM: 225 MG GI RATING: VERY LOW

Fabulous Fruit Trifle

YIELD: 9 SERVINGS

18 ladyfingers (about 4½ ounces), split open; or 8 slices (½-inch-thick) sponge cake or low-fat pound cake

Pudding
2 cups skim or low-fat milk
1 package (4-serving size) cook-and-serve vanilla pudding mix (sugar-free or regular)

Fruit Mixture
2 cups fresh sliced strawberries or peeled diced peaches or apricots
1 cup fresh or frozen (thawed) raspberries, blackberries, blueberries, or pitted dark sweet cherries

2 tablespoons sugar

2–3 tablespoons amaretto or orange liqueur

Topping

½ cup nonfat or low-fat vanilla yogurt (sugar-free or regular)

1½ cups nonfat or light whipped topping

3 tablespoons sliced toasted almonds (see page 78)

1. Use the milk to prepare the pudding according to package directions. Transfer to a covered container and refrigerate for several hours or until well chilled.

2. To make the fruit mixture, combine the ingredients in a medium bowl and toss to mix well. Set aside for 20 minutes to allow the juices to develop.

3. To assemble the trifle, arrange half of the ladyfingers or cake slices over the bottom of a 2½-quart glass bowl. Top first with half of the fruit mixture, then half of the pudding. Repeat the layers.

4. To make the topping, put the yogurt in a medium bowl and gently fold in the whipped topping. Swirl the mixture over the top of the trifle, cover, and chill for at least 2 hours. Sprinkle the almonds over the top just before serving.

Nutritional Facts (per serving)

CALORIES: 162   CARBOHYDRATES: 30 G   CHOLESTEROL: 26 MG   FAT: 2.5 G   FIBER: 2.2 G
PROTEIN: 4.4 G   SODIUM: 221 MG   CALCIUM: 121 MG   GI RATING: LOW

Tiramisu Trifle

YIELD: 9 SERVINGS

18 ladyfingers (about 4½ ounces), split open; or 8 slices (½-inch-thick) sponge cake
   or low-fat pound cake

¼ cup coffee liqueur

Pudding

2 cups skim or low-fat milk

1 package (4-serving size) cook-and-serve vanilla pudding mix (sugar-free or
   regular)

Fruit Mixture

2 cups sliced fresh strawberries or diced apricots (or 1 cup each)

1 cup fresh or frozen (thawed) raspberries

1 tablespoon sugar

Topping

1½ cups nonfat or light whipped topping

½ cup nonfat or low-fat vanilla yogurt (sugar-free or regular)

1 teaspoon cocoa powder (preferably Dutch processed cocoa), or 3 tablespoons
    shaved dark chocolate

3 tablespoons sliced toasted almonds (see page 78)

1. Use the milk to prepare the pudding according to package directions. Transfer to a covered container and refrigerate for several hours or until well chilled.

2. To make the fruit mixture, combine the ingredients in a medium bowl and toss to mix well. Set aside for 20 minutes to allow the juices to develop.

3. To assemble the trifle, arrange half of the ladyfingers or cake slices over the bottom of a 2½-quart glass bowl. Drizzle half of the liqueur over the ladyfingers or cake slices. Top with half of the fruit mixture and then half of the pudding. Repeat the layers.

4. To make the topping, put the whipped topping in a medium-sized bowl and gently fold in the yogurt. Swirl over the top of the trifle, cover, and chill for at least 2 hours. Just before serving, sift the cocoa or sprinkle the chocolate over the top of the trifle and sprinkle with the almonds.

Nutritional Facts (per serving)

CALORIES: 172 CARBOHYDRATES: 33 G CHOLESTEROL: 26 MG FAT: 2 G FIBER: 2.3 G
PROTEIN: 4.7 G SODIUM: 260 MG CALCIUM: 131 MG GI RATING: MODERATE

Black Forest Fudge Cake

YIELD 9 SERVINGS

½ cup unbleached flour

½ cup oat bran

¼ cup plus 2 tablespoons cocoa powder (preferably Dutch process cocoa)

⅔ cup sugar

½ teaspoon baking soda

⅛ teaspoon salt

12 ounces coarsely chopped frozen pitted dark sweet cherries (about 2½ cups), thawed

3 tablespoons canola oil

3 tablespoons fat-free egg substitute or 1 large egg, lightly beaten

1 teaspoon vanilla extract

⅓ cup chopped walnuts or pecans (optional)

1½ tablespoons powdered sugar (optional)

1. Place the flour, oat bran, cocoa, sugar, baking soda, and salt in a medium bowl, and stir to mix well. Add the cherries, including the juice that has accumulated during thawing, oil, egg, and vanilla extract, and stir to mix well. Set the batter aside for 10 minutes, then stir the batter again for 10 to 15 seconds. Fold in the nuts if desired.

2. Coat an 8-inch square baking pan with nonstick cooking spray, and spread the batter evenly in the pan. Bake at 350° F for 30 to 35 minutes, or just until a wooden toothpick inserted in the center of the cake comes out clean or coated with a few fudgy crumbs.

3. Let the cake cool in the pan to room temperature. If desired, sift the powdered sugar over the top of the cake just before cutting into squares and serving.

Nutritional Facts (per serving)

CALORIES: 199 CARBOHYDRATES: 34 G CHOLESTEROL: 0 MG FAT: 5.9 G FIBER: 4.6 G
PROTEIN: 5 G SODIUM: 114 MG CALCIUM: 8 MG GI RATING: MODERATE

Crisp Almond Cookies

For variety, substitute pecans, hazelnuts, or unsalted peanuts for the almonds.

YIELD: 36 COOKIES

1¾ cups sliced almonds

¾ cup sugar

2 egg whites brought to room temperature

Pinch salt

1 teaspoon vanilla extract

1. Combine 1½ cups of the almonds and ¼ cup of the sugar in the bowl of a food processor and process until the mixture is finely ground. Set aside.

2. Place the egg whites in a large glass bowl and add the salt. Beat with an electric mixer until soft peaks form when the beaters are raised. Still beating, slowly add the remaining ½ cup of sugar 1 tablespoonful at a time. Continue beating until all the sugar is mixed in and the mixture is thick and glossy. Beat in the vanilla extract.

3. Gently fold half of the ground almond mixture into the beaten egg whites, then fold in the remaining ground almond mixture.

4. Line 2 large cookie sheets with aluminum foil (do not coat with cooking spray). Drop rounded teaspoons of the egg white mixture onto the sheets, spacing them 1½ inches apart. Sprinkle about ⅓ teaspoon of the almond slices over each cookie, pressing them slightly onto the cookie to make them stick.

5. Bake at 350° F, switching the positions of the cookie sheets after 10 minutes, for 16 to 18 minutes or until the cookies are light golden brown. Turn the oven off and let the cookies sit in the oven with the door slightly ajar for 30 minutes. Then remove the cookie sheets from the oven and allow the cookies to cool on the pan to room temperature. Peel the cookies from the foil and serve immediately or store in an airtight container.

Nutritional Facts (per cookie)

CALORIES: 44 CARBOHYDRATES: 5 G CHOLESTEROL: 0 MG FAT: 2.4 G FIBER: 0.5 G
PROTEIN: 1.1 G SODIUM: 8 MG CALCIUM: 12 MG GI RATING: LOW

Maple Oatmeal Cookies

YIELD: 42 COOKIES

1⅓ cups quick-cooking (1-minute) oats
¾ cup whole-wheat pastry flour
⅔ cup sugar
½ teaspoon baking soda
½ teaspoon baking powder
½ teaspoon ground cinnamon
¼ cup maple syrup
1 large egg, lightly beaten
1 tablespoon water or orange juice
3 tablespoons canola oil
1 teaspoon vanilla extract
¾ cup chopped walnuts or pecans
½ cup plus 1 tablespoon chopped mixed dried fruit, apricots, raisins, or prunes

1. Combine the oats, flour, sugar, baking soda, baking powder, and cinnamon in a large bowl and stir to mix well. Add the maple syrup, egg, water or juice, canola oil, and vanilla extract and stir to mix well. Stir in the nuts and fruit.
2. Coat a large baking sheet with nonstick cooking spray and drop rounded teaspoonfuls of the dough onto the sheet, spacing them at least 1 inch apart. Flatten each cookie slightly with the tip of a spoon. Bake the cookies at 300° F for about 14 minutes or until the cookies have spread and appear dry around the edges. (They will not brown significantly during baking.)
3. Remove the cookies from the oven and cool on the sheet for 3 minutes. Then transfer the cookies to wire racks to cool completely. Serve immediately or transfer to an airtight container until ready to serve.

Nutritional Facts (per cookie)

CALORIES: 61 CARBOHYDRATES: 8 G CHOLESTEROL: 3 MG FAT: 2.6 G FIBER: 0.9 G PROTEIN: 1.4 G SODIUM: 22 MG CALCIUM: 9 MG GI RATING: MODERATE

Variation: Chocolate Oatmeal Cookies

Substitute Dutch processed cocoa powder for ¼ cup of the whole-wheat pastry flour, and substitute semisweet chocolate chips for the dried fruit.

Nutritional Facts (per cookie)

CALORIES: 67 CARBOHYDRATES: 8 G CHOLESTEROL: 3 MG FAT: 3.2 G FIBER: 0.9 G PROTEIN: 1.4 G SODIUM: 22 MG CALCIUM: 9 MG GI RATING: MODERATE

Frosted Grapes

YIELD: 4 SERVINGS

1 pound seedless green or red grapes

1. Wash the grapes with cool water and pat dry thoroughly with paper towels. Place the grapes in a plastic freezer bag and freeze for several hours or overnight.
2. Remove the grapes from the freezer and let sit for 1 to 2 minutes or until frosty on the outside before serving.

CALORIES: 85 CARBOHYDRATES: 21 G CHOLESTEROL: 0 MG FAT: 0.7 G FIBER: 1.2 G
PROTEIN: 0.8 G SODIUM: 2 MG CALCIUM: 13 MG GI RATING: LOW

Razzleberry Sundaes

YIELD: 4 SERVINGS

4 scoops (½ cup each) low-fat vanilla, chocolate, or cappuccino ice cream
1 cup fresh raspberries
¼ cup raspberry, amaretto, or hazelnut liqueur
2 tablespoons toasted chopped almonds or hazelnuts (see page 78); or shaved dark chocolate

1. Place one scoop of the ice cream into each of four 8-ounce dessert dishes.
2. Top the ice cream in each dish with a quarter of the raspberries and a tablespoon of the liqueur. Sprinkle some of the nuts or chocolate over the top and serve immediately.

Nutritional Facts (per serving)

CALORIES: 187 CARBOHYDRATES: 29 G CHOLESTEROL: 5 MG FAT: 3.9 G FIBER: 3.3 G
PROTEIN: 4 G SODIUM: 51 MG CALCIUM: 115 MG GI RATING: LOW

Peach-Almond Sundaes

For variety, substitute fresh apricots for the peaches.

YIELD: 4 SERVINGS

4 scoops (½ cup each) low-fat vanilla ice cream
1 cup diced, peeled fresh peaches
¼ cup amaretto liqueur
2 tablespoons toasted sliced almonds (see page 78)

1. Place one scoop of the ice cream into each of four 8-ounce dessert dishes.
2. Top the ice cream in each dish with a quarter of the peaches and a tablespoon of the liqueur. Sprinkle some of the nuts over the top and serve immediately.

Nutritional Facts (per serving)

CALORIES: 187 CARBOHYDRATES: 29 G CHOLESTEROL: 5 MG FAT: 3.9 G FIBER: 3.3 G

PROTEIN: 4 G SODIUM: 51 MG CALCIUM: 115 MG GI RATING: LOW

Ice Cream with Cherry-Brandy Sauce

YIELD: 4 SERVINGS

Sauce
¼ cup orange or cranberry juice
¼ teaspoon cornstarch
1 cup fresh or frozen pitted dark sweet cherries, halved
2 tablespoons brandy
1 tablespoon sugar

4 scoops (½ cup each) low-fat vanilla, chocolate, or cappuccino ice cream
2 tablespoons chopped walnuts or toasted chopped almonds (see page 78)

1. To make the sauce, combine 1 teaspoon of the juice and all the cornstarch in a small bowl and stir to mix well. Set aside. Put the cherries, remaining juice, brandy, and sugar in a 1-quart pot and bring to a boil over medium-high heat. Reduce the heat to medium-low, cover, and cook, stirring frequently, for about 5 minutes or until the cherries have released their juices and begin to break down. Cook uncovered, stirring frequently, for an additional 2 minutes or until the mixture is reduced by about one-fourth. Add the cornstarch mixture and cook, still stirring, for another minute or two or until the sauce thickens slightly and is reduced to ½ cup. Set the sauce aside for 5 minutes to cool slightly.

2. Place one scoop of the ice cream into each of four 8-ounce dessert dishes.

3. Top the ice cream in each dish with 2 tablespoons of the sauce. Sprinkle some of the nuts over the top, and serve immediately.

Nutritional Facts (per serving)

CALORIES: 189 CARBOHYDRATES: 29 G CHOLESTEROL: 5 MG FAT: 4.4 G FIBER: 2.2 G

PROTEIN: 4 G SODIUM: 50 MG CALCIUM: 112 MG GI RATING: LOW

Appendix: Glycemic Index Tables

This section presents a more extensive listing of foods than are presented in Chapter One. It includes the glycemic index values of numerous foods that have been published in the scientific literature plus information supplied by manufacturers.

This section lists the glycemic index of foods when compared to pure glucose, which has a GI of 100. When comparing foods, the following scale will help you put the GI in perspective:

- Very low GI = 39 or lower

- Low GI = 40–54

- Moderate GI = 55–69

- High GI = 70 or higher

In some studies, researchers use white bread as the reference food instead of glucose. This will cause the GI of a food to be different from the values shown in this appendix. If you should run across this situation, you can convert a GI based on white bread to a GI that uses glucose as the reference food by multiplying the white bread–based GI by 0.7.

The GI values assigned to foods should only be used as a *general* guide. Realize that factors like genetic variety, degree of ripeness, cooking time, and type of processing can cause some variation in the GI value of any given food. While most foods show very little variation in GI values when tested in different studies, some show quite a bit of variation. For instance, corn has tested as low as 46 and as high as 60 in different studies and carrots have tested as low as 49 and as high as 92. The GI of products like baked goods and cereals may vary from brand to brand and may change when manufacturers periodically reformulate their products.

Some of the GI values in this table represent the results of only one study, while others are averages of two or more studies. The values derived from an average of studies will be the most reliable—these are denoted by the (av) after the food listed. As more research is conducted and more manufacturers begin to have their products tested, knowledge about the glycemic index of foods will continue to expand.

When perusing this table, bear in mind that both glycemic index *and* the amount of carbohydrate that you eat contribute to your glycemic load. This means that if a food has a high GI, but is low in carbohydrate (like carrots), its impact on blood sugar and insulin levels will be much smaller than a food that has both a high GI and a high carbohydrate content (like jellybeans). Finally, remember that just because a food has a low GI does not necessarily make it a healthful choice. The following table includes approximate carbohydrate, fat, and calorie counts to help you choose foods that best fit your personal nutritional goals.

FOOD AND AMOUNT	GI	CARB(G)	FAT(G)	CALORIES
Breakfast Cereals				
All-Bran (av) (½ cup, 1 ounce)	42	20	1	50
Bran Buds (⅓ cup, 1 ounce)	58	24	0.5	80
Cheerios (1 cup, 1 ounce)	74	22	2	110
Coco Krispies (¾ cup, 1 ounce)	77	27	1	120
Corn Bran (¾ cup, 1 ounce)	75	23	1	90
Corn Chex (1 cup, 1 ounce)	83	26	0	110
Corn flakes (av) (1 cup, 1 ounce)	84	24	0	100
Cream of Wheat (3 tbsp dry)	66	25	0	120
Cream of Wheat, instant (3 tbsp dry)	74	25	0	120
Crispix (1 cup, 1 ounce)	87	25	0	110
Golden Grahams (1 cup, 1.4 ounces)	71	33	1.4	150
Grape-Nuts Nuggets (½ cup, 2 ounces)	67	47	1	210
Grape-Nuts Flakes (¾ cup, 1 ounce)	80	24	1	110
Just Right (1 cup, 2.1 ounces)	60	49	2	220
Life (¾ cup, 1.1 ounces)	66	25	1.5	120
Mueslix (av) (½ cup, 2.1 ounces)	56	45	3	210
Oat bran (½ cup dry, 1.4 ounces)	50	25	3	145
Quick-cooking oats (½ cup dry, 1.4 ounces)	65	27	3	150
Old-fashioned oats (av) (½ cup dry, 1.4 ounces)	49	27	3	150
Puffed wheat (av) (1¼ cups, ½ ounce)	74	11	0	50
Rice bran (¼ cup, 0.9 ounce)	19	9	6	119
Rice Chex (1¼ cups, 1.1 ounces)	89	27	0	120
Rice Krispies (1¼ cups, 1.2 ounces)	82	29	0	120
Shredded wheat (av) (1 cup, 1.7 ounces)	69	41	0.5	170
Special K (1 cup, 1.1 ounces)	54	23	0	110
Total whole grain flakes (¾ cup, 1 ounce)	76	23	1	110
Wheetabix (2 biscuits, 1.2 ounces)	75	28	1	120
Breads				
Bagel, white (small, 2.5 ounces)	72	38	1.1	195
Baguette (2 slices, 1 ounce)	95	15	0.9	78
Barley flour bread (av) (1 slice, 1 ounce)	66	15	1	80
Barley kernel bread (50 percent kernels) (1 slice, 1 ounce)	46	13	1	70

Food and Amount	GI	Carb(g)	Fat(g)	Calories
Bulgur bread (50 percent cracked wheat kernel) (1 slice, 1 ounce)	58	13	1	70
Chapati (av) (1 piece, 1.3 ounces)	57	20	2.5	120
Croissant (2.2 ounces)	67	28	16	260
Crumpet (2 ounces)	69	22	0.5	100
English muffin	60	26	1	131
Fruit loaf (wheat bread with dried fruit) (1 slice, 1.5 ounces)	47	22	4.3	134
Hamburger bun (1 bun, 1.5 ounces)	61	23	2.5	130
Kaiser roll (1 roll, 1.4 ounces)	73	22	4.3	133
Linseed (flax) rye bread (1 slice, 1.3 ounces)	55	17	2	100
Muffin, blueberry (1 muffin, 2 ounces)	59	30	6	185
Muffin, bran (1 muffin, 2 ounces)	60	34	6	199
Natural Ovens Happiness Bread (1 slice, 1.3 ounces)	63	15	0.5	70
Natural Ovens Hunger Filler Bread (1 slice, 1.1 ounces)	59	13	1	60
Natural Ovens 100 percent Whole Grain Bread (1 slice, 1.2 ounces)	51	14	0.5	60
Natural Ovens Natural Nutty Wheat Bread (1 slice, 1.2 ounces)	59	16	1	70
Oat bran (50 percent oat bran) (av) (1 slice, 1.1 ounces)	47	12	1.3	70
Pita bread (6-inch, 2 ounces)	57	31	0.5	130
Pumpernickel (whole grain) (1 slice, 1 ounce)	46	13	0.9	70
Rye flour bread (av) (1 slice, 1.1 ounce)	65	15	1	80
Rye kernel bread (80 percent kernels) (av) (1 slice, 1.2 ounces)	46	16	1	70
Cocktail rye bread (1 slice, ½ ounce)	58	7	0.5	36
Semolina bread (1 slice, 1 ounce)	64	14	1	80
Sourdough bread (1 slice, 1 ounce)	54	14	1	80
Sourdough rye bread (1 slice, 1 ounce)	57	14	1	80
Stuffing (from mix) (½ cup prepared)	74	22	8	178
Taco shells (1 shell, 0.6 ounce)	68	11	4	85
Waffles (plain) (1 waffle, 1.3 ounces)	76	15	3	98
White bread (av) (1 slice, 1 ounce)	70	15	1	80

FOOD AND AMOUNT	GI	CARB(G)	FAT(G)	CALORIES
Whole-wheat bread (av) (1 slice, 1 ounce)	69	15	1	80
Whole-wheat bread (stoneground) (1 slice, 1 ounce)	60	15	1	80

Crackers

Melba toast (3 pieces, ½ ounce)	70	11	0	50
Rice cakes (2 cakes, ⅔ ounce)	82	15	0.5	70
Ryevita whole grain crispbread (av) (2 slices, ⅔ ounce)	63	15	0	70
Kavli whole grain crispbread (3 slices, ½ ounce)	71	13	0	60
Saltines (5 crackers, ½ ounce)	74	11	2	70
Stoned Wheat Thins wheat crackers (2 crackers, ½ ounce)	67	10	1.5	60
Water crackers (av) (5 crackers, ½ ounce)	72	13	1.5	70

Grains

Barley (av) (½ cup cooked)	25	22	0.4	96
Buckwheat groats (av) (½ cup cooked)	54	17	0.5	77
Bulgur wheat (av) (½ cup cooked)	48	17	0.2	75
Cornmeal (3 tbsp dry, 1 ounce)	68	20	0.4	95
Couscous (½ cup cooked)	61	18	0.1	88
Millet (½ cup cooked)	71	18	1	94
Rice, basmati (½ cup cooked)	58	22	0.1	100
Rice, instant (½ cup cooked)	87	22	0.1	100
Rice, long grain brown (av) (½ cup cooked)	55	22	1	108
Rice, long grain white (av) (½ cup cooked)	56	22	0.1	100
Rice, long grain and wild (½ cup cooked)	54	21	0.2	95
Rice, parboiled (converted) (av) (½ cup cooked)	47	22	0.2	100
Rice, short grain white (av) (½ cup cooked)	88	27	0.2	120
Rice, wild (½ cup cooked)	57	18	0.3	83
Wheat berries (av) (½ cup cooked)	41	10	0.2	42

Pasta

Capellini (2 ounces dry)	45	42	1	210
Chinese beanthread (2 ounces dry)	26	48	0	190

Food and Amount	GI	Carb(g)	Fat(g)	Calories
Chinese rice vermicelli (2 ounces dry)	58	47	0	195
Egg fettuccine (2 ounces dry)	32	40	2.4	216
Linguine, thick (av) (2 ounces dry)	46	42	1	210
Linguine, thin (av) (2 ounces dry)	55	42	1	210
Macaroni (2 ounces dry)	45	42	1	210
Macaroni and cheese (boxed) (1 cup cooked)	64	48	17	390
Ravioli, meat (1¼ cups uncooked, 4 ounces)	39	46	9	330
Spaghetti (av) (2 ounces dry)	41	42	1	210
Spaghetti,, whole wheat (av) (2 ounces dry)	37	42	1	197
Spirali (2 ounces dry)	43	42	1	210
Star pastina (2 ounces dry)	38	42	1	210
Tortellini, cheese (¾ cup uncooked, 3 ounces)	50	39	6	250
Vermicelli (2 ounces dry)	35	42	1	210

Legumes

Food and Amount	GI	Carb(g)	Fat(g)	Calories
Baked beans (av) (½ cup)	48	25	2	134
Black-eyed peas (½ cup cooked)	42	18	0.5	100
Butter beans (av) (½ cup cooked)	31	18	0	80
Chickpeas (av) (½ cup cooked)	33	22	2	134
Chickpeas, canned (½ cup)	42	20	2	120
Kidney beans (av) (½ cup cooked)	27	20	0	110
Lentils, green (av) (½ cup cooked)	30	20	0.4	115
Lentils, red (av) (½ cup cooked)	26	20	0.4	115
Lima beans (½ cup cooked)	32	21	0.4	114
Navy beans (av) (½ cup cooked)	38	24	0.5	129
Pinto beans (½ cup cooked)	39	22	0.4	117
Pinto beans, canned (½ cup)	45	18	0.5	110
Soybeans (av) (½ cup cooked)	18	10	5.8	148
Split peas (½ cup cooked)	32	21	0.4	116

Vegetables

Food and Amount	GI	Carb(g)	Fat(g)	Calories
Beets (½ cup cooked)	64	8.5	0.2	37
Carrots (av) (½ cup cooked)	71	8	0.1	35
Corn, sweet (av) (½ cup cooked)	55	16	0.4	66
Lima beans, baby (½ cup cooked)	32	17	0.3	94
Parsnips (½ cup cooked)	97	15	0.2	63

Food and Amount	GI	Carb(g)	Fat(g)	Calories
Peas, green (av) (½ cup cooked)	48	11	0.2	62
Potatoes, baked (av) (1 medium, 4.5 ounces)	85	32	0.1	139
Potatoes, French fried (medium, 4 ounces)	75	43	20	370
Potatoes, instant (av) (½ cup cooked)	83	16	3.8	112
Potatoes, new (av) (3 medium, 4.5 ounces)	62	24	0.1	106
Pumpkin (½ cup cooked mashed)	75	6	0.1	25
Rutabaga (½ cup cooked cubes)	72	7	0.2	33
Sweet potatoes (av) (½ cup mashed)	54	24	0.1	103
Yam (½ cup cooked)	51	24	0.1	103

Fruits

Food and Amount	GI	Carb(g)	Fat(g)	Calories
Apple (av) (1 medium, 5.4 ounces)	36	22	0	80
Apple juice (av) (½ cup)	41	15	0.1	60
Apricots, canned light syrup (½ cup, 4.4 ounces)	64	21	0.1	80
Apricots, dried (av) (¼ cup)	31	20	0.1	77
Banana (av) (1 medium, 4.2 ounces)	53	27	0.5	108
Cantaloupe (¼ melon, 4.7 ounces)	65	12	0	50
Cherries (1 cup, 4.1 ounces)	22	19	1.1	84
Fruit cocktail, canned in juice (½ cup, 4.2 ounces)	55	14	0	5
Grapefruit (½ medium, 5.4 ounces)	25	16	0	
Grapefruit juice (½ cup)	48	11	0.1	8
Grapes (1 cup, 5.6 ounces)	43	28	0.9	13
Kiwi fruit (1 medium, 2.6 ounces)	52	12	0.5	50
Mango (1 cup slices, 5.8 ounces)	55	28	0.5	107
Orange (av) (1 medium, 5.3 ounces)	43	17	0.3	69
Orange juice (av) (½ cup)	57	13	0.3	56
Papaya (av) (1 cup cubes, 4.9 ounces)	58	14	0.2	55
Peach (1 medium, 3.5 ounces)	28	11	0.1	42
Peach, canned in heavy syrup (½ cup, 4.6 ounces)	58	26	0.1	96
Peach, canned in light syrup (½ cup, 4.4 ounces)	52	14	0.1	52
Peach, canned in natural juice (½ cup, 4.4 ounces)	30	14	0.1	55

Food and Amount	GI	Carb(g)	Fat(g)	Calories
Pear (av) (1 medium, 5.9 ounces)	36	25	0.7	97
Pear, canned in natural juice (½ cup, 4.4 ounces)	44	16	0.1	62
Pineapple (1 cup chunks, 5.5 ounces)	66	19	0.7	76
Plum (1 medium, 2.3 ounces)	24	9	0.4	36
Raisins (¼ cup)	64	29	0.2	109
Watermelon (1 cup cubes, 5.4 ounces)	72	11	0.7	50

Pizza

Food and Amount	GI	Carb(g)	Fat(g)	Calories
Pizza, cheese (2 slices, 7.6 ounces)	60	58	14	470

Soups

Food and Amount	GI	Carb(g)	Fat(g)	Calories
Black bean soup, canned (1 cup)	64	30	1.5	170
Lentil soup, canned (1 cup)	44	22	2	140
Split pea soup, canned (1 cup)	60	25	3	170
Tomato soup, canned (1 cup)	38	16	2	85

Dairy and Dairy Substitutes

Food and Amount	GI	Carb(g)	Fat(g)	Calories
Ice cream (av) (1 cup)	61	31	14	265
Ice cream, low-fat (1 cup)	50	36	4	200
Milk, chocolate (1 cup)	34	26	5	178
Milk, skim (1 cup)	32	12	0.4	85
Milk, whole (av) (1 cup)	27	11	8	150
Soymilk (1 cup)	31	13	8	158
Yogurt, low-fat with fruit and sugar (1 cup)	33	42	2.6	225
Yogurt, low-fat with fruit and aspartame (1 cup)	14	18	0.4	115

Beverages

Food and Amount	GI	Carb(g)	Fat(g)	Calories
Apple juice (½ cup)	41	15	0.1	60
Grapefruit juice (½ cup)	48	11	0.1	48
Orange juice (½ cup)	57	13	0.3	56
Soft drink (12 ounces)	68	35	0	140

Snack Foods

Food and Amount	GI	Carb(g)	Fat(g)	Calories
Corn chips (av) (1 ounce)	73	16	9.5	152
Peanuts (av) (¼ cup)	14	7	18	209
Popcorn, light microwave (3 cups)	55	13	2	71

Food and Amount	GI	Carb(g)	Fat(g)	Calories
Potato chips (av) (1 ounce)	54	15	10	108
Pretzels (1 ounce)	80	22	1	108

Sweets and Desserts

Food and Amount	GI	Carb(g)	Fat(g)	Calories
Banana bread (2 ounces)	47	31	6	185
Cake, angel food (1 ½ cake, 2 ounces)	67	33	0.5	146
Cake, banana (with sugar) (2 ounces)	47	30	5	170
Cake, banana (without sugar) (2 ounces)	55	24	8	170
Cake, pound (2 ounces)	54	28	11	220
Cake, sponge (2 ounces)	46	35	1.5	165
Cookies, arrowroot (5 cookies, 1 ounce)	66	18	4	110
Cookies, oatmeal (av) (2 cookies, 1.3 ounces)	55	25	6.5	162
Cookies, shortbread (2 cookies, 1 ounce)	64	19	7.2	150
Custard (½ cup)	43	15	6.6	148
Donut, cake-type (1 donut, 2.1 ounces)	76	24	19	280
Graham crackers (4 squares, 1 ounce)	74	22	2.8	118
Kudos whole-grain granola bars (chocolate chip) (1 bar, 1.3 ounces)	62	25	6	161
Pastry pie crust (⅛ crust)	59	11	8	121
Tapioca with milk (½ cup)	81	28	4	160
Vanilla wafers (7 cookies, 1 ounce)	77	21	4.4	122

Candy and Candy Bars

Food and Amount	GI	Carb(g)	Fat(g)	Calories
Chocolate (1 bar, 1.5 ounces)	49	26	13.5	225
Jellybeans (¼ cup, 1½ ounces)	80	40	0	156
Life Savers (4 candies, 0.56 ounce)	70	16	0	60
M&M's (peanut) (¼ cup, 1½ ounces)	33	26	11	220
Mars Bar (1 bar, 1.76 ounces)	62	31	11.5	233
Skittles (¼ cup, 1½ ounces)	70	37	2	170
Snickers Bar (1 bar, 2 ounces)	41	34	14	283
Twix Cookie Bars (caramel) (1 bar, 2 ounces)	44	37	14	283

Sugars and Sweeteners

Food and Amount	GI	Carb(g)	Fat(g)	Calories
Fructose (av) (1 tablespoon)	23	12	0	48
Honey (1 tablespoon)	58	17	0	64
Sucrose (white sugar) (av) (1 tablespoon)	65	12	0	48

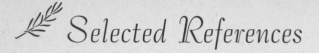 Selected References

Glycemic Index General

Brosnan, J. T. "Comments on metabolic needs for glucose and the role of gluconeogenesis." *European Journal of Clinical Nutrition* 1999;53(suppl 1);S107–11.

FAO/WHO Expert Consultation, April 14–18, 1997. "Carbohydrates in Human Nutrition." *Food and Agricultural Organization Food and Nutrition Paper 66.* Rome: FAO;1998. (Available online at fao.org/es/esn/carboweb/carbo.htm)

Gustafsson, K., Asp, N., Hagander, B., and Nyman, M. "Dose-response effects of boiled carrots and effects of carrots in lactic acid in mixed meals on glycemic response and satiety." *European Journal of Clinical Nutrition* 1994;48:386–96.

Macdonald, I. A. "Carbohydrate as a nutrient in adults: range of acceptable intakes." *European Journal of Clinical Nutrition* 1999;53(suppl 1);S101–6.

Wolever, T. "Dietary carbohydrates and insulin action in humans." *British Journal of Nutrition* 2000;83(suppl 1):S97–102.

Wolever, T., and Bolognesi, C. "Prediction of glucose and insulin responses of normal subjects after consuming mixed meals varying in energy, protein, fat, carbohydrate, and glycemic index." *Journal of Nutrition* 1996;126:2807–12.

Wolever, T., Jenkins, D., Jenkins, A., and Josse, R. G. "The glycemic index: methodology and clinical implications." *American Journal of Clinical Nutrition* 1991;54:846–54.

Wolever, T., Nguyen, P. M., Chiasson, J. L., Hunt, J. A., Josse, R. G., Palmason, C., Rodger, N. W., Ross, A., Ryan, E. A., and Tan, M. H. "Determinants of diet glycemic index calculated retrospectively from diet records of 342 individuals with non-insulin-dependent diabetes mellitus." *American Journal of Clinical Nutrition* 1994;59:1265–69.

Glycemic Index of Foods

Bjorck, I., Granfeldt, Y., Liljeberg, H., Tovar, J., and Asp, N. "Food properties affecting the digestion and absorption of carbohydrates." *American Journal of Clinical Nutrition* 1994;59(suppl):699S-705S.

Brand, J. C., Nicholson, P. L., Thorburn, A.W., and Truswell, A. S. "Food processing and the glycemic index." *American Journal of Clinical Nutrition* 1985;42:1192–96.

Brand-Miller, J., Pang, E., and Bramall, L. "Rice: a high or low glycemic index food?" *American Journal of Clinical Nutrition* 1992;56:1034–36.

Brand-Miller, J., Pang, E., and Broomhead, L. "The glycaemic index of foods containing sugars: comparison of foods with naturally-occurring v. added sugars." *British Journal of Nutrition* 1995;73:613–23.

Brand-Miller, J. C., Wang, B., McNeil, Y., and Swan, V. "The glycaemic index of more breads, breakfast cereals, and snack products." *Proceedings of the Nutrition Society of Australia* 1997;21:144.

Brighenti, F., Castellani, G., Casiraghi, M. C., Leopardi, E., Crovetti, R., and Testolin, G. "Effect of neutralized and native vinegar on blood glucose and acetate responses to a mixed meal in healthy subjects." *European Journal of Clinical Nutrition* 1995;49:242–47.

Cunnane, S., Gangull, S., Menard, C., Liede, A., Hamadeh, M., Chen, Z., Wolever, T., and Jenkins, D. "High alpha-linolenic acid flaxseed: some nutritional properties in humans." *British Journal of Nutrition* 1993;69:443–53.

Foster-Powell, K., and Brand-Miller, J. "International tables of glycemic index." *American Journal of Clinical Nutrition* 1995;62:871S–93S.

Holm, J., and Bjorck, I. "Bioavailability of starch in various wheat-based bread products: evaluation of metabolic responses in healthy subjects and rate and extent of in vitro starch digestion." *American Journal of Clinical Nutrition* 1992;55:420–29.

Holt, S., Brand-Miller, J., and Petocz, P. "An insulin index of foods: the insulin demand generated by 1000-KJ portions of common foods." *American Journal of Clinical Nutrition* 1997;66:1264–76.

Jenkins, D., Wesson, V., Wolever, T., Jenkins, A., Kalmusky, J., Guidici, S., Csima, A., Josse, R., and Wong, G. "Wholemeal versus wholegrain breads: proportion of whole or cracked grain and the glycaemic response." *British Medical Journal* 1988;297:958–60.

Jenkins, D. A., Wolever, T., Jenkins, A. L., Giordano, C., Giudici, S., Thompson, L. U., Kalmusky, J., Josse, R. G., and Wong, G. S. "Low glycemic response to traditionally processed wheat and rye products: bulgur and pumpernickel bread." *American Journal of Clinical Nutrition* 1986;43:516–20.

Liljeberg, H. G., Lonner, C. H., and Bjorck, I. M. "Sourdough fermentation of addition of organic acids or corresponding salts to bread improves nutritional properties of starch in healthy humans." *Journal of Nutrition* 1995;125(6):1503–11.

Ross, S. W., Brand, J. C., Thorburn, A. W., and Truswell, A. S. "Glycemic index of processed wheat products." *American Journal of Clinical Nutrition* 1987;46:631–35.

Soh, N. L., and Brand-Miller, J. "The glycaemic index of potatoes: the effect of variety, cooking method and maturity." *European Journal of Clinical Nutrition* 1999;53:249–54.

Wolever, T. M., Jenkins, D. J., Kalmusky, J., Giordano, C., Giudici S., Jenkins, A. L., Thompson, L. U., Wong, G. S., and Josse, R. G. "Glycemic response to pasta: effect of surface area, degree of cooking, and protein enrichment." *Diabetes Care* 1986;9(4):401–4.

Wolever, T. M., Katzman-Relle, L., Jenkins, A. L., Vuksan, V., Josse, R. G., and Jenkins, D. A., "Glycaemic index of 102 complex carbohydrate foods in patients with diabetes." *Nutrition Research* 1994;14(5):651–69.

Glycemic Index, Carbohydrates, and Weight Loss

Agus, M., Swain, J. F., Larson, C. L., Eckert, E. A., and Ludwig, D. S. "Dietary composition and physiologic adaptations to energy restriction." *American Journal of Clinical Nutrition* 2000;71:901–7.

Holt, S. H. A., and Brand-Miller, J. "Particle size, satiety and the glycaemic response." *European Journal of Clinical Nutrition* 1994;48:496–502.

Kabir, M., Rizkalla, S., Quignard, A., Guerre-Millo, M., Boillot, J., Ardouin, B., Luo, J., and Slama, G. "A high glycemic index starch diet affects lipid storage-related enzymes in normal and to a lesser extent in diabetic rats." *Journal of Nutrition* 1998;128:1878–83.

Ludwig, D. S., Majzoub, J. A., Ahmad, A. Z., Dallal, G., Blanco, I., and Roberts, S. B. "High glycemic index foods, overeating, and obesity." *Pediatrics* 1999;103(3):261–66.

Ludwig, D. S., Periera, M. A., Kroenke, C. H., Hilner, J. E., Van Horn, L., Slattery, M. L., and Jacobs, D. R. "Dietary fiber, weight gain, and cardiovascular disease risk factors in young adults." *Journal of the American Medical Association* 1999;282;1539–46.

Ludwig, D. S. "Dietary glycemic index and obesity." *Journal of Nutrition* 2000;130:280S–283S.

Morris, K. L., and Zemel, M. B. "Glycemic index, cardiovascular disease, and obesity." *Nutrition Reviews* 1999; 57(9):273–76.

Roberts, S. B. "High-glycemic index foods, hunger, and obesity: Is there a connection?" *Nutrition Reviews* 2000;58(6):163–69.

Slabber, M., Barnard, H. C., Kuyl, J. M., Dannhauser, A., and Schall, R. "Effects of a low-insulin-response, energy-restricted diet on weight loss and plasma insulin concentrations in hyperinsulinemic obese females." *American Journal of Clinical Nutrition* 1994;60:48–53.

Insulin Resistance General

Despres, J. P., Lamarche, B., Mauriege, P., Cantin, B., Dagenais, G. R., Moorjani, S., and Lupien, P. J. "Hyperinsulinemia as an independent risk factor for ischemic heart disease." *New England Journal of Medicine* 1996;334(15):952–57.

Fukagawa, N. K., Anderson, J. A., Hagerman, G., Young, V. R., and Minaker, K. L. "High-carbohydrate, high-fiber diets increase peripheral insulin sensitivity in healthy young and old adults." *American Journal of Clinical Nutrition* 1990;52:524–28.

Joannie, J. L., Auboiron, S., Raison, J., Basdevant, A., Bornet, F., and Guy-Grand, B. "How the degree of unsaturation of dietary fatty acids influences the glucose and insulin responses to different carbohydrates in mixed meals." *American Journal of Clinical Nutrition* 1997;65(5):1427–33.

Lakka, H. M., Lakka, T. A., Tuomilehto, J., Sivenius, J., and Salonen, J. "Hyperinsulinemia and the risk of cardiovascular death and acute coronary cerebrovascular events in men." *Archives of Internal Medicine* 2000;160:1160–68.

Marshall, J. A., Bessesen, D. H., and Hamman, R. F. "High saturated fat and low starch and fibre are associated with hyperinsulinaemia in a non-diabetic population: The San Luis Valley diabetes study." *Diabetologia* 1997;40:430–38.

Meigs, J. B., Mittleman, M. A., Nathan, D. M., Tofler, G. H., Singer, D. E., Murphy-Sheehy, P. M., Lipinska, I., D'Agostino, R. B., and Wilson, P. W. "Hyperinsulinemia, hyperglycemia, and impaired hemostasis: The Framingham offspring study." *Journal of the American Medical Association* 2000;283:221–28.

Reaven, G. M. "Banting lecture 1988. Role of insulin resistance in human disease." *Diabetes* 1988;37: 1595–1607.

Reaven, G. M. "Pathophysiology of insulin resistance in human disease." *Physiological Reviews* 1995; 75(3):473–86.

Riccardi, G., and Rivellese, A. A. "Dietary treatment of the metabolic syndrome—the optimal diet." *British Journal of Nutrition* 2000;83(suppl 1):S143–48.

Smith, U. "Carbohydrates, fat, and insulin action." *American Journal of Clinical Nutrition* 1994;59(suppl):686S–89S.

Vessby, B. "Dietary fat and insulin action in humans." *British Journal of Nutrition* 2000;83 (suppl 1):S91–96.

Insulin Resistance and Body Weight

Folsom, A. R., Vitelli, L. L., Lewis, C. E., Schreiner, P. J., Watson, R. L., and Wagenknecht, L. E. "Is fasting insulin concentration inversely associated with rate of weight gain? Contrasting findings from the CARDIA and ARIC study cohorts." *International Journal of Obesity and Related Metabolic Disorders* 1998;22(1):48–54.

Gould, A. J., Williams, D. E. M., Byrne, C. D., Hales, C. N., and Wareham, N. J. "Prospective cohort study of the relationship of markers of insulin resistance and secretion with weight gain and changes in regional adiposity." *International Journal of Obesity and Related Metabolic Disorders* 1999;23(12):1256–61.

Hanson, C. W., Bagardus, C., and Pratley, R. E. "Long-term changes in insulin action and insulin secretion associated with gain, loss, regain and maintenance of body weight." *Diabetologia* 2000;43: 36–46.

Hoag, S., Marshall, J. A., Jones, R. H., and Hamman, R. F. "High fasting insulin levels associated with lower rates of weight gain in persons with normal glucose tolerance: The San Luis Valley diabetes study." *International Journal of Obesity and Related Metabolic Disorders* 1995;19(3)175–80.

Hodge, A. M., Dowse, G. K., George, K., Alberti, M. M., Tuomilehto, J., Gareeboo, H., and Zimmet, P. Z. "Relationship of insulin resistance to weight gain in nondiabetic Asian, Indian, Creole, and Chinese Mauritians." *Metabolism* 1996;45(5):627–33.

McLaughlin, T., Abbasi, F., Carantoni, M., Schaaf, P., and Reaven, G. "Differences in insulin resistance do not predict weight loss in response to hypocaloric diets in healthy obese women." *Journal of Clinical Endocrinology and Metabolism* 1999;84:578–81.

Schwartz, M. W., Boyko, E. J., Kahn, S. E., Rasvussin, E., and Bogardus, C. "Reduced insulin secretion: An independent predictor of body weight gain." *Journal of Clinical Endocrinology and Metabolism* 1995;80:1571–76.

Segal, K. R., Landt, M., and Klein, S. "Relationship between insulin sensitivity and plasma leptin concentration in lean and obese men." *Diabetes* 1996;45;988–91.

Sigal, R. J., El-Hashimy, M., Martin, B. C., Soeldner, J. S., Krolewski, A. S., and Warram, J. H. "Acute postchallenge hyperinsulinemia predicts weight gain: a prospective study." *Diabetes* 1997;46(6): 1025–29.

Swinburn, B. A., Nyomba, B. L., Saad, M. F., Zurto, F., Raz, I., Knowier, W. C., Lillioja, S., Bogardus, C., and Ravussin, E. "Insulin resistance associated with lower rates of weight gain in Pima Indians." *Journal of Clinical Investigation* 1991;88:168–73.

Wing, R. R. "Insulin sensitivity as a predictor of weight regain." *Obes Res* 1997;5(1):24–29.

Zavaroni, I., Zuccarelli, A., Gasparini, P., Massironi, P., Barilli, A., and Reaven, G. "Can weight gain in healthy, nonobese volunteers be predicted by differences in baseline plasma insulin concentration?" *Journal of Clinical Endocrinology and Metabolism* 1998;83:3498–500.

Glycemic Index, Carbohydrates, and Diabetes

Brand-Miller, J. C. "Importance of glycemic index in diabetes." *American Journal of Clinical Nutrition* 1994;59(suppl):747S–52S.

Chandalia, M., Garg, A., Lujohann, D., von Bergmann, K., Grundy, S., and Brinkley, L. J. "Beneficial effects of high dietary fiber intake in patients with type 2 diabetes mellitus." *New England Journal of Medicine* 2000;342(19):1392–98.

Jarvi, A. E., Karlstrom, B. E., Granfeldt, Y. E., Bjorck, I. E., Asp, N. G., and Vessby, B. O. "Improved glycemic control and lipid profile and normalized fibrinolytic activity on a low-glycemic index diet in type 2 diabetic patients." *Diabetes Care* 1999;22:10–18.

Liljeberg, H., and Bjorck, I. "Effects of a low-glycemic index spaghetti meal on glucose tolerance and lipaemia at a subsequent meal in healthy subjects." *European Journal of Clinical Nutrition* 2000. 54(1):24–28.

Luscombe, N. D., Noakes, M., and Clifton, P. M. "Diets high and low in glycemic index versus high monounsaturated fat diets: effects on glucose and lipid metabolism in NIDDM." *European Journal of Clinical Nutrition* 1999;53(6):473–78.

Salmeron, J., Ascherio, A., Manson, J. E., Stampfer, M. J., Colditz, G. A., Wing, A. L., and Willet, W. C. "Dietary fiber, glycemic load, and risk of non-insulin-dependent diabetes mellitus in women." *Journal of the American Medical Association* 1997;277:472–77.

Salmeron, J., Ascherio, A., Rimm, E. B., Codlitz, G. A., Spiegelman, D., Jenkins, D. J., Stampfer, M. J., Wing, A. L., and Willet, W. C. "Dietary fiber, glycemic load, and risk of NIDDM in men." *Diabetes Care* 1997;20(4):545–50.

The Diabetes and Nutrition Study Group (DNSG) of the European Association for the Study of Diabetes (EASD), 1999. "Recommendations for the nutritional management of patients with diabetes mellitus." *European Journal of Clinical Nutrition* 2000;54(4):353–55.

Uusitupa, M. "Fructose in the diabetic diet." *American Journal of Clinical Nutrition* 1994;59 (suppl):753S–57S.

Glycemic Index, Carbohydrates, and Heart Disease

Epstein, F. H. "Hypertension and associated metabolic abnormalities—the role of insulin resistance and the sympathoadrenal system." *New England Journal of Medicine* 1996;334(6):374–81.

Festa, A., D'Agostino, R., Howard, G., Mykkanen, L., Tracy, R. P., and Haffner, S. M. "Chronic subclinical inflammation as part of the insulin resistance syndrome." *Circulation* 2000;102:42.

Frost, G., Keogh, B., Smith, D., Akinsanya, K., and Leeds, A. "The effect of low-glycemic carbohydrate on insulin and glucose response in vivo and in vitro in patients with coronary heart disease." *Metabolism* 1996;45(6):669–72.

Frost, G., Leeds, A., Trew, G., Margara, R., and Dornhorst, A. "Insulin sensitivity in women at risk of cornary heart disease and the effect of a low glycemic diet." *Metabolism* 1998;47(10):1245–51.

Frost, G., Leeds, A., Dore, C., Madeiros, S., Brading, S., and Dornhorst, A. "Glycaemic index as a determinant of serum HDL-cholesterol concentration." *Lancet* 1999;353:1045–48.

Jenkins, D., Wolever, T., Kalmusky, J., Giudici, S., Giordano, C., Wong, G., Bird, J., Patten, R., Hall, M., and Buckley, G. "Low glycemic index carbohydrate foods in the management of hyperlipidemia." *American Journal of Clinical Nutrition* 1985. 42(4):604–17.

Liu, S., Willett, W., Stampfer, M., Hu, F., Franz, M., Sampson, L., Hennekens, C., and Manson, J. "A prospective study of dietary glycemic load, carbohydrate intake, and risk of coronary heart disease in U.S. women." *American Journal of Clinical Nutrition* 2000;71(6);1455–61.

Luscombe, N. D., Noakes, M., and Clifton, P. M. "Diets high and low in glycemic index versus high monounsaturated fat diets: effects on glucose and lipid metabolism in NIDDM." *European Journal of Clinical Nutrition* 1999;53:473–78.

Reaven, G. M. "The role of insulin resistance and hyperinsulinemia in coronary heart disease." *Metabolism* 1992;41(suppl 1):16–19.

Stampfer, M. J., Hu, F. B., Manson, J. E., Rimm, E. B., and Willett, W. C. "Primary prevention of coronary heart disease in women through diet and lifestyle." *New England Journal of Medicine* 2000;343:16–22.

Glycemic Index, Carbohydrates, and Cancer

Bostick, R. M., Potter, J. D., Kushi, L. H., Sellers, T. A., Steinmetz, K. A., McKenzie, D. R., Gapstur, S. M., and Folsom, A. R. "Sugar, meat, and fat intake, and non-dietary risk factors for colon cancer incidence in Iowa women (United States)." *Cancer Causes and Control* 1994;5(1):38–52.

De Stefani, E., Deneo-Pellegrini, H., Mendilaharsu, M., Ronco, A., and Carzoglio, J. C. "Dietary sugar and lung cancer: a case control study in Uruguay." *Nutrition and Cancer* 1998;31(2):132–37.

Del Giudice, M. E., Fantus, I. G., Ezzat, S., McKeown-Eyssen, G., Page, D., and Goodwin, P. J. "Insulin and related factors in premenopausal breast cancer risk." *Breast Cancer Research and Treatment* 1998;47(2):111–20.

Franceschi, S., Favero, A., Parpinel, M., Giacosa, A., and La Vecchia, C. "Italian study on colorectal cancer with emphasis on influence of cereals." *European Journal of Cancer Prevention* 1998;7(suppl 2):S19–23.

Franceschi, S., Favero, A., Decarli, A., Negri, E., La Vecchia, C., Ferraroni, M., Russo, A., Salvini, S., Amadori, D., Conti, E., Montella, M., Giacosa, A. "Intake of macronutrients and risk of breast cancer." *Lancet* 1996;347:1351–56.

Giovannucci, E. "Insulin and colon cancer." *Cancer Causes and Control* 1995;6(2):164–79.

Hankinson, S. E., Willett, W. C., Colditz, G. A., Hunter, D. J., Michaud, D. S., Deroo, B., Rosner, B., Speizer, F. E., and Pollak, M. "Circulating concentrations of insulin-like growth factor-1 and risk of breast cancer." *Lancet* 1998.351:1393–96.

Josefson, D. "High insulin levels linked to deaths from breast cancer." *British Medical Journal* 2000;320:1496.

Kaaks, R. "Nutrition, hormones, and breast cancer: is insulin the missing link?" *Cancer Causes Control* 1996;7(6):605–25.

Kim, Y. I. "Diet, lifestyle, and colorectal cancer: is hyperinsulinemia the missing link?" *Nutrition Reviews* 1998;56(9):275–79.

Slattery, M. L., Benson, J., Berry, T. D., Duncan, D., Edwards, S. L., Caan, B. J., and Potter, J. D. "Dietary sugar and colon cancer." *Cancer Epidemiology, Biomarkers, and Prevention* 1997;6(9):677–85.

Stoll, B. A. "Biological mechanisms in breast cancer invasiveness: relevance to preventive interventions." *European Journal of Cancer Prevention* 2000;9(2):73–79.

———. "Adiposity as a risk determinant for postmenopausal breast cancer." *International Journal of Obesity and Related Metabolic Disorders* 2000. 24(5):527–33.

———. "Western nutrition and the insulin resistance syndrome: A link to breast cancer." *European Journal of Clinical Nutrition* 1999;53:83–87.

Volkers, N. "Diabetes and Cancer: Scientists search for a possible link." *Journal of the National Cancer Institute* 2000;92(3):192.

Glycemic Index, Carbohydrates, and Polycystic Ovary Syndrome

Berga, S. L. "The obstetrician-gynecologist's role in the practical management of polycystic ovary syndrome." *American Journal of Obstetrics and Gynecology* 1998;179(6 Pt 2):S109–13.

Diamanti-Kandarakis, E., and Zapanti, E. "Insulin sensitizers and antiandrogens in the treatment of polycystic ovary syndrome." *Annals of the New York Academy of Science* 2000;900:203–12.

Holte, J. "Polycystic ovary syndrome and insulin resistance: thrifty genes struggling with over feeding and sedentary lifestyle?" *Journal of Endocrinology Investigations* 1998;21(9):589–601.

Huber-Bucholz, M. M., Carey, D. G., and Norman, R. J. "Restoration of reproductive potential by lifestyle modification in obese polycystic ovary syndrome: role of insulin sensitivity and luteinizing hormone." *Journal of Clinical Endocrinology and Metabolism* 1999;84(4):1470–74.

Kidson, W. "Polycystic ovary syndrome: a new direction in treatment." *Medical Journal of Australia* 1998;169(10):537–40.

Lefbvre, P., Bringer, J., Renard, E., Boulet, F., Clouet, S., and Jaffiol, C. "Influences of weight, body fat patterning and nutrition on the management of PCOS." *Human Reproduction* 1997;12(suppl 1):72–81.

Legro, R. S. "Polycystic ovary syndrome: current and future treatment paradigms." *American Journal of Obstetrics and Gynecology* 1998;179(6 Pt 2):S101–S8.

Pasquali, R., Casimirri, F., and Vicennati, V. "Weight control and its beneficial effect on fertility in women with obesity and polycystic ovary syndrome." *Human Reproduction* 1997. 12(suppl 1):82–87.

Protein and Body Weight

Alford, B. B., Blankenship, A. C., and Hagen, R. D. "The effects of variations in carbohydrate, protein, and fat content of the diet upon weight loss, blood values, and nutrient intake of adult obese women." *Journal of the American Dietetic Association* 1990; 90(4);534–40.

Baba, N. H., Sawaya, S., Torbay, N., Habbal, Z., Azar, S., and Hashim, S. A. "High protein vs. high carbohydrate hypoenergetic diet for the treatment of obese hyperinsulinemic subjects." *International Journal of Obesity and Related Metabolic Disorders* 1999;23(11):1202–6.

Golay, A., Allaz, A. F., Morel, Y., Tonnac, N., Tankova, S., and Reaven, G. "Similar weight loss with low- or high-carbohydrate diets." *American Journal of Clinical Nutrition* 1996;63:174–78.

Golay, A., Eigenheer, C., Morel, Y., Kujawski, P., Lehmann, T., and do Tonnac, N. "Weight loss with high or low carbohydrate diet?" *International Journal of Obesity* 1996;20:1067–72.

Hill, J. O., Melanson, E. L., and Wyatt, H. T. "Dietary fat intake and regulation of energy balance: implications for obesity." *Journal of Nutrition* 2000;130:284S–288S.

Horton, T. J., Brachey, D. H., Reed, G. W., Peters, J. C., and Hill, J. O. "Fat and carbohydrate overfeeding in humans: different effects on energy and storage." *American Journal of Clinical Nutrition* 1995;62:19–29.

Larosa, J. C., Fry, A. G., Muesing, R., and Rosing, D. R. "Effects of high-protein, low-carbohydrate dieting on plasma lipoproteins and body weight." *Journal of the American Dietetic Association* 1980;77:264–69.

Piatti, P. M., Monti, L. D., Magni, F., Fermo, I., Baruffaldi, L., Nasser, R., Santambrogio, G., Librenti, M. C., Galli-Kienle, M., Pontiroli, A. E., and Pozza, G. "Hypocaloric high-protein diet improves glucose oxidation and spares lean body mass: Comparison to hypocaloric high-carbohydrate diet." *Metabolism* 1994;43(12)1481–7.

Skov, A. R., Toubro, S., Ronn, B., Holm, L., and Astrup, A. "Randomized trial on protein vs carbo-hydrate in ad libitum fat reduced diet for the treatment of obesity." *International Journal of Obesity and Related Metabolic Disorders* 1999;23(5):528–36.

Worthington, B. S., and Taylor, L. E. "Balanced low-calorie vs. high-protein-low-carbohydrate re-ducing diets." *Journal of the American Dietetic Association* 1974; 64(1):47–55.

Yost, T., Jensen, D., Haugen, B., and Eckel, R. "Effect of dietary macronutrient compostion on tissue-specific lipoprotein lipase activity and insulin action in normal weight subjects." *American Journal of Clinical Nutrition* 1998;68:296–302.

Weight Loss Maintenance

Coakley, E. H., Rimm, E. B., Colditz, G., Kawachi, I., and Willet, W. "Predictors of weight change in men: Results from the health professionals follow-up study." *International Journal of Obesity and Related Metabolic Disorders* 1998;22(2);89–96.

Grodstein, F., Levine, R., Troy, L., Spencer, T., Colditz, G. A., and Stampfer, M. J. "Three-year follow-up of participants in a commercial weight loss program. Can you keep it off?" *Archives of Internal Medicine* 1996;156(12):1302–6.

Klem, M. L., Wing, R. R., McGuire, M. T., Seagle, H. M., and Hill, J. O. "A descriptive study of indi-viduals successful at long-term maintenance of substantial weight loss." *American Journal of Clini-cal Nutrition* 1997;66:239–46.

McGuire, M. T., Wing, R. R., Klem, M. L., Seagle, H. M., and Hill, J. O. "Long-term maintenance of weight loss: do people who lose weight through various weight loss methods use different behav-iors to maintain their weight?" *International Journal of Obesity and Related Metabolic Disorders* 1998;22(6):572–77.

Pavlou, K. N., Krey, S., and Steffee, W. P. "Exercise as an adjunct to weight loss and maintenance in moderately obese subjects." *American Journal of Clinical Nutrition* 1989;49:1115–23.

Sarlio-Lahteenkorva, S., Rissanen, A., and Kaprio, J. "A descriptive study of weight loss mainte-nance: 6 and 15 year follow-up of initially overweight adults." *International Journal of Obesity and Related Metabolic Disorders* 2000;24:116–25.

Schoeller, D. A., Shay, K., and Kushner, R. F. "How much physical activity is needed to minimize weight gain in previously obese women?" *American Journal of Clinical Nutrition* 1997;66:551–56.

Sherwood, N. E., Jeffery, R. W., French, S. A., Hannan, P. J., and Murray, D. M. "Predictors of weight gain in the pound of prevention study." *International Journal of Obesity and Related Metabolic Dis-orders* 2000;24:395–403.

Shick, S. M., Wing, R. R., Klem, M. L., McGuire, M. T., Hill, J. O., and Seagle, H. "Persons successful at long term weight loss and maintenance continue to consume a low-energy, low-fat diet." *Journal of the American Dietetic Association* 1998;98:408–13.

Exercise

Anderson, R. E., Wadden, T. A., Bartlett, S. J., Zemel, B., Verde, T. J., and Franckowiak, S. C. "Effects of lifestyle activity vs structured aerobic exercise in obese women." *Journal of the American Medical Association* 1999;281(4):335–40.

Blundell, J. E., and King, N. A. "Effects of exercise on appetite control: loose coupling between energy expenditure and energy intake." *International Journal of Obesity and Related Metabolic Disorders* 1998;22(suppl 2):S21–S29.

Dunn, A. L., Marcus, B. H., Kampert, J. B., Garcia, M. E., Kohl, H. W., and Blair, S. N. "Comparison of lifestyle and structured interventions to increase physical activity and cardiorespiratory fitness." *Journal of the American Medical Association* 1999;281(4):327–34.

Saris, W. H. M. "Fit, fat, and fat free: the metabolic aspects of weight control." *International Journal of Obesity and Related Metabolic Disorders* 1998;22(suppl 2):S15–21.

General Nutrition

Anderson, J. W., and Hanna, T. J. "Whole grains and protection against coronary heart disease: what are the active components and mechanisms?" (editorial) *American Journal of Clinical Nutrition* 1999;70:307–8.

Flegal, K. M., Carroll, M. D., Kuczmarski, R. J., and Johnson, C. L. "Overweight and obesity in the United States: prevalence and trends, 1960–1994." *International Journal of Obesity* 1998;22:39–47.

Liu, S., Stampfer, M. J., Hu, F. B., Giovannucci, E., Rimm, E., Manson, J. E., Hennekens, C. H., and Willet, W. C. "Whole grain consumption and risk of coronary heart disease: results from the Nurse's Health Study." *American Journal of Clinical Nutrition* 1999;70:412–19.

Mokdad, A. H., Serdula, M. K., Dietz, W. H., Bowman, B. A., Marks, J. S., and Koplan, J. P. "The spread of the obesity epidemic in the United States, 1991–1998." *Journal of the American Medical Association* 1999; 282:1519–22.

Slavin, J. L., Martini, M. C., Jacobs, D. R., and Marquart, L. "Plausible mechanisms for the protectiveness of whole grains." *American Journal of Clinical Nutrition* 1999;70(suppl):459S–63S.

U.S. Department of Agriculture, Center for Nutrition Policy and Promotion. "Is total fat consumption really decreasing?" *Nutrition Insight* 5; April 1998.

U.S. Department of Agriculture, Economic Research Service, Agriculture Information Bulletin No. 750. Frazao, E., ed. "America's Eating Habits: Changes and Consequences."

Willet, W. C. "The dietary pyramid: does the foundation need repair?" *American Journal of Clinical Nutrition* (editorial) 1998;68:218–19.

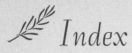 Index